The Cognitive Neuropsychology of Alzheimer-type Dementia

The Cognitive Neuropsychology of Alzheimer-type Dementia

Edited by

ROBIN G. MORRIS
Department of Psychology,
Institute of Psychiatry, London

Oxford New York Tokyo
OXFORD UNIVERSITY PRESS
1996

Oxford University Press, Great Clarendon Street, Oxford OX2 6DP
Oxford New York
Athens Auckland Bangkok Bombay
Calcutta Cape Town Dar es Salaam Delhi
Florence Hong Kong Istanbul Karachi
Kuala Lumpur Madras Madrid Melbourne
Mexico City Nairobi Paris Singapore
Taipei Tokyo Toronto
and associated companies in
Berlin Ibadan

Oxford is a trade mark of Oxford University Press

Published in the United States
by Oxford University Press Inc., New York

A catalogue record for this book is available from the British Library

Library of Congress Cataloging in Publication Data

Cognitive neuropsychology of Alzheimer-type dementia / edited by Robin G. Morris. – 1st ed.
Includes bibliographical references.
1. Cognition disorders in old age – Pathophysiology. 2. Senile dementia – Pathophysiology. 3. Alzheimer's disease – Pathophysiology. 4. Cognitive neuroscience. I. Morris, Robin, 1958–.
[DNLM: 1. Dementia – physiopathology. 2. Dementia – psychology. 3. Alzheimer's Disease – physiopathology. 4. Alzheimer's Disease – psychology. 5. Neuropsychology. 6. Cognition Disorders – physiopathology. WM 220 C676 1996]
RC524.C64 1996 616.8'3 – dc20 96–22542

ISBN 0 19 852343 2

Typeset by Palimpsest Book Production Limited, Polmont, Stirlingshire

Printed in Great Britain by Bookcraft (Bath) Ltd
Midsomer Norton, Avon

To Lorna, Rebecca, and Jonathan

Preface

Cognitive neuropsychology seeks to analyse those impairments in human cognitive function that arise from damage to the brain. The focus is on establishing the functional architecture of cognition *per se*, sometimes deliberately ignoring the neurobiological substrate. Thus breakdown of basic cognitive functions, such as attention, memory, language, and thought can be studied in detail without even considering the physiological cause. As the discipline has matured, however, the linkage between the mind and the brain has resurfaced, particularly with the advent of more advanced neuroimaging techniques. It is within this general background that the recent neuropsychology of the dementias has been conducted, doing much to dispel the myth that all dementias constitute 'global impairments in mental function'. For example, the 'flag-ship' dementia, Alzheimer's disease, is associated with distinct and characteristic changes in different aspects of cognition, some of which are demonstrably not impaired. Furthermore, even in such a well-established cause of dementia, different types are emerging, accompanied by various cognitive manifestations of the disease. Thus the aim of the cognitive neuropsychological approach is to tease apart the different consequences of the disease using this powerful framework.

With this aim in view, the first section of the book focuses on the theoretical issues and research methodology that guides research in the area. This includes a justification of the modular approach in relation to dementia, and tackles the difficulty of researching a disease that is progressive in nature, also illustrating the appropriateness of single case study methodology. The main body of the book covers different mental functions as defined by cognitive psychology. The aim is not to be comprehensive, but to focus on areas where more rapid progress has been made. Thus, for example, areas such as attention, executive processes, episodic and semantic memory have all been subject to substantial theoretical development in relation to Alzheimer's disease in the last few years. A more specific development has been relating cognitive impairments to changes in brain functioning, using the parallel approaches of neuropathology, neuroimaging, and neurochemistry. Hence, there is a section focusing on these areas, attempting to integrate the previous research. Finally, the book considers the implications of cognitive impairment to the management of dementia, including developments in techniques for assessment, rehabilitation, and psychopharmacological treatment. These approaches have tended to develop separately but recent developments have tended to redress this imbalance, with the theoreticians beginning to take a greater interest in the practical application of their research.

Overall, the book is intended to draw together recent developments in the neuropsychology of Alzheimer's disease in a way that will appeal to professionals with an academic or clinical interest in the disorder. As such, it is aimed at cognitive psychologists, clinical psychologists, neurologists, psychiatrists, and the growing number of neuroscientists who are investigating the neurobiology of Alzheimer's disease but wish to understand how they may relate to cognitive changes.

London R. G. M.
April 1996

Contents

Contributors

Sarah K. Agnew, Department of Psychology, Institute of Psychiatry, London SE5 8AF, UK.

Lars Bäckman, Department of Psychology, University of Gothenburg, Gothenburg, Sweden; and Section of Psychology, Stockholm Gerontology Research Centre and Department of Clinical Neuroscience, Division of Geriatric Medicine, Karolinska Institute, Stockholm, Sweden.

James T. Becker, Neuropsychology Research Program, Departments of Psychiatry and Neurology, University of Pittsburgh Medical Center, Pittsburgh, PA, USA.

Meryl A. Butters, Brain Injury Program, Departments of Psychiatry and Neurology, University of Pittsburgh Medical Center, Pittsburgh, PA, USA.

H. Branch Coslett, Department of Neurology, Temple University, Philadelphia, PA, USA.

H. Valerie Curran, Clinical Health Psychology, University College London, Gower St, London WC1E 6BT, UK.

Sergio Della Sala, Department of Psychology, University of Aberdeen, King's College, Old Aberdeen AB9 2UB, UK.

V. Olga B. Emery, Department of Psychiatry, Dartmouth Medical School, One Medical Center Drive, Lebanon, NH 03756, USA.

Christine Fennema-Notestine, Departments of Psychology and Cognitive Science, University of California, San Diego, CA, USA.

Morris Freedman, Behavioral Neurology Program and Rotman Research Institute of Baycrest Center for Geriatric Care, Department of Medicine (Neurology), Mount Sinai Hospital and University Of Toronto, Ontario, Canada.

Elaine Funnell, Department of Psychology, Royal Holloway College, University of London, Egham, Surrey TW20 0EX, UK.

Colin Gray, Department of Psychology, University of Aberdeen, King's College, Old Aberdeen AB9 2UB, UK.

John D. W. Greene, Department of Neurology, Addenbrooke's Hospital, Hills Rd, Cambridge CB2 2QQ, UK.

Agneta Herlitz, Section of Psychology, Stockholm Gerontology Research Centre and Department of Clinical Neuroscience, Division of Geriatric Medicine, Karolinska Institute, Stockholm, Sweden.

John R. Hodges, University Neurology Unit, Addenbrooke's Hospital, Hills Rd, Cambridge CB2 2QQ, UK.

Daphne Kidron, Behavioral Neurology Program and Rotman Research Institute of Baycrest Center for Geriatric Care, Department of Medicine (Neurology), Mount Sinai Hospital and University of Toronto, Ontario, Canada.

Michael D. Kopelman, Academic Unit of Psychiatry, United Medical and Dental Schools of Guy's and St Thomas's Hospitals, St Thomas's Campus, London SE1 7EH, UK.

Oscar L. Lopez, Neuropsychology Research Program, Departments of Psychiatry and Neurology, University of Pittsburgh Medical Center, Pittsburgh, PA, USA.

Jane L. Mathias, Department of Psychology, University of Adelaide, Adelaide, SA 5005, Australia.

Edgar Miller, Department of Psychology (Clinical Section), University of Leicester, Leicester LE1 7RH, UK.

Robin G. Morris, Department of Psychology, Institute of Psychiatry, London SE5 8AF, UK.

Marcus Richards, Section of Old Age Psychiatry, Institute of Psychiatry, De Crespigny Park, Denmark Hill, London SE5 8AF, UK.

Eleanor M. Saffran, Department of Speech—Language—Hearing, Temple University, Philadelphia, PA, USA.

David P. Salmon, Department of Neurosciences (0948), University of California, San Diego, 9500 Gilman Drive, La Jolla, CA 92093–0948, USA.

Bob Woods, School of Psychology, University of Wales, Bangor, Gwynedd LL57 2DG, UK.

Abbreviations

ACh	acetylcholine
AChE	acetylcholinesterase
AD	Alzheimer-type dementia
ADA	Alzheimer's Disease Association
ADAS	Alzheimer's Disease Assessment Scale
adFAD	autosomal dominant familial Alzheimer's disease
ADL	activities of daily living
AERP	auditory event-related potential
ALS	Articulatory Loop System
APP	amyloid precursor protein
APP	amyloid precursor protein gene
ARC	annual rate of deterioration
ARIMA	autoregressive integrated moving average
ARM	articulatory rehearsal mechanism
BDS	Blessed Dementia Scale
BZ	benzodiazepine
CANTAB	Cambridge Automated Neuropsychological Test Automated Battery
CDR	Clinical Dementia Rating scale
CES	Central Executive System
ChAT	choline acetyltransferase
CNS	central nervous system
CSF	cerebrospinal fluid
CT	computerized tomography
CVLT	California Verbal Learning Test
DRS	Dementia Rating Scale
EEG	electroencephalogram
EP	evoked potential
ERP	Event Related Potential
FDG	fluorodeoxyglucose
fMRI	functional magnetic resonance imaging
FVEP	flashing-light visual evoked potential
GABA	gamma-aminobutyric acid
HD	Huntington's disease
HMPAO	hexamethyl-propylene amine oxime
IMC	Information Memory – Concentration Test
IMP	inositol 5′-monophosphate
MDRS	Mattis Dementia Rating Scale
MID	multi-infarct dementia

MMSE	Mini-Mental State Examination
MODA	Milan Overall Dementia Assessment
MRI	magnetic resonance imaging
MSQ	Mental Status Questionnaire
NART	National Adult Reading Test
NFT	neurofibrillary tangles
NGF	nerve growth factor
NINCDS	National Institute of Neurological and Communicative Disorders and Stroke
OMD	organic mental deterioration
OUCH	Organised Unitary Content Hypothesis
PD	Parkinson's disease
PDP	parallel distributed processing
PET	positron emission tomography
PRVEP	reverse checkerboard presentation visual evoked potential
PSS	phonological short-term store
rCBF	regional cerebral blood flow
RO	Reality Orientation
RT	reaction time
SAD	sporadic Alzheimer's disease
SAS	supervisory attentional system
SP	scopolamine
SPET	single photon emission tomography
SPMSQ	Short Portable Mental Status Questionnaire
SPT	subject-performed task
Tc	technetium
THA	tetrahydroaminoacridine (tacrine)
TSC	Test for Syntactic Complexity
VEP	visual evoked potential
VSSP	Visuospatial Scratchpad
WAB	Western Aphasia Battery
WAIS-R	Wechsler Adult Intelligence Scale—Revised
WKS	Wernicke–Korsakoff's syndrome
WMS	Wechsler Memory Scale

I. Theoretical background

ONE

A cognitive neuropsychology of Alzheimer-type dementia

Robin G. Morris

INTRODUCTION

The aim of this chapter is to introduce the concept of Alzheimer-type dementia (AD), and outline briefly the theoretical and methodological issues involved in studying the syndrome. Alzheimer's disease takes its name from the now famous neuropathologist, Alöis Alzheimer, who described the histological characteristics of the disease in a 51-year-old patient with generalized cognitive impairment in the late nineteenth century (Alzheimer 1907; see Förstl and Levy 1991). It is now known to be the most common cause of dementing illness, and research into the disease has captured the imagination of neurobiologists, neurologists, and neuropsychologists during the last 20 years.

DIAGNOSIS AND TERMINOLOGY

Despite this, *in vivo*, the diagnosis of Alzheimer's disease is presumptive without the use of a post-mortem examination, the reason being that no certain biological marker of the disease exists. Even with a post-mortem analysis, considerable overlap is found between the brains of normal elderly people and those with the diagnosis of Alzheimer's disease, in terms of the defining neuropathological features (see Chapter 13). In life, the diagnostic schemes are essentially based on the demonstration of cognitive decline in the absence of possible causes and rigorous implementation of procedures such as the National Institute of Neurological and Communicative Disorders and Stroke, and the Alzheimer's Disease Association (NINCDS–ADRDA) criteria have produced accuracy rates of approximately 80% (McKhann *et al.* 1984; Tierney *et al.* 1988). It is for this reason that various presumptive terms have been applied, which acknowledge the relative inaccuracy of diagnosis and treat the condition partly as a syndrome. These include, for example, senile dementia of the Alzheimer-type (SDAT), dementia of the Alzheimer-type (DAT) and Alzheimer-type dementia (AD). In this book the latter term and abbreviation is used consistently, the exception being the chapter on neurobiological aspects where it has been more convenient to revert to referring to Alzheimer's disease. AD can be defined variously, but the main procedures take their lead from the NINCDS–ADRDA criteria that there should be specific neuropsychological deficits in at least two areas of functioning, for example memory, language, or praxis, and deterioration should be progressive; and diagnosis should be supported by neurological and electroencephaological examination.

By applying these criteria, steady progress has been made in defining AD and understanding the neurolopsychological deficits. This has led to what Morris (1994) has described as a 'patchwork of theories' covering different aspects of cognition in AD. These studies have been conducted under the umbrella of what can broadly be termed 'Cognitive Neuropsychology' where this term refers to the use of the techniques and theories that stem from cognitive psychology to understand the deficits in mental functioning that follow brain injury (McCarthy and Warrington 1990). Cognitive psychology has provided a wide range of theoretical frameworks and techniques with which to study dementia that go far beyond the traditional neuropsychological psychometric approach. By careful dissection of different aspects of functioning it has been possible to dispel the myth that all aspects of cognition in AD are uniformally impaired, something that used to dull enthusiasm for research in this area. Indeed, a theme running through the various chapters on cognition in the second section is that cognitive studies of AD can even provide insights into the cerebral organization of cognitive skills and abilities, the more radical aim of cognitive neuropsychology. These approaches, which provide the theoretical backdrop to the book, are reviewed briefly in this chapter.

ONE ALZHEIMER-TYPE DEMENTIA OR MORE?

In understanding AD, the degree of patient heterogeneity has always been an issue, and there is now considerable cognitive evidence to support different patterns of cognitive decline (Capitani *et al.* 1988). Asymmetric patterns of impairment in cerebral metabolism have been detected which map on to more specific neuropsychological deficits. For example patients with right hypometabolism have been shown to be accompanied by more pronounced visuospatial impairment. Conversely, verbal neuropsychological deficits are correlated with left hemisphere hypometabolism (Haxby *et al.* 1988). The pattern of dysfunction can change over time, for example the metabolic asymmetries becoming more pronounced.

As well as metabolic asymmetries, AD patients can present with predominant cognitive deficits in different domains of functioning. These include a dissociation between 'executive' and 'episodic' memory deficits. Becker *et al.* (1992) were able to isolate subgroups of AD patients who showed extreme impairments in these types of functioning, one group who were impaired on measures of problem solving, cognitive resource allocation, and shifting mental sets, the other who were impaired on tests of long-term memory. A follow-up study of a larger group of patients showed the same differentiation and this has also been observed by Baddeley *et al.* (1991). They point out that this is not some statistical artefact, due to some patients falling at the extreme end of a particular scale by chance, since arbitary 'syndromes' requiring a particular combination of scores did not produce particular patterns.

The heterogeneity must reflect the different way in which the disease process is damaging the brain, but also the premorbid characteristics of the patients and how these interact with cognitive impairment. There is also increasing evidence that Alzheimer's disease will split into different aetiologies and as this becomes clearer it may lead to a refinement in neuropsychological research. A current example is patients described as having Lewy body variants of Alzheimer's disease, who, in the past, may have been grouped together with AD patients for the purposes of neuropsychological investigation. These patients can present with marked fluctuations in cognitive functioning (Perry *et al.* 1990) and there is the suggestion that, compared to 'typical' AD, visuospatial functioning, attention, and verbal fluency are more affected (Hansen *et al.* 1990). There is also the finding of different neuropsychological profiles in familial cases of AD as reviewed by Agnew in Chapter 15.

Heterogeneity within AD and between different subtypes might suggest the need to abandon group studies, and, indeed, the arguments for using single case methodology are put by Funnell in Chapter 2. Nevertheless, there is probably sufficient commonality between patients for group studies to provide a useful description of cognitive functioning in AD as a syndrome. In addition, by studying patients in groups, paradoxically it is possible to identify 'focal' deficits in subgroups of patients as illustrated above. It may be that the number of subgroups of AD will increase as more is understood about the disease, and this will revise some of our ideas about cognitive dysfunction. The chapters below, however, illustrate the usefulness of a multifaceted approach to AD, in certain instances studying individual patients in great detail, whilst in other instances exploring the characteristics of groups.

FUNCTIONAL ARCHITECTURE OF THE MIND

One of the main tenets of cognitive psychology is that mental processes can be split into specific modules or structures that function semi-autonomously. This notion, which can be traced back, for example, to the nineteenth-century aphasiologist Lichtheim, identifies specific centres that process information which have a network of communicative links. The series of boxes represent the modules and the lines between them represent the flow of information or, in certain instances, the coordinating mechanisms that bind the processes together. In more recent times, the different components are described as being part of a 'functional architecture' which is identified by a combination of studying normal subjects and neuropsychological impairment (McCarthy and Warrington 1990).

Such theorizing is commonplace in neuropsychology and there are many examples in this book of how it has been applied to AD. For example, in Chapter 4 I describe how the Working Memory Model has been used to further the understanding of short-term memory impairment in AD. In this case, the cognitive structures include the Central Executive System (CES), the Articulatory Loop System (ALS), and the Visuospatial Scratchpad (VSSP). The modularity of the system is supported by preservation of the ALS, with a contrasting impairment in the CES as indicated by a series of studies by Morris (1994) and by Baddeley and colleagues (Baddeley *et al.* 1991). Another example, is provided by Greene and Hodges in Chapter 8, who base their theorizing on Valentine *et al.*'s (1991) model of face and name recognition, which includes separate face and name recognition units, that are linked to what are termed person identity nodes. In AD it is suggested that the deficit in face recognition involves primarily disruption of 'semantic knowledge of famous persons' in other words, the person identity node, rather than the face and name recognition units.

The models described above are supported by the well-known theoretical concepts of dissociation and double dissociation (Shallice 1979). The former refers to a deficit in one measure of function, with relative preservation of another. As with other forms of brain damage, this type of finding in AD does not necessarily suggest a distinct processing is involved because each test of function may simply have differential sensitivities to a more general deficit. In AD, this is always a possibility and limits the extent to which data from this patient group can be used to develop modular theories of cognition. The more powerful method of double dissociation, however, can be used in this context and there are various examples stemming from AD studies. To use one of the same examples cited above, the preservation of the ALS and inferred impairment in executive functioning shows a mirror reversal in patients with selective verbal short-term memory deficits and adds to the evidence that these functions are dissociated in relation to working memory (Morris and Baddeley 1988). Another example is the comparison between procedural memory and episodic memory outlined by Salmon in Chapter 7. AD patients show impaired episodic memory and learning, but unimpaired motor learning. This contrasts markedly with patients with Huntington's chorea who show marked motor learning deficits.

MODULARITY VERSUS CONNECTIONISM

Nevertheless, the extent to which cognitive systems can be split up into modular systems is hotly disputed. An extreme view, espoused, for example, by Fodor (1983), is that each module processes material in isolation and simply transfers information onwards, but without computations being affected by other information. This has been termed information encapsulation and the theorizing behind it 'the locality assumption'. The view has been strongly criticized by those who take a more interactive view of the brain and can model cognitive functioning or dysfunction using connectionist approaches (Farah and McClelland 1991). Despite this, at a gross level, modularity is widely accepted and accords with what is known about the functional architecture of the brain, namely that there is some degree of differentiation of functioning. In relation to AD the debate is of interest because it determines what type of approach is adopted for explaining deficits. Approaches to AD reflect these differences, with some taking the 'box' and 'arrow' approach, as indicated above, and others using a more connectionist framework (see, for example, Morris 1994).

Studies of AD may even inadvertently inform this debate. For example the strongest evidence for information encapsulation perhaps is the existence of unimpaired modules in the presences of widespread cognitive decline. A more extreme connectionist approach would have difficulty in accounting for this finding because interactive processing would tend to produce a global deficit. In AD, however, there are many examples of preserved 'modules', metaphorically surrounded by damage to other parts of the system. For example, Moscovitch and Umilta (1990) point to the fact that some AD patients, despite gross intellectual deficits, are able to repeat and read grammatically incorrect sentences (Schwartz *et al.* 1979). The selective preservation of the articulatory loop system in AD is another example, contrasting with impairments in all other aspects of the working memory system (Morris 1994).

Despite evidence for modular deficits in AD the neurobiology of AD points overwhelmingly towards widespread deterioration of neuronal systems, with damage throughout the association neocortex and loss connectivity between brain regions (De Lacoste and White 1993; Leuchter *et al.* 1992; Morris 1994). Although parallel distributed processing (PDP) models primarily concern a description of cognition, they are buttressed by neurobiological plausibility, the 'nodes' used as the building blocks of the network being analagous to neurones. The type of networks described in PDP models mirror neurobiological networks or systems. In this sense AD provides a model for what would happen if the network is lesioned in a distributed fashion, rather than in one location. It is therefore perhaps not surprising that cognitive systems, such as semantic memory, that have been modelled successfully using a PDP framework can by impaired by a wide range of lesions (Small 1995). Perhaps neurodegenerative disorders such as AD should be considered more closely in terms of understanding connectionist systems.

RELATIONSHIPS WITH NEUROBIOLOGY

Using a cognitive approach, the brain can be treated as a 'black box' with no recourse to thinking about the internal workings at a physiological level (Shallice 1979). This approach has provided many insights into neuropsychological impairment as well as indicating what the brain *does* in a functional sense. Nevertheless, by studying different types of brain damage it has been possible to map cognitive structures on to brain regions or systems. Functional neuroimaging is adding to this process very rapidly, with the advantage of exploring brain and behaviour relationships in normal brains. In relation to AD, the challenge is that the damage is so widespread both neuropathologically and neuropharmacologically that it is difficult to disentangle the different contributory factors to neuropsychological impairment. Despite this a great deal of progress has been made in this area, as indicated in Part III of this book, provided it is borne in mind that no single pathological event is implicated. One area which has been relatively neglected in AD has been exploring the relationship between neurobiological and cognitive neuropsychological functioning. Where this has happened, it has yielded interesting results, for example the Parasuraman *et al.* (1992) studies of the mechanism of selective attention, combining cognitive tasks with neuroimaging. This type of approach points the way for future research in the field.

REFERENCES

Alzheimer, A. (1907). Über eine eigenartige Erkrankung der Hirnrinde. *Allgemeine Zeitschrift für Psychiatrie und psychiatrisch-gerichtlich Medizine*, **64**, 146–8.

Baddeley, A. D., Bressi, S., Della Sala, S., Logie, R., and Spinnler, H. (1991). The decline of working memory in Alzheimer's disease. *Brain*, **114**, 2521–42.

Becker, J. T., Bajulaiye, O., and Smith, C. (1992). Longitudinal analysis of a two-component model of the memory deficit in Alzheimer's disease. *Psychological Medicine*, **22**, 437–45.

Capitani, E., Della Sala, S., Lucchelli, F., Soave, P., and Spinnler, H. (1988). Perceptual attention in aging and dementia measured by Gottschaldt's hidden figure test. *Journal of Gerontology*, **43**, 157–63.

De LaCoste, M. C. and White, C. L. (1993). The role of cortical connectivity in Alzheimer's disease pathogenesis: A review and model system. *Neurobiology of Aging*, **14**, 1–16.

Farah, M. J., and McClelland, J. L. (1991). A computational model of semantic memory impairment: Modality specificity and emergent category-specificity. *Journal of Experimental Psychology: General*, **120**, 339–57.

Fodor, J. A. (1983). *The modularity of the mind*. Bradford Books/MIT Press, Cambridge.

Förstl, H. and Levy, R. (1991). Foreword to the translation of 'On certain peculiar diseases of old age' (by Alois Alzheimer). *History of Psychiatry*, **ii**, 71–4.

Hansen, L., Salmon, D., Galasko, D. *et al.* (1990). The Lewy body variant of Alzheimer's disease: A clinical and pathological entity. *Neurology*, **40**, 1–8.

Haxby, J. V., Grady, C. L., Koss, E., Horwitz, B., Shapiro, M., Friedland, R. P., *et al.* (1988). Heterogenous anterior – posterior metabolic patterns in dementia of the Alzheimer's type. *Neurology*, **38**, 1853–63.

Leuchter, A. F., Newton, T. F., Cook, I. A., Walter, D. O., Rosenberg-Thompson, S., and Lachenbruch, P. A. (1992). Changes in brain functional connectivity in Alzheimer-type and multi-infarct dementia. *Brain*, 115, 1543–61.

McCarthy, R. A. and Warrington, E. K. (1990). *Cognitive neuropsychology: A clinical introduction*. Academic Press, San Diego, CA.

McKhann, G., Drachman, D., Folstein, M., Katzman, R., Price, D., and Stadlan, M (1984). Clinical diagnosis of Alzheimer's disease: report of the NINCDS—ADRDA Work Group. *Neurology*, **34**, 939–44.

Morris, R. G. (1994). Recent developments in the neuropsychology of dementia. *International Review of Psychiatry*, **6**, 85–107.

Morris, R. G. and Baddeley, A. D. (1988). Primary and working memory functioning in Alzheimer-type dementia. *Journal of Experimental and Clinical Psychology*, **51**, 757–66.

Moscovitch, M. and Ulmita, C. (1990). Modularity and neuropsychology: Modules and central processes in attention and memory. In *Modular deficits in Alzheimer-type dementia*, (ed. M. F. Schwartz). pp. 1–59. Bradford Books/MIT Press, Cambridge.

Parasuraman, R., Greenwood, P. M., Haxby, J. V., and Grady, C. L. (1992). Visuospatial attention in dementia of the Alzheimer's type. *Brain*, **115**, 711–33.

Perry, R. H., Irving, D., Blessed, G., Fairbairn, A., and Perry, E. K. (1990). Senile dementia of Lewy body type. A clinically and neuropathologically distinct form of Lewy body dementia in the elderly. *Journal of Neurological Science*, **95**, 119–39.

Schwartz, M. F., Marin, O. S. M., and Saffran, E. M. (1979). Dissociations of language function in dementia. A case study. *Brain and Language*, **7**, 277–306.

Shallice, T. (1979). Case study approach in neuropsychological research. *Journal of Clinical Neuropsychology*, **1**, 183–211.

Small, T. (1995). The real functional architecture is gray, wet and slippery. *Behavioural and Brain Sciences*, **17**, 81–2.

Tierney, M. C., Fisher, R. H., Lewis, A. J., Zorzitto, M. J., Snow, W. G., Reid, D. W. *et al.* (1988). The NINCDS-ADRDA work group criteria for the clinical diagnosis of probable Alzheimer's disease: a clinicopathologic study of 57 cases. *Neurology*, **38**, 359–64.

Valentine, T., Bredart, S., Lawson, R., and Ward, G. (1991). What's in a name? Access to information from people's names. *European Journal of Cognitive Psychology*, **3**, 147–76.

TWO

The single case study and Alzheimer-type dementia

Elaine Funnell

INTRODUCTION: THE CASE FOR THE SINGLE CASE STUDY APPROACH

Most investigations into the cognitive deficits in Alzheimer-type dementia (AD) have studied groups of subjects in order to answer such questions as, 'What is the nature of the naming/memory/attention disorder in this syndrome'? The purpose is to draw up a profile of characteristics based on theory which can be used to aid in the diagnosis of AD, monitoring decline, and helping in the development of neurorehabilitation approaches.

This approach has the advantage of being able to generalize in relation to AD, but it is based on the assumption of patient homogeneity, which as the previous chapter has suggested is not necessarily present. The arguments in favour of studying individual AD patients have been outlined in detail by Myrna Schwartz (1987). She provides evidence that the generally accepted stages model of AD, which propose that memory loss and personality change mark the onset, followed by the development of more focal symptoms, such as aphasia, apraxia, agnosia, cannot be sustained when individuals with deviating patterns are taken into account. She describes a number of individuals, each of whom has a different type of focal cognitive disorder, which is disproportionately compromised compared to other cognitive skills, and argues that 'there is no generalization about the inevitable ordering of symptoms in primary progressive dementia that has not been contradicted by reports in the literature.' She notes further that:

> The notion that there is a typical profile may well derive from the standard practice of excluding patients who fail to conform to a priori conceptions of how diseases of the Alzheimer type should manifest themselves . . . Given the sizeable accumulation of data attesting to the fact that such focal representations are not inconsistent with DAT [AD], and indeed, even with histologically verified Alzheimer's disease, such practices can no longer be countenanced.

Searching for the defining cognitive features of neurological disorders is not unique to the study of AD. The study of aphasia was dominated for many years by a similar approach, in which individuals with aphasia were grouped according to the locus of the lesion (anterior or more posterior) and then subjected to investigations of particular aspects of language processing (such as spelling) in the expectation that different patterns of performance would be revealed across the two groups. But a century of such research has yielded no theoretical understanding of the nature of the underlying cognitive processes responsible for the deficits observed. Gurd and Marshall (1991) note that the study of groups selected on the basis of non-cognitive criteria, or on cognitive groupings which entail varieties of patterns of symptoms, such as aphasia or dementia, is 'inherently unreliable'. Martin (1990) observes that 'Our understanding of Alzheimer's disease will be hampered if we insist on maintaining research practices that by their very nature can potentially obscure fundamental characteristics of the entity that they seek to describe.'

MODULAR SYSTEMS

Clinicians have long been aware from studies of individual subjects with localized neurological disorders (such as those that arise through stroke or tumour) that brain damage can separate cognitive processes into broad modality-specific domains, producing, for example, specific impairments of language (aphasia), visual space (visual neglect), object recognitive disorders (agnosia), and disorders in assembling movements and forming ideas (apraxia). But it is only relatively recently, following careful investigations into the nature of the cognitive deficits underlying particular disorders, for example the classic studies of disorders of *short-term memory* (Warrington and Shallice 1969) and *oral reading* (Marshall and Newcombe 1973), that theoreticians have become aware of the complexity of the cognitive systems underlying the ability to carry out particular cognitive tasks.

These studies of specific processing deficits suggested that cognitive systems are composed of a collection of processing modules which together produce normal skilled performance, but which give rise to a range of distinctly different cognitive disorders if particular components of the system are damaged. The belief in the modular nature of such systems, which is argued to be essential for the efficient processing of information in complex systems (Marr 1976; Shallice 1981), was influenced by the information processing approach to cognitive theory that was developing at the time, and which has become increasingly influential over the past 20 years. Existing modular theories, such as the logogen model (Morton 1979), were elaborated to account for particular patterns of cognitive disorder (e.g. Morton and

Patterson 1980) and new modular theories were developed to account for normal and abnormal performance in processing domains (such as face processing) where no such models had previously existed (e.g. Bruce and Young 1986). As an example of a simple modular theory, Fig. 2.1 illustrates the basic processing modules thought to be involved in object naming.

However, it soon became clear that when modular systems are damaged they can give rise to a large variety of different finegrain behavioural symptoms, making it virtually impossible to find identical patterns of cognitive deficit across individuals. This, in turn, has meant that attempts to characterize precisely the symptom complex of a particular cognitive disorder across a group of subjects has proved to be impossible. Consequently, the search for cognitive syndromes has been abandoned (Coltheart 1984; Ellis 1987).

Instead of syndromes, individual patterns of performance are explained by locating the deficits that give rise to each disorder within a model of the modular processing system underlying *normal* performance. In this way, a unified account of all possible combinations of symptoms can, in principle, be achieved. For example Fig. 2.1 illustrates a very simple model of picture naming composed of three basic units: (1) a set of structural codes describing the object's visual appearance; (2) a set of semantic codes providing information about category membership and semantic associations with the object, such as where the object might be found, how it might be used, etc.; and (3) a set of phonological codes representing the spoken names of the object. Naming disorders of visually presented objects could arise if any one of these three components was damaged, but each could be explained with reference to the same processing model, thus providing a framework with which to account for all disorders observed. As Coltheart (1984) writes:

> If no two patients in a group exhibit identical constellations of symptoms, then each patient requires an individual explanation. This does not prevent one from making generalisations across patients, but the generalisations do not take the form of claiming that there exists a single syndrome which many patients exhibit. Instead, these generalisations take the form of claiming that there exists a single model of the relevant cognitive system which can offer interpretations of the various sets of symptoms exhibited by various different patients.

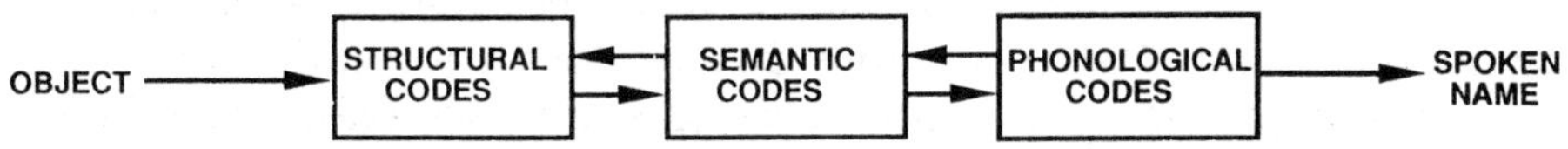

FIG. 2.1 A simple model of the processes involved in confrontation naming.

This approach is the essence of cognitive neuropsychology, a method and theory which combines clinical neuropsychology and cognitive psychology (Coltheart 1984), and with which this book is concerned.

SINGLE CASE STUDIES OF COGNITIVE IMPAIRMENTS ASSOCIATED WITH DEMENTIA

At present, the assessment of individuals with suspected dementia most commonly uses a dementia scale (e.g. Mattis 1973), which provides an overall score reflecting the *severity* of the disorder. These tests are quick to carry out, and for the most part probably give an accurate assessment of the severity of the dementia. However, in some cases the results of such tests are likely to be misleading since they tap heavily into verbal memory skills and may therefore underestimate the cognitive abilities of individuals with predominately verbal disorders. they may also fail to pick up the cognitive decrements of individuals whose verbal skills are intact, but who may have other severe impairments, such as visual processing impairments, giving a misleadingly favourable impression of cognitive function in these cases. Although more complex text batteries generally assess a variety of different cognitive domains, and are potentially more informative, the generally small number of items included in the different sections of the test prevents reliable comparisons across tasks.

Over the years, clinical and cognitive neuropsychologists have developed a variety of tests designed to expose different cognitive disorders and to pinpoint the nature of the underlying cognitive deficit or deficits. If we take a hypothetical subject with a problem with naming objects as an example, then, by using the Graded Naming Test (McKenna and Warrington 1980) and selected tests from the Birmingham Object Recognition Battery (Riddoch and Humphreys 1993) it would be possible to determine whether a subject had a visual processing disorder, a naming disorder, or both. When these tests are used with other well-established clinical tests, such as the Wisconsin Card Sorting Test (Nelson 1976) which taps cognitive operations such as planning, problem solving, and attention, we can go a long way towards revealing the degree and nature of the cognitive function available to a subject in those cognitive domains for which we have well worked-out theories.

The use of tests designed to examine very specific cognitive functions allows one to ask, 'What cognitive deficits does this individual have?' Rather than providing an overall score of severity on a dementia scale, the use of specific cognitive tests provides a profile of the individual's actual cognitive function in particular tasks. Only a handful of detailed studies of the cognitive disorders of individuals with dementing disorders have taken this approach, but each study has shown modular patterns of breakdown in performance in which some cognitive functions involved in a task are impaired, while others appear to be either relatively or entirely spared (e.g. Holland *et al* 1985; Schwartz *et al* 1979; Warrington 1975; Whitaker 1976). A recent publication of a selection of detailed case studies of the cognitive disorders of a series of individual subjects has testified further to the range of modular deficits that can be observed in AD (Schwartz 1990).

LONGITUDINAL STUDIES OF COGNITIVE DECLINE

The types of tests mentioned briefly above can be used to establish the pattern of an individual's cognitive impairments at any particular stage in the course of the disease. However, unless the tests are repeated regularly, they cannot capture the nature of any changes in cognitive abilities occurring over time. Repeated testing is therefore essential if the characteristics of the cognitive decline are to be monitored so that the following aspects can be determined: (1) the rate and regularity of the decline; (2) the consistency with which particular pieces of information (for example particular names, particular concepts) are lost or retained over repeated tests; (3) the nature of the information that is lost; and (4) what happens to a piece of information between the time it is available and the time at which it appears to be irrevocably lost. Answers to these questions will not only provide information about the cognitive disorder of the subject, but will also tell us more about the representation and loss of knowledge in cognitive systems.

SOME EXAMPLES OF SINGLE CASE STUDIES OF NAMING DISORDERS ASSOCIATED WITH DEMENTIA

In order to explain the single case study approach to cognitive decline in dementia in more concrete terms, I shall describe briefly the study of the naming disorders observed in three subjects: Mrs K (referred to as Mary in previous reports), Mrs P, and Mrs C, each of whom developed a progressive cognitive disorder of insidious onset, during middle age. In each case, the behavioural symptoms, and lack of clinical signs associated with other causes of dementia, were consistent with a probable diagnosis of Alzheimer's disease, although in the case of the second individual, the behavioural characteristics also fitted the historical diagnosis of Pick's disease (Hodges *et al.* 1992). Table 2.1 provides some brief details about each subject.

TABLE 2.1 Details of three single case studies

Subject's name	Age (years)	Presenting symptoms	Scans (CT/SPECT)	Previous reports
Mrs K	58	Disorders of naming, spelling, and arithmetic	Left temporal/ parietal hypometabolism	Funnell and Hodges 1991; Funnell 1992
Mrs P	62	Disorders of naming and comprehension	Focal atrophy left temporal lobe	Hodges *et al.* 1992; Funnell and Hodges 1996
Mrs C	47	Disorders of naming and memory	No signs	Funnell and Hodges 1996

Two different types of naming test are usually used to identify naming disorders associated with dementia: confrontation naming tests, in which a series of pictures of objects are presented for naming; and category fluency tests, in which the subject is asked to generate names to a given category (for example animals or fruits). When tests of both types were presented to the first two subjects, Mrs K and Mrs P, they were both impaired on both types of naming test, but the third subject, Mrs C, had severe problems only with verbal category fluency, on tests of confrontation naming her performance was normal (she scored in the bright normal range on the demanding Graded Naming Test, McKenna and Warrington 1980). Whether or not one concludes that Mrs C has a naming deficit clearly depends upon which type of naming test is presented, and suggests that tests of confrontation naming and verbal fluency can make rather differing demands on underlying cognitive operations.

Category fluency tests are argued to require the use of problem-solving strategies for planning and carrying out the recall of items from memory and for keeping a record of the items already recalled (Estes 1974), and would appear to involve the use the supervisory system of the central executive (Shallice 1988). If Mrs C's naming difficulty in category fluency tasks were due to a problem with some aspect of executive function, then she should also show problems on tests (such as the Wisconsin Card Sorting Test) which specifically tap such functions. This turned out to be the case: Mrs C had severe problems with such tasks, in particular, she appeared to have a problem with sustaining ideas and plans. For example she would forget during the task what she should be doing, and in language tasks, such as describing the activities in a picture, she would begin sentences and then stop, often in the middle of words (see Funnell and Hodges 1996 for more details). Thus Mrs C's naming disorder did not appear to be a language disorder *per se*, but arose from a disorder of executive functions affecting only those language tasks that required its services. By contrast, confrontation naming tasks reduce the demand upon executive functions by presenting the individual items directly to the subject for naming and by requiring only the activation of an associated schema for the recalling the specific name.

As it happens, Mrs K and Mrs P, whose naming abilities were impaired on both confrontation and verbal category fluency tests, had no problems on tasks of attention and planning. Their naming deficits, which differed between them, arose for other reasons which can be explained with reference to the model of naming shown in Fig. 2.1. This model predicts that a disorder of naming could arise from damage to various components: from a problem arising in access to, or within, processes involved in recognizing pictures (that is, the structural codes); from a problem arising in access to, or within, processes involved in understanding words and pictures (that is, the semantic codes); or from a problem arising in access to, or within, processes involved in finding the name (namely, the phonological codes); or from any combination of these deficits.

Specific cognitive tests established that neither subject had problems with the visual processing of pictured objects, suggesting that the naming disorder occurred at stages down-line from the pictogens, with processes concerned with either the comprehension of objects and their names, or with the retrieval of spoken names. One way to distinguish between these different areas of possible deficit is to ask subjects to match spoken or written words to pictures, or to define the meanings of spoken words. Subjects who cannot do these tasks would appear to have a comprehension disorder which would also affect object naming.[1] On the other hand, if a subject is able to match words to pictures successfully, but cannot then name the pictures, the problem would appear to lie with processes involved in finding a name.

When the naming disorders of Mrs K and Mrs P were investigated using these tests, it was found that Mrs K had a specific disorder of access to word forms in the phonological codes, while Mrs P had a disorder which affected the semantic codes, making it difficult to understand names and to identify objects. Thus although the naming abilities of these two patients showed severe impairments on both confrontation and category fluency tests, the underlying cognitive deficits were quite different. When the deficits of the three subjects are indicated on the model of naming, to which a component has

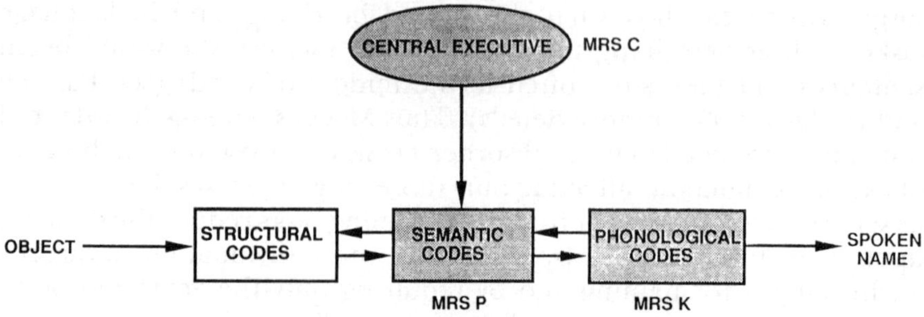

FIG. 2.2 A simple model of the processes involved in confrontation naming and category fluency, indicating the locations of the cognitive deficits underlying the naming disorders of the three subjects.

been added to represent processes involved in executive function (see Fig. 2.2), it is clear that the naming disorders of each of the these three subjects arise from deficits to different processing components. Details of further methods used in support of these conclusions can be found in the publications referred to in Table 2.1.

COGNITIVE CHANGES OVER TIME

Longitudinal studies of each subject's naming showed that, in every case, verbal fluency scores declined, Mrs C's to a point at which she could produce the name of only three animals, which she then repeated, although her confrontation naming remained at a normal level over this time period. Interestingly, in earlier tests she had produced a wider variety of animal names in category fluency tasks than had the other two subjects, who were confined to producing names of the most familiar animals.

A study of the decline of Mrs K's specific word-finding problem showed that particular names dropped out at a fast and constant rate from her vocabulary, failing to reappear at subsequent tests. For a while, it seems that these names could be prompted into activity if the first sound of the object's name was provided for her, but, later on, cues failed to produce these names, suggesting that the strength of the cognitive representations of the names had faded beyond a point at which they could be accessed. Although at the time this study was carried out no variable could be found which predicted the time course with which particular words disappeared from Mrs K's vocabulary (see Funnell and Hodges 1991), a later study has shown that measures of the age at which different words are thought to be acquired in life did predict the pattern of names lost over time from Mary's vocabulary, showing that words learned later were more likely to disappear first (Hirsh and Funnell 1995).

Longitudinal studies of Mrs P's comprehension of word meanings showed a regular, but fairly slow, decline over time. Concepts for less familiar objects such as *sword* and *syringe,* were affected before concepts for more familiar objects, such as *dog* and *church.* Affected concepts gradually broadened in meaning and became confused with the concepts of objects belonging to the same semantic category; for example, less familiar animals could not be distinguished from other less familiar animals. Eventually, for some items, no vestiges of meaning appeared to remain, a pattern of semantic breakdown that has been reported elsewhere (Funnell 1992; Hodges *et al.* 1995; Schwartz *et al.* 1979).

IMPLICATIONS OF SINGLE CASE STUDIES FOR QUALITY OF LIFE AND MANAGEMENT

Knowing about the underlying cognitive deficits of a particular subject can provide important information for the individual and family concerned about the nature of the cognitive problem or problems, the expected rate of decline, and the likely extent of the effects of a particular disorder upon cognition in general. Even from the study of a restricted task such as object naming, quite a lot can be learned. For instance, the naming ability of the first subject, Mrs K, declined at a regular and very fast rate, so that after only three presentations of any particular naming test, it was possible to predict accurately the point at which Mrs K would be unable to name any items on that test. Secondly, it was possible to predict that, so long as the disorder was restricted to the recall of spoken word forms, Mrs K should continue to understand the words she failed to name, and so take part in conversation. Unfortunately, as it happened, Mrs K later developed a rapidly progressing semantic disorder so that she eventually became unable either to produce or comprehend names (Funnell 1992).

Mrs P's comprehension disorder declined gradually over five years of assessment. Over the first year no decline was apparent, but over several years a steady decline became observable at a rate which predicted that conceptual ability would not be detectable at a point seven years after assessment began. Mrs P's ability to comprehend the names of objects could be predicted by how common the object was, and it proved to be possible to improve her comprehension and naming ability by reintroducing her to some concepts which she appeared to have partially forgotten (Funnell 1996). The fact that recent experience seemed to strengthen her memory for particular concepts suggested that keeping her involved in everyday tasks, outings, and social activities should help to maintain her conceptual base. It also suggested that verbal communication would be improved if the vocabulary used to converse with her mapped on to more common concepts, since these were more likely to be preserved. At present, five years after initial assessment, Mrs P continues to run the house and to cook (although earlier interests in dressmaking activities have waned), and to attend activities outside the home. Interestingly, her inability to identify many common objects and object names in standard testing situations has not affected her ability to use these objects in everyday life (a phenomenon which is currently under investigation).

Of the three subjects, the third individual, Mrs C, had the most fundamental problems. Her naming disorder on the category fluency task arose from a disorder to executive control processes involved in problem solving and planning: in particular, she appeared to have difficulty in sustaining attention to a plan once initiated. This disorder increasingly affected spontaneous speech, which requires the use of processes involved with forming ideas and turning ideas into words, which became severely impoverished, even though she quite clearly understood most of what was being said to her and what was happening around her. Executive control processes are used in all tasks that require planning or problem solving, and it was noticeable that Mrs C's ability to initiate and carry out household tasks also became increasingly impaired. It appears that a progressive disorder affecting central mental operations can have particularly far-reaching effects upon cognition.

NOTE

1. This account overlooks the possibility that comprehension deficits could arise from loss of memory for the surface forms of the words used in the comprehension tests. This omission (and others) has been made to help make plain the general issues involved in the single case study approach and to avoid the confusions which could arise if a complete account were given here of all the procedures and assumptions involved.

REFERENCES

Bruce, V. and Young, A. W. (1986). Understanding face recognition. *British Journal of Psychology*, **77**, 305–27.

Coltheart, M. (1984). Editorial. *Cognitive Neuropsychology*, **1**, 1–8.

Ellis, A. W. (1987). Intimations of modularity, or, the modularity of mind: Doing cognitive neuropsychology without syndromes. In *The cognitive neuropsychology of language* (ed. M. Coltheart, G. Sartori, and R. Job). Lawrence Erlbaum Associates, London.

Estes, W. K. (1974). Learning theory and intelligence. *American Psychologist,* **29**, 740–9.

Funnell, E. (1992). Progressive loss of semantic memory in a case of Alzheimer's disease. *Proceedings of the Royal Society of London,* **B249**, 287–91.

Funnell, E. (1996). A case of forgotten knowledge. In *Broken memories* (ed. R. Campbell and M. Conway), pp.225–36. Blackwell, Oxford (in press).

Funnell, E. and Hodges, J., R. (1991). Progressive loss of access to spoken word forms in a case of Alzheimer's disease. *Proceedings of the Royal Society of London,* **B243**, 173–9.

Funnell, E. and Hodges, J. R. (1996). Deficits of semantic memory and executive control: Evidence for differing effects upon naming in dementia. *Aphasiology* (In press).

Gurd, J. and Marshall, J. C. (1991). Neuropsychology: Cognitive status in progressive neurological illness. *Current Opinion in Psychiatry,* **4**, 612–15.

Hirsh, K. W. and Funnell, E. (1995). Those old, familiar things: Age of acquisition, familiarity and lexical access in progressive aphasia. *Journal of Neurolinguistics,* **9**, 23–32.

Hodges, J. R., Graham, N., and Patterson, K. (1995). Charting the progression in semantic dementia: implications for the organisation of semantic memory. *Memory,* **3**, 463–95.

Hodges, J. R., Patterson, K. E., Oxbury, S., and Funnell, E. (1992). Semantic dementia. *Brain,* **115**, 1783–806.

Holland, A. L., McBurney, D. H., Moossy, J., and Reinmuth, O. M. (1985). The dissolution of language in Pick's disease with nerofibrillary tangles: A case study. *Brain and Language,* **24**, 36–58.

Kay, J., Lesser, R., and Coltheart, M. (1992). *PALPA.* Lawrence Erlbaum Associates, London.

McKenna, P. and Warrington, E. K. (1980). *The Graded Naming Test.* Nelson, Windsor.

Marr, D. (1976). Early processing of visual information. *Philosophical Transactions of the Royal Society of London,* **B275**, 483–524.

Marshall, J. C. and Newcombe, F. (1973). Patterns of paralexia: a psycholinguistic approach. *Journal of Psycholinguistic Research,* **2**, 175–99.

Martin, A. (1990). Neuropsychology of Alzheimer's disease: The case for subgroups. In *Modular deficits in Alzheimer-type dementia* (ed. M. F. Schwartz), pp.143–176. MIT, Cambridge, Mass.

Mattis, S. (1973). *Dementia Rating Scale.* NFER-Nelson, Windsor.

Morton, J. (1979). Facilitation in word recognition: Experiments causing change in the logogen model. In *Processing of visible language* (ed. P.A. Kolers M.E. Wrolstad, and H. Bouma), pp.259–68. Plenum Press, New York.

Morton, J. and Patterson, K. E. (1980). A new attempt at an interpretation, or, an attempt at a new interpretation. In *Deep dyslexia* (ed. M. Coltheart, K. Patterson, and J.C. Marshall), pp.91–118. Routledge & Kegan Paul, London.

Nelson, H. E. (1976). A modified card sorting test sensitive to frontal lobe defects. *Cortex,* **51**, 353–61.

Riddoch, M. J. and Humphreys, G. (1993). *Birmingham Object Recognitive Battery*. Lawrence Erlbaum Associates, Hove.

Schwartz, M. F. (1987). Focal cognitive deficits in dementia of the Alzheimer type. *Neuropsychology*, **1**, 27–35.

Schwartz, M. F. (1990). *Modular deficits in Alzheimer-type dementia*. Cambridge, MIT Books, Mass.

Schwartz, M. F., Marin, O. S. M., and Saffran, E. M. (1979). Dissociations of language function in dementia: A case study. *Brain and Language*, **7**, 277–306.

Schwartz, M. F., Saffran, E. M., and Marin, O. S. M. (1980). Fractionating the reading process in dementia: evidence for word specific print-to-sound impairments. In *Deep dyslexia* (ed. M. Coltheart, K. Patterson, and J.C. Marshall), pp. 259–69. Routledge & Kegan Paul, London.

Shallice, T. (1981). Neurological impairment of cognitive processes. *British Medical Bulletin*, **37**, 187–92.

Shallice, T. (1988). *From neuropsychology to mental structure*. Cambridge University Press, Cambridge.

Warrington, E. K. and Shallice, T. (1969) The selective impairment of auditory verbal short-term memory. *Brain*, **92**, 885–96.

Warrington, E. K. (1975). The selective impairment of semantic memory. *Quarterly Journal of Experimental Psychology*, **27**, 197–9.

Whitaker, H. (1976). A case of the isolation of the language function. In *Studies in Neurolinguistics* II, (ed. H. Whitaker and H.A. Whitaker), pp. 1–58. Academic Press, New York.

THREE

Charting decline in dementia

Colin Gray and Sergio Della Sala

INTRODUCTION

Expressions such as 'dotage' and 'second childhood', which date back at least to the time of Galen (see Spinnler and Della Sala 1988 for a review), are metaphors which mask the existence of a number of distinct conditions to which the generic term *dementia* is now applied. The more specific term *organic mental deterioration* (OMD) denotes a progressive functional impairment arising from a degenerative disease of the brain over and above vascular accident or metabolic disorder. In keeping with the title of the book, the present chapter is concerned with Alzheimer-type dementia (AD), a form of OMD which, while mainly a disease of the elderly, can occasionally affect people in their forties and fifties (Bachman *et al.* 1992). AD is a terminal condition which leads inexorably to a state of total cognitive debilitation and death (Adams and Victor 1989).

The current state of knowledge of the natural history of the disease, its nosology and progress derive largely from studies carried out only within the past ten years or so (e.g. Becker 1988; Becker *et al.* 1994; Botwinick *et al.* 1986; Katzman *et al.* 1988*a*). Such work was made possible by the availability, for the first time, of substantial numbers of patients in whom the course of the disease could be studied. A number of pharmacological investigations have been conducted with a view to ameliorating the effects of the disease (see Chapter 18). Other work has concentrated upon the progressive impairment of cognition for the purpose either of obtaining a global rating of dementia (often in relation to significant clinical events, or endpoints, e.g. Berg *et al.* 1988; Kraemer *et al.* 1994), or of developing a more fine-grained normative sequencing across a range of specified cognitive functions (Becker *et al.* 1994).

The need for further research

Despite the dramatic increase in our knowledge of the natural history of AD yielded by recent studies, some of the most important questions have yet to be answered unequivocally. There has been, for example, much dispute about the trajectory of the disease, the rate of progress (especially in relation to age of onset), and whether AD is a single condition or a set of closely related disorders. Sometimes, there are striking discrepancies between the results of different studies, as when Katzman *et al.* (1988*a*) failed to find evidence for an effect of age of onset on rate of decline, whereas Jacobs *et al.* (1994) found strong evidence for such an effect. There is also disagreement about the relationship between age of onset and language functions, some finding no relationship (Selnes *et al.* 1988), others finding greater language impairment with late onset (Bayles 1991), and still others finding greater language impairment with early onset (Filley *et al.* 1986).

Aim of this chapter

Underlying many of these disputes and discrepancies are methodological considerations of research strategy and measurement. The purpose of this chapter is to identify those aspects of research procedure that we believe are most crucial, and to indicate ways in which the progress of the disease can be monitored accurately from its earliest manifestations to the final stages.

METHODOLOGICAL CONSIDERATIONS

The course of AD typically runs for between six and twelve years (Spinnler and Della Sala 1988, p. 264). Despite the comparative brevity of this period, there are important methodological parallels with developmental studies of healthy cognitive functioning over the greater part of the lifespan. The charting of the trajectory of OMD, however, presents additional problems relating to measurement, patient selection, and subject attrition.

In this section, we shall consider general research strategy, measuring instruments, (including their reliability, validity, and the cognitive functions they appear to be tapping), a number of problems in the tracking of decline, and some aspects of the statistical analysis of the data.

Research strategy: cross-sectional and longitudinal research

When studying either age-related changes in cognition or progressive cognitive decline associated with AD, the researcher has available either (or both) of two strategies: (1) *cross-sectional*, whereby all measurements of any individual are taken at one point in time; (2) *longitudinal*, in which the same individuals are measured, on the same variables, at several points during the course of the study. There are, of course, 'hybrid' designs, which combine some of the features of (1) and (2): for instance an individual tested on one variable could be tested on another at a later point. The cross-sectional and longitudinal approaches do not always yield the same answer to the same question. For example when applied to age-related changes in intelligence, cross-sectional work has indicated a decline after the age of 30 years, whereas longitudinal studies indicate a sustained level of performance lasting into late middle age (Baltes *et al.* 1976).

Since the merits and demerits of cross-sectional and longitudinal research have already been discussed exhaustively elsewhere (e.g. Spector 1981), only one or two remarks are germane here. The cross-sectional strategy affords control over various important properties of the sample, notably the size, and (to some degree) representativeness on crucial demographic variables. Moreover, *some* of the potentially confounding secular influences that bedevil the interpretation of longitudinal studies (see Spector 1981) cannot arise when all the data are gathered at the same time. Furthermore, the biases exacerbated by uneven subject attrition in longitudinal research (see below) are likely to be less marked in cross-sectional research; although it may be difficult to recruit some types of subject (for example elderly people with a university education).

The hypothesis that two conditions A and B are independent is confirmed by finding the *double dissociation* pattern in a set of data, whereby not only can A occur with or without B but also B can occur with or without A, thus establishing that neither variable is a necessary or a sufficient condition for the other. In a cross-sectional study with 55 patients, Baddeley *et al.* (1991*a*) found a double dissociation between long-term memory (as measured by learning performance) and short-term (span) memory: that is, some patients were poor on span but better on learning, which is characteristic of short-term amnesia; but others showed the reverse pattern, as in global amnesia. The infrequency of such cases, however, illustrates one of the principal advantages of cross-sectional work: larger samples increase the likelihood of finding cases for infrequent cells in a two-way classification, as in the Baddeley *et al.* study.

It should not be supposed, however, that cross-sectional research is entirely immune to the confounding effects of secular influences. An intelligence test which is used to compare subjects in different age groups on supposedly pure measures of native spatial ability, attention, and concentration may favour those who have had their childhood in the computer age, with its super-abundance of games requiring precisely those abilities: such children, that is to say, are sophisticated with respect to the cognitive demands of some types of test item content.

In the field of AD research, the great problem with cross-sectional studies is that the statistics they yield often give rise to highly misleading expectations about the course of deterioration in the individual patient. Even among those carefully diagnosed as AD patients, a marked heterogeneity of cognitive deficits can be found, at least in the early stages of the disease (Baddeley *et al.* 1991*b*; Becker 1988; Capitani *et al.* 1986; Della Sala *et al.* 1986; Martin *et al.* 1986; Spinnler and Della Sala 1988).

Correlation does not imply causation. Therefore, since most psychological hypotheses assert that one variable has a causal effect upon another, or that one cognitive function organizes or drives another, cross-sectional research is ill-suited to hypothesis testing. Longitudinal research can bring more powerful evidence to bear upon such questions of cognitive structure and causality.

Recent studies of the trajectories of decline, in individual patients, on an array of cognitive tasks have permitted the testing of hypotheses about cognitive architecture. For example Hodges *et al.* (1995) studied a patient with semantic dementia over a period of two years, with a view to resolving competing theories of semantic organization. They found evidence of the preservation of knowledge applicable to general categories, while item-specific information was lost, a pattern which they prefer, however, to interpret in terms of a network concept, rather than a structural hierarchy.

Using dual methodology, Baddeley *et al.* (1991*b*) sought support for the hypothesis that, in AD patients (in contrast with amnesics), many aspects of cognitive deterioration arise from a deficit in the controlling central executive component of working memory. With dual task methodology, a potential confounding variable is the greater demand that dual tasks may make upon the limited general processing capacity of AD patients. By following a longitudinal strategy, whereby patients served as their own controls, Baddeley *et al.* were able to show not only that dual task performance deteriorated while single task performance was maintained, but also that the rate of deterioration co-varied with whether single or dual task performance was required, rather than simply upon level of task difficulty.

Measuring instruments

A first diagnosis of AD is, at best, a provisional statement, a suspicion rather than a confident categorization. The course of diagnosis as a whole follows a 'cascade schedule' (Spinnler and Della Sala 1988), comprising three stages of progressively finer filtering: (1) a preliminary enquiry into the patient's personal history of difficulties that are suggestive of dementia; (2) formal neuropsychological testing; (3) a neurological examination, supplemented by CT scanning, to exclude other kinds of dementia. At stage 1, the presence of the syndrome of dementia is (provisionally) established; at stage 2, a provisional diagnosis of the specific disease condition of AD is made; at stage 3, possible alternatives are excluded by neurological screening.

The measuring instruments used to chart the progress of cognitive decline in AD have been of two general types; namely, brief screening instruments, which yield global scores, and test batteries, which permit a fine-grained analysis of patterns of presentation and decline.

Screening instruments

Among the most widely used screening tests in the USA are the Blessed Information Memory–Concentration Test (IMC) (Katzman *et al.* 1988*a*; Thal *et al.* 1986), the Mini-Mental State Examination (MMSE) (Folstein *et al.* 1975; Galasko *et al.* 1990), the Cognitive Capacity Screening Examination (CCSE) (Jacobs *et al.* 1977), the Mental Status Questionnaire (MSQ) (Kahn *et al.* 1960), the Short Portable Mental Status Questionnaire (SPMSQ) (Pfeiffer 1975), and the Dementia Rating Scale (DRS) (Mattis 1976). Other screening instruments are the Clinical Dementia Rating (CDR) (Hughes *et al.* 1982; Berg *et al.* 1984), the Global Deterioration Scale (GDS) (Reisberg 1982), the Milan Overall Dementia Assessment (MODA) (Brazzelli *et al.* 1994), and the CAMDEX (Roth *et al.* 1986).

The MMSE yields a score varying from 0 to 30, progressing in steps of one unit (values greater than 23 are taken to indicate that the patient is not impaired). Scores on the DRS vary, in half-unit steps, from 0 to 17. Anything higher than 17 is taken to indicate dysfunction. The CDR examines six kinds of cognitive ability, and rates each on a scale from 0 (normal) to 3 (severely impaired). The GDS, on the other hand, identifies 7 main stages of progressively severe impairment. The difference in the nominal ranges of these four tests illustrates a major difficulty with the comparison of results from different studies: mental impairment is measured on a variety of different scales with varying number of points. Moreover, while some tests (for instance the MMSE) are measures of performance level, with higher scores indicating higher levels of functions, others (for example the CDR, the GDS, the DRS, and the IMC) express the severity of cognitive impairment as an error score. So it is that what some authors describe as a 'floor effect' on one test is dubbed a 'ceiling effect' on another. Hereafter, to avoid confusion, we shall use the terms 'ceiling' and 'floor' in the conceptual, rather than the numerical, sense to refer to the highest and lowest performance plateaux, respectively.

Other potential difficulties with translation, however, are less easily remedied. When measurements are made on an *interval scale*, as in physics, chemistry, or engineering (Stevens 1946), it is a straightforward matter to transform measurements from one unit to another, as when using the formula C/(F-32)=5/9 to convert temperature units from degrees Celsius to degrees Fahrenheit or vice versa. But considerable difficulties can arise with attempts to effect similar translations with ratings that are aggregates of highly heterogeneous items (in this case varying mixtures of cognitive and practical enquiries).

While some conversion algorithms are available (e.g. Thal *et al.* 1986), the markedly different compositions of some pairs of tests would render such an exercise highly questionable, even though the use of each scale may be well justified by the linear summative scaling model (Nunnally 1978, p. 83), and both tests may have good psychometric properties.

Screening instruments vary considerably in the composition of the items they contain. The MMSE has a rather perfunctory coverage of cognition. The CAMDEX, on the other hand, contains a subscale concerned exclusively with cognitive functioning. The MODA has an even larger cognitive component (85% of items); but there are also items testing everyday coping skills, included to improve the validity of the test and extend its applicability to more severely demented patients.

Reliability and validity

In psychometric theory (Nunnally 1978), a measuring instrument must meet two requirements: it must be (1) reliable, and (2) valid. The first of these is a necessary, but not a sufficient, condition for the second. A reliable instrument is one which, given that the measured characteristic does not change, gives consistent results when different people measure the same target on different occasions. A mental measuring instrument must also be valid: that is it must measure what it is supposed to measure. As with reliability, there are several practical interpretations of validity; and an instrument that is 'valid' in one interpretation may not be so in another.

Reliability of the tests used in Alzheimer research

A number of studies have established that the MMSE, the CCSE, the DRS, the MSQ, and the SPMSQ all have adequate inter-rater reliability; and good test–retest reliability has been established for MMSE, the DRS, and the SPMSQ (Nelson *et al.* 1986). The CDR and the MODA also show good levels of reliability (Brazzelli *et al.* 1994; Galasko *et al.* 1991).

Haxby *et al.* (1992) compared the signal-to-noise ratio for the WAIS IQ (Wechsler 1965, 1981), DRS, and MMSE by dividing the mean rate of decline by the standard error of the measurement. Using this measure, they showed that the WAIS IQ, which takes considerably longer to administer than the DRS and MMSE, achieves a higher signal-to-noise ratio than the shorter measuring instruments, presumably because it takes the largest behavioural sample.

Interpretations of validity in Alzheimer research

In Alzheimer research the term *validity* is used in several different senses: (1) accuracy of diagnosis; (2) measuring the severity of the condition; (3) tracking the course of the disease; (4) estimating the time to arrive at a specified endpoint; (5) predicting the rate of decline. These are quite distinct interpretations of validity: an instrument that is valid either as a diagnostic instrument or as a measure of severity is not necessarily good for 'tracking' the progress of the disease (see Galasko *et al.* 1991).

An important aspect of the first of these usages is incremental validity (Nelson *et al.* 1986), that is the extent to which the use of a screening test improves upon the diagnostic accuracy of clinical examinations. In our view, however, it is in the context of follow-up testing, rather than more extensive cross-sectional examination, that the biggest improvements in diagnostic validity are to be obtained (see below).

Validity of diagnostic instruments

The status of AD as a distinct disease entity, separable from other forms of dementia and with a demonstrable basis in deterioration of the central nervous system, is no longer seriously questioned. Histological examination reveals a set of features (such as fibrillary tangles and plaques) which, though none is specific to AD, occur in a pattern which is highly characteristic of the condition (Selkoe 1988) (see Chapter 13).

The diagnosis of AD is, nevertheless, subject to error. There are several reasons for this, the principal being that there are no *in vivo* neurological markers upon which the diagnostician can place reliance. In the 1980s, studies of neuropathology showed that diagnosis was confirmed at post mortem in only 80–85% of cases (Joachim *et al.* 1988; Wade *et al.* 1987). Present day diagnosis, however, may be considerably more accurate than this (Mendez *et al.* 1992). Moreover, a valid *in vivo* marker may be just around the corner (e.g. Scinto 1994). At the moment, however, it is safe to assume that any study inevitably includes, in addition to genuine AD patients, some who are suffering from other forms of dementia (whether of vascular or of metabolic origin); in fact, some of the symptoms of psychiatric disturbance (such as manic-depressive illness) are very similar to the impaired cognition of patients in the early stages of AD.

Incremental validity in diagnosis

Having noted the satisfactory reliability of five common measuring instruments, Nelson *et al.* (1986) nevertheless conclude that none of the tests increases the level of diagnostic accuracy beyond that achieved by clinical examinations alone. This, they suggest, is because 'The tests reviewed do not detect many types of cognitive deficit that may bear critically on differential diagnosis and case management' (p. 73). Moreover, when they carried out their review, little consideration had been given to demographic or other variables. As a result, the tests showed unacceptably high false-negative rates.

From the diagnostic point of view, improvements in validity may result from longitudinal research into trajectories of performance on a variety of cognitive functions. The establishment of normative sequencing permits the identification, in an individual patient, of unusual onset of the kind that, nevertheless, eventually leads to an 'Alzheimer-like' pattern at a later stage (Della Sala *et al.* 1986).

The effective use of subsequent retesting (e.g. Brazzelli *et al.* 1994). To strengthen the incremental diagnostic validity of a cognitive screening test is another demonstration of the power of longitudinal research to resolve questions that lie beyond the reach of the cross-sectional approach.

Validity of tests used to chart the progress of AD

Despite the unmistakable signature of AD at autopsy, the various histopathological features, when considered individually, are neither peculiar to AD nor do they necessarily correlate with degree of cognitive deterioration during OMD. For example Galasko *et al.* (1991) have reviewed work on the behaviour of a number of measures that are usually taken at autopsy: plaque and tangle counts, levels of choline acetyltransferase, neurone counts, and nucleolar size. It was found, for example, that scores on the IMC test (number of errors) at the stage of diagnosis correlated positively with the number of plaques and choline acetyltransferase at autopsy, an association which obtained both in AD patients and in normal controls (Blessed *et al.* 1968; Katzman *et al.* 1983). The MMSE has also been found to correlate with the number of plaques at autopsy (Martin *et al.* 1987). While such findings validate the IMC and MMSE as rough tests of severity of neuropathology, however, the histopathological features concerned show little evidence of covarying with the severity of OMD as the disease progresses. In one of the few bioptic studies reported in the literature, Mann *et al.* (1988) found, as the disease progressed in five

AD patients, no increase in the plaque and tangle counts, despite obvious cognitive deterioration (though neurone and nucleolar counts did show progressive worsening). Moreover, Katzman *et al.* (1988*b*) reported a group of non-demented elderly people who, autoptically, met Khachaturian's (1985) pathological critera for AD. These findings, together with the claim that education may afford a resource buffer which preserves competence level, despite neuropathological changes (Stern *et al.* 1992), cast doubt upon the tracking validity of pathological features.

From the reports of studies that are available in the literature, electro-physiological and radiographic measures do not compare well with 'behavioural' criteria or test performance as tools for monitoring the progress of AD. As with the neuropathological features, changes on such *in vivo* neuro-physiological and anatomical measures may not be reflected in changes in cognitive performance, and the former may be insensitive to significant deterioration in performance levesl (Galasko *et al.* 1991).

The best 'trackers' would appear to be neurophysiological instruments that have been supported by the necessary psychometric research on their reliability. It has been shown, for example, that the WAIS-R performs well as a tracker, probably because it takes a larger sample of cognitive functioning than do briefer instruments such as the MMSE; on the other hand, it contains no measure of the ability to commit new information to long-term memory or to orient oneself in time and space (Haxby *et al.* 1992). The DRS test, is also reliable, valid and a good tracker (Jacobs *et al.* 1994); although it has been suggested that its memory and orientation items may not be sufficiently sensitive to detect changes in functions that have already shown impairment on the occasion of the first testing (Haxby *et al.* 1992, p. 587).

Problems in tracking the decline in Alzheimer's disease

In this subsection we shall consider some recurrent problems which have made it difficult to build up a coherent picture of the progress of AD: floor and ceiling effects limit a test's range of usefulness; selection of the patient sample is more than a matter of diagnosis and presents a number of dilemmas; practice effects can distort the disease's measured trajectory; and the performance of a tracker test may well depend upon which of a number of possible endpoints has been chosen for the study.

Floor and ceiling effects: widening the psychometric window

Many measuring instruments show floor and/or ceiling effects, rendering them insensitive to variation of function either at the initial or final stages of the disease. Both the IMC and the MMSE have the disadvantage that scores on them reach floor level (expressed, in the case of the IMC, as a maximum number or errors) at quite an early stage in the progress of AD. The DRS, however, reaches floor level at a much later stage and is therefore more suitable for use with severely demented patients (Salmon *et al.* 1990).

Performance on some of the more specialized items in neuropsychological tests soon reaches floor level, rendering such tests unsuitable for measuring deterioration during the final stages of the course of OMD. It is desirable, however, to have brief screening instruments that measure deterioration throughout the course of the disease. The 'psychometric window' can be widened by including a number of very simple items, resulting in a non-zero aggregate score even in severely deteriorated patients (Brazzelli *et al.* 1994).

There are also reports of ceiling effects when screening tests have been used with patients in the early stages of AD. For example Katzman *et al.* (1988*a*) found that the IMC showed a ceiling effect (expressed as a minimum number of errors) when the error scores were below 24. It may be that the most commonly used tests are insufficiently sensitive to the sorts of cognitive (especially linguistic) failures that might be noticeable to patients' relatives or emerge in a sensitive clinical interview.

A modified version of the MMSE, the nMMS, has been developed by Mayeux *et al.* (1981). As well as the 30 items in the standard MMSE, the nMMS contains forwards and backwards digit span, calculations, questions on the current president of the USA and his four predecessors, and confrontation naming of items from the Boston Naming Test (Goodglass and Kaplan 1972). Despite this more extensive cognitive coverage, however, the nMMS may still not pick up the first signs of language impairment, to which the relatives of patients are known to be sensitive (Haxby *et al.* 1992).

Selection of the patient sample

Many considerations determine the selection of the patient sample: the goal of study, the plan for the statistical analysis of the data, the patients' initial level of performance, and the choice of endpoint.

In view of doubt associated with the diagnosis of AD in its early stages, the practice of retaining, in the patient sample, a number of questionable cases has much to recommend it. Even if some of those patients must subsequently be dropped from the present study, their data may not only help to enhance subsequent diagnostic accuracy but also afford insights into the neuropsychological nature of AD in comparison with other forms of OMD and dementia.

A good study would detail inclusion criteria to permit comparisons with other work and meta-analysis, as well as eventually permitting detection of false-positives and-negatives. For example Summers *et al.* (1986) excluded a subject who was positive on the Shilling test despite the fact that cobalamin deficiency may not cause dementia (though it can produce neuropsychiatric symptoms) (Lindenbaum *et al.* 1988). To include the case is to risk a false-positive, but to exclude it is to increase the risk of a false-negative. We recommend the retention of such cases, with a full explanation of the dilemma.

But diagnosis (and the maximization of its validity) are by no means the only considerations in the selection of the patient sample. If it is intended to measure each patient in the study on several occasions over a period of time, it is necessary to consider the patient's initial scores on whatever screening instruments are to be used. Should a patient be near floor level on the first occasion of testing, subsequent testing is unlikely to provide further useful information.

In view of the remarks on incremental validity in diagnosis, the researcher should be mindful of the advantages of achieving a sample that is representative of the population with respect to demographic variables such as age, sex, and level of education (Crawford *et al.* 1995; Gray *et al.* 1992).

Practice effects

When a patient is measured repeatedly on the same variable, practice effects are a potential confounding variable, which may flatten the trajectory of measured performance. A case in point is a longitudinal study by Galasko *et al.* (1993), in which the scores of 39 patients tested four times on the MMSE and the IMC showed evidence of a short-term practice effect.

Endpoints

An important practical issue is the extent to which an aggregate score on a screening instrument can predict how long before continuous nursing is required and institutionalization must be considered. Much reported research is endpoint-oriented in this way.

Even from this important practical point of view, the interpretation of the results of various endpoint studies is problematic. There are several reasons for this: different studies have used different endpoints, different measuring instruments have been used, and the ambient social and nursing provision at different locations varies enormously. Any of these factors can affect the time taken by a patient to reach an endpoint.

In terms of deepening our understanding of the neuropsychology of AD, endpoints have the added disadvantage that, since they depend on such extraneous factors as local administrative policy and provision, family circumstances, and so on, the reaching of one cannot be expected to have a precise neuropsychological interpretation; moreover, the behaviour of an *aggregate* measure, even one calculated from subscores on broad categories of items, does not add to the fine-grained knowledge that is now so urgently required.

Measuring the rate of decline

The rate at which deterioration progresses in AD has been the subject of many investigations, both in its own right as an important aspect of the disease and in relation to such questions as whether it is age-related (Capitani *et al.* 1990; Jacobs *et al.* 1994), differs between different ethnic groups (Katzman *et al.* 1988*a*), or varies between supposedly different kinds of AD (Martin *et al.* 1986).

The problems of interpreting research on endpoints was touched upon in the preceding section. A measure of annual rate of deterioration (ARC), which does not relate to arbitrary clinical events or administrative decisions, is now regarded by many as a more useful target for prediction. This view is supported by recent work indicating that rate of decline may be constant for a given individual patient (Haxby *et al.* 1992; Jacobs *et al.* 1994). The observed change is obtained by simple subtraction from the previous year's score. Conceptually simple as this measure seems, however, it is worth noting that reports of observed change in various studies are expressed in units of the scales used, and so may not be comparable across studies. Raw difference scores have the additional disadvantage of being correlated with patients' initial scores on a test: a given simple difference, therefore, has different meanings for high and low initial scorers. For this reason, it is often better to work with residual difference scores, which are residuals from regression of the raw differences upon the baseline score differences (e.g. see Lucca *et al.* 1993).

A major consideration is that of the reliability of estimates of rate of decline (van Belle *et al.* 1990). As those authors point out, a difference in a variable measured on two occasions is a reflection of several factors: 'aging, the natural history of the disease, response to treatment and measurement, non-standard conditions, different observers, and statistical artifacts' (p. 589).

From psychometric theory, van Belle *et al.* show that the reliability of the rate measure depends upon the length of the period of the study, not upon the frequency of testing within the period. The reliability of changes, therefore, can be increased by extending the interval between measurements. While the reliability was estimated at just over 0.7 after a minimum period of study of 1.5 years, both the MMSE and the DRS scales were found to provide unreliable estimates of change if the period of observation was less than one year. For such short periods, therefore, these screening instruments should be combined with other measures of cognitive change. It is pointed out, however, that screening can tolerate a lower level of reliability of changes than can staging tests (van Belle *et al.* 1990, p. 595).

For growth-curve analysis of the sort undertaken by van Belle *et al.* patients with three or more test scores are required in order to obtain estimates of the residual variability.

Statistical considerations

New methods

The computer revolution of recent years has added immeasurably to the selection of statistical tools that are available for research. The researcher's arsenal now includes, as well as the traditional parametric non-parametric, an array of powerful multivariate methods such as multiple regression and path analysis, as well as a number of techniques that can handle qualitative variables.

The traditional Pearson correlation has been used to attempt to tease out causal relationships among variables on which there are longitudinal data, by studying the patterns of cross-lagged correlations. This mode of analysis, however, provides a limited basis for inference (Asher 1976; Markus 1979). The potential of longitudinal studies for resolving important questions of causality is more fully exploited by techniques such as path analysis (Bentler 1992; Everitt 1984). The use of path analysis, as available in computing packages such as LISREL and EQS, is now widespread. These methods are applicable to data sets from both cross-sectional and longitudinal studies (see Cuttance and Ecob 1987, who illustrate the use of the methods with both kinds of study).

Some cautions and caveats

This imposing panoply of new statistical ordnance, however, should not blind the user to some fundamental aspects of statistical testing and the nature of the data sets yielded by studies of AD.

The assumptions of statistical models The making of a formal statistical test always presupposes that the data have been generated according to an interpretation (usually in the form of an equation) known as a statistical model. The models underlying well-known statistical tests such as analysis of variance, t-tests, and multivariate methods make varyingly strict specifications which are often not satisfied by the data from longitudinal studies of AD.

The data from a longitudinal study constitute a time series. In recent years, great advances have been made in the analysis of time series data, and these new methods have been put to good use in such subjects as economics, which generates data of the sort the techniques of time series analysis were intended to handle. For long series of measurements, the autoregressive integrated moving average (ARIMA) is sensitive to trends and discontinuities. Unfortunately, studies of decline during AD yield too few measurements for the application of ARIMA, which requires a minimum of 50 data points (McDowall *et al.* 1980).

The importance of adequate statistical power

The power of a statistical test is the probability that the null hypothesis, if false, will be rejected. With small samples, this probability may be very low, which means that an insignificant result is impossible to interpret. But sample size is not the only determinant of power: marked individual differences can inflate error terms and lead to insignificance.

The traditional Fisherian hypothesis-testing procedure creates the danger of falsely accepting the null hypothesis as, for example, in the case of Boller *et al.* (1991) and Ortof and Crystal (1989) who found no significant relationship between age at onset and rate of decline. It has been remarked, however, that since in both sets of data there is a marked tendency for early-onset subjects to decline more rapidly, this negative conclusion may have been based upon tests of insufficient power (Jacobs *et al.* 1994).

The problem of subject attrition

In a project extending over much of the course of AD, a marked diminution of available subjects is inevitable. For example in the study of Baddeley *et al.* (1991*b*), the sample available for the first testing session comprised 28 AD patients. By the third session, however, this number had dropped to 15.

Two problems can arise with subject attrition. The more obvious is that, as the samples diminish in size, formal statistical tests lose power. There is also the possibility, however, that those subjects who remain available throughout the study and contribute to the final sample of data are from a special subgroup of the original population. To ascertain whether this is so, one might compare these survivors with the casualties on variables measured at the beginning of the study. This was done in the study of Baddeley *et al.* who concluded that 'The subgroups of "survivors" did not appear to differ demographically from the other patients, nor did they differ in level of performance on any of the wide range of psychometric and neuropsychological measures taken on these subjects' (p. 2525). That is certainly true of the survivors and casualties of the second session. It can be seen from their Table 1, however, that on the Ravens PM, the survivors at stage 3 averaged 19.5, whereas the drop-outs averaged 12.5. This pattern is also evident in the data from the Token Test and the Street CT. Comparisons with normative data led Baddeley *et al.* to conclude that 'the surviving AD patients were affected by a relatively mild and slow progressive form of the disease. While they showed few differences from the non-surviving patients on the initial test, it would be unwise to assume that they are a typical sample of all AD patients' (p. 2526).

Handling missing values

It is rare (and in studies of AD virtually impossible) to have a complete multivariate data set: almost inevitably, there will be some subjects for whom values are available on some variables (or trials), but not on others. A common stage in many multivariate methods is the construction of a correlation matrix (R), a rectangular array whose columns (and rows) contain the correlation between one variable and each of the others in the study. When some data are missing, however, the researcher wishing to construct the R-matrix is faced with a dilemma: does one perform the analysis *casewise*, that is, including only those subjects for whom there are values on *all* the variables (so all the correlations refer to the same sample of subjects); or does one consider the variables in *pairwise* fashion, including all subjects for whom data on both variables are available (which can mean that different correlations are based on data from non-identical samples of subjects)?

The choice between the pairwise and casewise approaches is not a simple one, and depends upon a number of considerations, both substantive and statistical. Each approach has advantages and disadvantages. For example while the pairwise approach has the satisfying property of making use of all the data from a study, there may be a severe statistical drawback. A matrix is said to be positive semidefinite when each of its eigenvalues (which, in the present context, can be interpreted as variances) is either positive or zero. The problem with the pairwise deletion strategy is that it *may* (though it does not always do so) result in an ill-conditioned matrix, that is one with negative eigenvalues, with consequent problems for the interpretation of the statistics in, say, a path analysis. For example the contribution of a variable to the variance of the DV may be greatly exaggerated.

There are several variants of the casewise approach (resulting in the loss of data from varying numbers of subjects) and they may result in different final path models. In choosing which missing value strategy to adopt, a crucial question is whether missing values can be considered as 'random gaps' in the data. Rarely would the missing values in AD research data meet those specifications.

SOME SUBSTANTIVE ISSUES

Modelling the trajectory of AD: linear and non-linear approaches

A recurrent finding in the longitudinal studies has been the apparent differences among patients in their profiles of progress of the disease, leading some to suspect that there may be different varieties of AD (Martin *et al.* 1986). Some interpetations of the disease's course, however, raise the possibility that at least some of this variation may have arisen because the patients studied were at different points on the disease's trajectory.

Brooks *et al.* (1993) have called into question the widely held assumption that the decline of cognitive functions (or, at any rate, performance on the tests used to monitor those functions) is linear throughout the progress of the disease (Fig. 3.1a). Instead, they argue, the disease trajectory, as measured by instruments such as the MMSE, typically follows what they term a 'trilinear' trajectory, beginning with a relatively stable initial plateau phase, followed by a second phase of marked linear decline, and ending in a second plateau, representing a final phase of relative stability (Fig. 3.1b). Others, however, have found that their data show a bilinear trajectory, whereby an initial plateau phase is followed by a period of steady decline (e.g. Haxby *et al.* 1992). Stern *et al.* (1994), however, claim that the annual rate of change in cognitive subscale scores on the ADAS follows a quadratic trajectory, with slower deterioration for mildly and severely demented patients than for those with moderate dementia.

In support of their model, Brooks *et al.* (1993) compare linear with

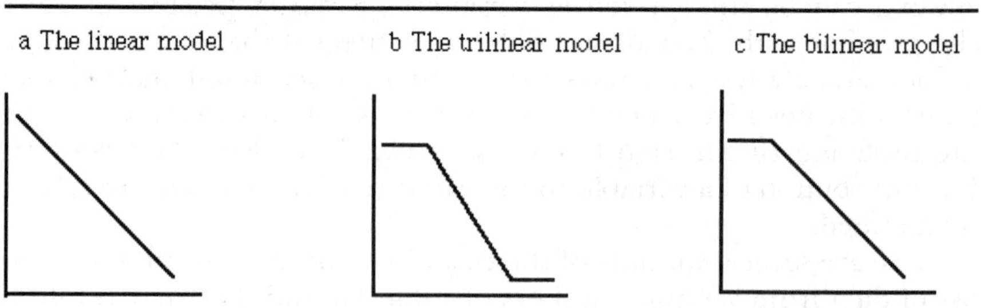

FIG. 3.1 Three hypothetical trajectories of decline in Alzheimer's disease.

trilinear analysis of data from 80 AD patients and find that the trilinear model gives a better fit to the data: that is, the trilinear model is better able to predict the patients' real scores on the MMSE than is the linear model. The trilinear model is a 'better fit' according to the *least squares* criterion, by which the sum of the squares of the differences between the true scores (y) on the MMSE and the estimates from the model (y') is as small as possible. The best-fitting model, that is, minimizes $\Sigma\ (y - y')^2$.

A word of caution may be appropriate here. The practice of fitting a mathematical model *a posteriori* to a set of data is not without risk. Any set of points (x, y) can be predicted more accurately by fitting more complex functions; in fact, if there is only one value y for each value x, *perfect* prediction of p points (x, y) is possible from a polynomial of degree (p–1). The improvement, however, may be statistically insignificant and hence not robust to a replication of the study with new patients.

Non-linearity of the trajectory of AD would have important implications for the interpretation of the findings of longitudinal studies. If the scores of patients at various stages in the profile of progression (some on a slope, others at a plateau) are combined, the averages yielded by statistical analysis are unlikely to be optimally representative of any of the patients in the study.

If, on the other hand, the profile of decline is indeed non-linear, agreement has yet to be achieved on its precise nature. The discrepancies reported in the literature may arise from the different measuring instruments used by the investigators concerned. In view of the foregoing discussion of floor and ceiling effects, it is important to make a clear distinction between *measured* decline and the deterioration of brain functioning underlying such decline. The inherent limitations of psychological measurement confine direct study exclusively to the former.

Age and rate of decline

There has been much dispute over the question of whether there are different varieties of AD, some (particularly those with early onset) being characterized by a more rapid rate of progress (Martin *et al.* 1986). A cross-sectional study by Capitani *et al.* (1990) showed early onset to be associated with more severe impairment. In view of the rapidity of the progression of other organic diseases (such as cancer) in younger patients, the suspicion that this also occurs in AD is entirely reasonable. Unfortunately there are several studies that fail to support the hypothesis. Huff *et al.* (1987) found a relationship between age and rate of decline; but they found the rate to be higher in patients with late onset. Katzman *et al.* (1988*a*) failed to confirm that there is *any* relationship between age of onset and rate of decline. And while Haxby *et al.* (1992) did find a very rapid rate of decline in their two patients with early onset, they found no relationship between age and rate of decline after the age of 50. At present, therefore, the picture is inconclusive.

At this stage it would be highly desirable to resolve the controversy in the literature over whether age is a factor in rate of decline at all, and if so, the direction of the relationship. The question of whether the age-rate link would confirm the existence of a distinct presenile form of AD is, it will be noted, quite a separate issue: to pursue the analogy with cancer in the young, rapidity of the progress of a disease does not, of itself, demonstrate that it is a distinct condition.

The effects of institutionalization

There has been much discussion of whether transferring AD patients to an institution (as opposed to trying to maintain them in their own homes) actually accelerates the progress of the disease. In a study comparing (among other groups) AD patients in nursing homes with those in community care, Katzman *et al.* (1988*a*) failed to obtain supporting evidence for the hospitalization hypothesis and concluded that 'the rate of change of mental status score is independent of whether the patient is in a nursing home or in the community' (p. 388). While it is true that such debilitating conditions as depression are much more prevalent in institutions for the elderly, this may arise because 'depressed people are more likely to be admitted to institutions in the first place' (Lindsey and Murphy 1989). The available evidence, deriving from studies in which demographic variables were adequately controlled, would support the view that the AD patient's terminal decline is determined very largely by biological processes, rather than social factors.

Level of education

Some researchers have found evidence for a lower prevalence of AD in those with a high level of education (for reviews, see Friedland 1993 and Katzman 1993). It has been suggested that education 'may provide a reserve that compensates for the neuropathological changes of AD' (Stern *et al.* 1992, p. 371) and that 'lower education may be a marker for decreased cerebral reserve capacity placing individuals at greater risk for displaying impairment' (Becker *et al.* 1994, p. 592).

This hypothesis is cogently argued and well worth further investigation. It is important to establish, however, that the putative education effect is not merely an artefact of methodology. Some studies have used screening tests that may well present less of a challenge to highly educated testees in the early stages of AD, whose first performance on them may therefore fail to show any deficit. Such false-negatives would have a strong effect upon the records of relative incidence of AD patients in the top educational categories at any time, giving the appearance of later onset in the well educated.

If there is such a bias, it can be reduced by using instruments for which there are normative data on appropriate demographic variables. Such data are available for the MODA (Brazzelli *et al.* 1994). Other sources of bias, however, can only be satisfactorily solved in the context of a longitudinal study, with pre-set testing times for all those patients provisionally included. Such additional control is yet another of the many advantages afforded by longitudinal research.

CONCLUSIONS

This chapter has identified a number of considerations which are of crucial importance when designing a longitudinal study of the progress of AD. Provided future studies are designed with these in mind, they should yield data that clarify some current issues, such as whether there are different subtypes of Alzheimer's disease, with varying patterns of progress.

When choosing an appropriate battery of tests, it is important to distinguish those measures that are optimally sensitive to change over a relatively short period from those designed for global assessment and diagnosis: a good screening test is not necessarily good at tracking decline.

For the statistical analysis of the data to be informative, the initial sample should be as large as possible, since massive patient attrition is almost inevitable in a study covering a large part of the course of the disease. A criterion for selection should have sufficient scope for further deterioration on the measuring instruments available. To permit the calculation of such useful statistics as signal-to-noise ratios, subjects should be tested on at least three occasions.

While there is reason to question the widely held assumption that the progress of the disease follows a linear path, non-linear profiles can arise from floor and ceiling effects resulting from insensitivity of tests at either extreme of their scales. In this respect, it is known that some tests are much more sensitive than others. Nevertheless, it is important to try to ensure that subjects are compared over corresponding sections of their performance profiles, so that one subject on a performance plateau is not compared with another in a phase of decline.

Tests should be selected carefully with a view to permitting a sufficiently fine-grained analysis of cognitive performance. Several of the most widely used tests have insufficient coverage of linguistic and other cognitive functions to detect the earliest signs of deterioration. Strengthening the cognitive component should not only improve the accuracy of diagnosis but also yield insights into the cognitive architecture and pattern of decline. At all times, care should be taken to check that the distributional assumptions of the formal statistical tests are tenable. It may be necessary to use tests that make few distribution assumptions. It is also worth bearing in mind that, with small samples especially, statistics such as the mean and the standard deviation can give a highly misleading impression of the level and spread of a sample of data. This is also true of incautious use of the Pearson correlation with a small bivariate data set.

Several striking inconsistencies in the findings reported in the literature may be clarified by consideration of the different methods and measurements used by the research teams concerned. It is recommended that, in general, reports should include much more information about the sources of the subjects, their demographic and other characteristics, and the criteria used for inclusion of subjects in the study.

ACKNOWLEDGEMENT

The authors wish to thank Dr Annalena Venneri for commenting on this chapter at various stages in its preparation.

REFERENCES

Adams, R. D., and Victor, M. (1989). *Principles of neurology*. McGraw-Hill, New York.

Alzheimer, A. (1977). A unique illness involving the cerebral cortex: A case report from the mental institution in Frankfurt am Main. Translated in *Neurological classics in modern translation* D. A. Rottenburg and F. H. Hochberg, pp.41–4). Hafner, New York. (Originally published in 1907.)

American 'Psychiatric Association. (1987). *Diagnostic and statistical manual of mental disorders, DSM-III-R*, (3rd edn, revised), American Psychiatric Association, Washington, DC.

American Psychiatric Association (1994). *Diagnostic and statistical manual of mental disorders, DSM-IV* (4th edn), American Psychiatric Association, Washington, DC.

Asher, H. B. (1976). *Causal modeling*, Sage University Paper series on Quantitative Applications in the Social Sciences, 07–003. Sage, Beverly Hills, CA.

Bachman, D. L., Wolf, P. A., Linn, R., *et al.* (1992). Prevalence of dementia and probable senile dementia of the Alzheimer type in the Framingham Study. *Neurology*, **42**, 115–19.

Baddeley, A. D., Della Sala, S., and Spinnler, H. (1991*a*). The two component hypothesis of memory deficit in Alzheimer's disease. *Journal of Clinical and Experimental Neuropsychology*, **13**, 372–80.

Baddeley, A. D., Bressi, S., Della Sala, S., *et al.* (1991*b*). The decline of working memory in Alzheimer's disease. *Brain*, **114**, 2521–42.

Baltes, P. B., Reese, H. W., and Nesselroade, J. R. (1976). *Life-span developmental psychology: introduction to research*, Wadsworth Publishing Company, Monterey, CA.

Bayles, K. A. (1991). Age at onset of Alzheimer's disease: Relation to language dysfunction. *Archives of Neurology*, **48**, 155–9.

Becker, J. T. (1988). Working memory and secondary memory deficits in Alzheimer's disease. *Journal of Clinical and Experimental Neuropsychology*, **10**, 739–53.

Becker, J. T., Boller, F., Lopez, O. L., *et al.* (1994). The natural history of Alzheimer's disease. *Archives of Neurology*, **51**, 585–94.

Bentler, P. M. (1992) *EQS: Structural equations program manual.* BMDP Statistical Software, Los Angeles, CA.

Berg, L., Danziger, W. L., Storandt, M., *et al.* (1984). Predictive features in mild senile dementia of the Alzheimer type. *Neurology*, **34**, 563–9.

Berg, L., Miller, J. P., Storandt, M., *et al.* (1988). Mild senile dementia of the Alzheimer type: 2. Longitudinal assessment. *Annals of Neurology*, **23**, 477–84.

Blessed, G., Tomlinson, B. E., and Roth, M. (1968). The association between quantitative measures of dementia and of senile change in the cerebral grey matter of elderly subjects. *British Journal of Psychiatry*, **114** 797–811.

Boller, F., Becker, J. T., Holland, A. L., *et al.* (1991). Predictors of decline in Alzheimer's disease. *Cortex*, **27**, 9–17.

Botwinick, J., Storandt, M., and Berg, L. (1986). A longitudinal, behavioral study of senile dementia of the Alzheimer type. *Archives of Neurology*, **43**, 1124–7.

Brazzelli, M., Capitani, E., Della Sala, S. *et al.* (1994). A neuropsychological instrument adding to the description of patients with suspected dementia: The 'Milan Overall Dementia Assessment'. *Journal of Neurology, Neurosurgery and Psychiatry*, **57**, 1510–17.

Brooks, J. O., Kraemer, H. C., Tanke, E. D., *et al.* (1993). The methodology of studying decline in Alzheimer's disease. *Journal of the American Geriatric Society*, **41**, 623–8.

Capitani, E., Della Sala, S., and Spinnler, H. (1986). Neuropsychological approach to dementia. In K. *Neurology*, (ed. Poeck, H. J. Freund and H. Gaensehirt), pp. 61–9. Springer, Heidelberg.

Capitani, E., Della Sala, S., and Spinnler, H. (1990). Controversial neuropsychological issues in Alzheimer's disease: Influence of onset-age and hemispheric asymmetry of impairment. *Cortex*, **26**, 133–45.

Coolican, H. (1994). *Research methods and statistics in psychology*, (2nd edn), Hodder and Stoughton, London.

Crawford, J. R., Gray, C. D., and Allan, K. M. (1995). The WAIS-R(UK): Basic psychometric properties in an adult UK sample. *British Journal of Clinical Psychology*, **34**, 237–50.

Cuttance, P. and Ecob, R. (1987). *Structural modelling by example.* Cambridge University Press, Cambridge.

Della Sala, S., Nichelli, P., and Spinnler, H. (1986). An Italian series of patients with organic dementia. *Italian Journal of Neurological Sciences*, **7**, 27–41.

Everitt, B. S. (1984). *An introduction to latent variable models*, Chapman & Hall, London.

Filley, C. M., Kelly, J., and Heaton, R. K. (1986). Neuropsychologic features of early-and late-onset Alzheimer's disease. *Archives of Neurology*, **43**, 574–6.

Folstein, M. F., Folstein, S. E., and McHugh, P. H. (1975). Mini-mental state: A practical method for grading the cognitive state of patients for the clinician. *Journal of Psychiatric Research*, **12**, 189–98.

Friedland, R. P. (1993). Epidemiology, education, and the ecology of Alzheimer's disease. *Neurology*, **43**, 246–9.

Galasko, D., Kaluber, M. R., Hofstetter, C. R., *et al.* (1990). The Mini Mental State Examination in the early diagnosis of Alzheimer's disease. *Archives of Neurology*, **47**, 49–52.

Galasko, D., Corey-Bloom, J., and Thal, L. J. (1991). Monitoring progression in Alzheimer's disease. *Journal of the American Geriatric Society*, **39**, 932–941.

Galasko, D., Abramson, I., Corey-Bloom, J., *et al.* (1993). Repeated exposure to the Mini-Mental State Examination and the Information-Memory-Concentration Test results in a practice effect in Alzheimer's disease. *Neurology*, **43**, 1559–63.

Goodglass, H., and Kaplan, E. (1972). *Assessment of aphasia and related disorders.* Lea & Febiger, Philadelphia.

Gray, C., Chisholm, D., Smith, P. *et al.* (1992). The role of the child psychiatric ward in health care: Experiences with different types of admission over a period of twenty-one years. *Irish Journal of Psychological Medicine*, **9**, 17–23.

Haxby, J. V., Raffaele, K., Gillette, J., *et al.* (1992). Individual trajectories of cognitive decline in patients with dementia of the Alzhheimer type. *Journal of Clinical and Experimental Neuropsychology*, **14**, 575–592.

Hodges, J. R., Graham, N., and Patterson, K. (1995). Charting the progression in semantic dementia: Implications for the organisation of semantic memory. *Memory*, **3**, 463–95.

Huff, F. J., Growdon, J. H., Gorkin, S., *et al.* (1987). Age at onset and rate of progression of Alzheimer's disease. *Journal of the American Geriatric Society*, **35**, 27–30.

Hughes, C. P., Berg, L., Danziger, W. L., *et al.* (1982). A new clinical scale for the stageing of dementia. *British Journal of Psychiatry*, **140**, 566–72.

Jacobs, J. W., Bernhard, M. R., Delgado, A., *et al.* (1977). Screening for organic mental syndromes in the medically ill. *Annals of Internal Medicine*, **86**, 40–6.

Jacobs, D., Sano, M., Marder, K., *et al.* (1994). Age at onset of Alzheimer's disease: Relation to pattern of cognitive dysfunction and rate of decline. *Neurology*, **44**, 1215–20.

Jachim, C. L., Morris, J. H., Selkoe, and D. J. (1988). Clinically diagnosed Alzheimer's disease: Autopsy results in 150 cases. *Annals of Neurology*, **24**, 50–6.

Kahn, R. L., Goldfarb, A. I., Polack, M., *et al.* (1960). Brief objective measures for the determination of mental status in the aged. *American Journal of Psychiatry*, **117**, 326–8.

Katzman, R. (1993). Education and the prevalence of dementia and Alzheimer's disease. *Neurology*, **43**, 13–20.

Katzman, R., Brown, T., Fuld, P., *et al.* (1983). Validation of a short Orientation-Memory-Concentration Test of cognitive impairment. *American Journal of Psychiatry*, **140**, 734–9.

Katzman, R., Brown, T., Thal, L. J., *et al.* (1988*a*). Comparison of rate of annual change of mental status score in four independent studies of patients with Alzheimer's disease. *Annals of Neurology*, **24**, 384–9.

Katzman, R., Terry, R., De Teresa, R., *et al.* (1988*b*). Clinical, pathological and neurochemical changes in dementia: A subgroup with preserved mental status and numerous neocortical plaques. *Annals of Neurology*, **23**, 138–44.

Khachaturian, Z. S. (1985). Diagnosis of Alzheimer's disease. *Archives of Neurology*, **42**, 1097–105.

Kraemer, H. C., Tinklenberg, J., and Yesavage, J. A. (1994). 'How far' vs 'How fast' in Alzheimer's disease. *Archives of Neurology*, **51**, 275–9.

Lindenbaum, J., Healton, E. B., Savage, D. G., *et al.* (1988). Neuropsychiatric disorders caused by cobalamin deficiency in the absence of anemia or macrocytosis. *New England Journal of Medicine*, **318**, 1720–8.

Lindsey, J., and Murphy, E. (1989). Dementia, depression and subsequent institutionalization—the effect of home support. *International Journal of Geriatric Psychiatry*, **4**, 3–9.

Lucca, U., Comelli, M., Tettamanti, M., *et al.* (1993). Rate of progression and prognostic factors in Alzheimer's disease: A prospective study. *Journal of the American Geriatric Society*, **41**, 45–9.

McDowall, D., McCleary, E., Meidinger, E., *et al.* (1980). *Interrupted time series analysis*, Sage University Paper series on Quantitative Applications in the Social Sciences, 07–021. Sage, Beverly Hills, CA.

Mann, D. M. A., Marcyniuk, B., Yates, P. O., *et al.* (1988). The progression of the pathological changes of Alzheimer's disease in frontal and temporal neocortex examined both at biopsy and at autopsy. *Neuropathology and Applied Neurobiology*, **14**, 177–95.

Markus, G. B. (1979). *Analyzing panel data*, Sage University Paper series on Quantitative Applications in the Social Sciences, 07–018. Sage Publications, Beverly Hills.

Martin, A., Brouwers, P., Lalonde, F., *et al.* (1986). Towards a behavioral typology of Alzheimer's patients. *Journal of Clinical and Experimental Neuropsychology*, **8**, 594–610.

Martin, E. M., Wilson, R. S., Penn, M. D., *et al.* (1987). Cortical biopsy results in Alzheimer's disease: correlation with cognitive deficits. *Neurology*, **37**, 1201–4.

Mattis, C. (1976). Mental status examination for organic mental syndrome in the elderly patient. In *Geriatric psychiatry: A handbook for psychiatrists and primary care physicians*, (ed. L. Bellak and T. B. Karasu), pp. 77–121. Grune and Stratton, New York.

Mayeux, R., Stern, Y., Rosen, J., *et al.* (1981). Depression, intellectual impairment and Parkinson's disease. *Neurology*, **31**, 645–50.

Mendez, M. F., Mastri, A. R., Sung, J. H., *et al.* (1992). Clinically diagnosed Alzheimer's disease: Neuropathological findings in 650 cases. *Alzheimer's Disease and Associated Disorders*, **8**, 35–43.

Morris, R. G. (1994). Recent developments in the neuropsychology of dementia. *International Review of Psychiatry*, **6**, 85–107.

Nelson, A., Fogel, B. S., and Faust, D. (1986). Bedside cognitive screening instruments: A critical assessment. *Journal of Nervous and Mental Disease*, **174**, 73–83.

Nunnally, J. C. (1978). *Psychometric theory*, (2nd edn). McGraw-Hill, New York.

Ortof, E. and Crystal, H. A. (1989). Rate of progression of Alzheimer's disease. *Journal of the American Geriatric Society*, **37**, 511–14.

Pfeiffer, E. (1975). A short portable mental status questionnaire for the assessment of organic brain deficit in elderly patients. *Journal of the American Geriatric Society*, **23**, 433–41.

Reisberg, B., Ferris, S. H., de Leon, M. J., *et al.* (1982). The Global Deterioration Scale (GDS): An instrument for the assessment of primary degenerative dementia (PDD). *American Journal of Psychiatry*, **139**, 1136–9.

Roth, M., Tym, E., Mountjoy, C. Q., *et al.* (1986). CAMDEX: A standardized instrument for the diagnosis of mental disorder in the elderly with special reference to the early detection of dementia. *British Journal of Psychiatry*, **148**, 698–709.

Rubin, D. B. (1976). Inference and missing data. *Biometrika*, **63**, 581–92.

Salmon, D. P., Thal, L. J., Butters, N., *et al.* (1990). Longitudinal evaluation of dementia of the Alzheimer type: a comparison of 3 standardized mental status examinations. *Neurology*, **40**, 1225–30.

Scinto, L. F., Daffner, K. R., Dressler, D., *et al.* (1994). A potential noninvasive neurobiological test for Alzheimer's disease. *Science*, **266**, 1051–4.

Selkoe, D. J. (1988). Protein chemistry of neurofibrillary bundles and myeloid plaques in Alzheimer's disease: Relation to cytoskeleton. In *Ageing and the brain*, (ed. R. D. Terry), pp. 165–81. Raven Press, New York.

Selnes, O. A., Carson, K., Rovner, B., *et al.* (1988). Language dysfunction in early-and late-onset possible Alzheimer's disease. *Neurology*, **38**, 1053–6.

Spagnoli, A., Lucca, U., Menasce, G., *et al.* (1991). Long-term acetyl-L-carnitine treatment in Alzheimer's disease. *Neurology*, **41**, 1726–32.

Spector, P. E. (1981). *Research designs.* Sage University Paper series on Quantitative Applications in the Social Sciences, 07–023. Sage, Beverly Hills.

Spinnler, H., and Della Sala, S. (1988). The role of clinical neuropsychology in the neurological diagnosis of Alzheimer's disease. *Journal of Neurology*, **235**, 258–71.

Stern, Y., Alexander, G. E., Prohovnik, I., *et al.* (1992). Inverse relationship between education and parietotemporal perfusion deficit in Alzheimer's disease. *Annals of Neurology*, **32**, 371–5.

Stern, R. G., Mohs, R. C., Davidson, M. *et al.* (1994). A longitudinal study of Alzheimer's disease: Measurement, rate and predictors of cognitive deterioration. *American Journal of Psychiatry*, **151**, 390–6.

Stevens, S. S. (1946). On the theory of scales of measurement. *Science*, **103**, 677–80.

Summers, W. K., Majovski, L. V., Marsh, G. M., *et al.* (1986). Oral tetrahydroamin-ocridine in long-term treatment of senile dementia, Alzheimer type. *New England Journal of Medicine*, **315**, 1241–5.

Thal, L. J., Grundman, M., and Golden, R. (1986). Alzheimer's disease: A correlational analysis of the Blessed information – memory – concentration test and the mini-mental state exam. *Neurology*, **36**, 262–4.

Wade, J.P.H., Mirsen, T. R., Hachinski, V. C., *et al.* (1987). The clinical diagnosis of Alzheimer's disease. *Archives of Neurology*, **44** 24–9.

Wechsler, D. (1955). *Manual for the Wechsler Adult Intelligence Scale.* Psychological Corporation, New York.

Wechsler, D. (1981). *Manual for the Wechsler Adult Intelligence Scale – Revised.* Psychological Corporation, New York.

II. Neuropsychological functioning

FOUR

Attentional and executive dysfunction

Robin G. Morris

INTRODUCTION

The ability to coordinate sequence cognitive operations is an important feature of everyday mental activity. For example in most activities several tasks have to be carried out in sequence, transferring attention between them at the appropriate time. Incoming sensory information has to be 'sifted' and the correct stream of information given priority in terms of processing. The cognitive processes that facilitate this type of mental functioning can be subsumed under the headings 'attention' or 'executive functioning', hence the title of the chapter.

Attention can be split broadly into three main areas to be considered: (1) *sustained attention*, the ability to attend to a particular sensory input or set or sensory inputs for long time period; (2) *selective attention*, the selection process by which one stream of sensory imput is attended to, screening out other competing inputs; (3) *divided attention*, in which attention is split between more than one input or task, involving such processes as sequencing, allocation of processing resources, and time sharing between tasks. The latter falls under the rubric of executive functioning in the more specialist sense used in this chapter, following the use of the term by Baddeley and colleagues (Baddeley 1992; Baddeley and Hitch 1974).

SUSTAINED ATTENTION

It has been observed that impairments in attention frequently accompany different forms of brain damage (Mattis 1976). These, however, should be distinguished from the gross impairment in attention that accompanies confusional states. In Alzheimer-type dementia (AD), the patient is essentially 'alert' and able to take in information from their surroundings to a certain level of efficiency, certainly at the early stages.

This clinical notion of 'alertness' perhaps most readily translates into the cognitive concept of vigilance, the ability to detect a stimulus and respond readily (Allport 1989). This is typically assessed using tasks in which a target occurs infrequently and unpredictably and has to be discriminated from other unpredictable items, the type of activity, for example, needed when scanning a moving crowd of people over a long time period to detect a person. *Vigilance* in this sense is known to decline over time, but not more so for normal older adults (Parasuraman and Giambra 1991). The rate of decline is made more rapid by degrading the stimulus, for example, by adding random noise to a visual stimulus, or by introducing a secondary task. This has been interpreted as being because the noise or distraction increases the demands on central processing resources, which tend to decline more rapidly over time (Parasuraman *et al.* 1991). In AD there is some evidence for a gross preservation of vigilance using this type of paradigm. For example Lines *et al.* (1991) required subjects to listen to a train of short tones, indicating the number by pointing to a choice array of numbers (1–15). To test the 'vigilance' component they had to push a button when a target digit appeared on a visual display unit (VDU). The AD patients were no worse than control subjects, with the same detection rate throughout.

One potential criticism of this experiment was the low levels of errors made by both groups of subjects and the lack of decline in performance over time which might suggest that the test was generally insensitive (Parasuraman and Haxby 1993). However, the lack of impairment at least points towards no gross impairment. Also, a similar version of the task had been found to be sensitive to the effects of the anticholinergic drug scopolamine (Brok *et al.* 1988). Berardi *et al.* (1992) reports that if the subsidiary task is made even more demanding this does produce a decrement in AD patients, but this is perhaps less surprising, since if any task is made sufficiently complex or difficult it is likely to record a deficit with this group of patients.

Overall, therefore, 'vigilance' shows no striking deficit at least in early AD. Congruent results have been found when investigating the ability to maintain states of readiness to respond for very short periods, perhaps milliseconds. This ability has been termed tonic alertness and is more related to the mobilization of cognitive resources in the 'direction' of an *expected* stimulus. Nebes and Brady (1993) required subjects to press one of two keys according to the position of a 'square' presented either at the top or the bottom of a VDU. Phasic attention was induced by presenting a warning tone, which normally speeds the response, with optimal effect when presented approximately 300 ms before the squares. AD patients were found to be slower overall to respond, but the degree of benefit due to the tone was the same as in the control subjects. They also found that the changes in speed of responses associated with varying the distance between the tone and the squares was the same in both subjects, further supporting the notion that phasic attention is also unimpaired.

SELECTIVE ATTENTION

The ability to shift attention between different sensory inputs has also been studied in AD. This ability can be fractionated in several different ways, probably relying on different cognitive mechanisms. For example the shift of attention between two locations in a visual field is differentiated from switching between the salient dimensions of a multidimensional stimulus, such as on the Stroop test, or between mental tests as in the case of the Trail Making test where the subject has to alternate between letters and numbers. Clinical tasks such as the Stroop test and Trail Making show clear deficits in patients with AD (Grady *et al.* 1988; Haxby *et al.* 1989).

Visual selective attention

Attentional shifts in spatial tasks have been studied in the context of a model that splits the process into their constituent components (Posner *et al.* 1984*a*). Specifically, this includes engaging or focusing attention on a location, disengaging attention, and shifting (or moving) to another location. These component processes can be studied experimentally to pinpoint a specific type of deficit. There is substantial evidence that this type of attention is controlled by the posterior cortical parietal region (LaBerge 1990; Posner *et al.* 1984*b*) (see also Chapter 13). A preliminary study by Freed *et al.* (1989) used a version of the Posner (1980) selective attention task. The subject has to press a response key whenever an 'X' appears in the left or right of the VDU. A visual warning signal is used in the form of an arrow which in 80% of trials points towards the location of the X (valid cue), but in 20% points in the opposite direction (invalid cue). Normally, the valid cue speeds the response, whilst the invalid cue produces a slower response. The explanation is that the cue shifts the attention of the subject to the location, engaging attention in the correct position if valid, but taking it away from the target if invalid. Freed *et al.* (1989) found the pattern of results to be normal in AD patients apart from a subgroup who had reduced levels of noradrenergic metabolites in the cerebrospinal fluid. These tended, paradoxically, to respond more rapidly to invalid rather than valid cues.

A more extensive study has been conducted by Parasuraman *et al.* (1992), leading to different results. Freed *et al.* (1989) had used long durations between the cue and the target (2000 and 3000 ms). Parasuraman *et al.* (1992) increased the range from 200 to 2000, investigating facilitation or inhibition at the short durations. A letter discrimination task was also used in which subjects either had to respond to a single letter or decide whether it was a vowel or a consonant. This manipulation was to facilitate visuospatial attention at a higher level rather than responding to simple luminance or visual 'energy' detection. They found that AD patients showed the normal advantage with a valid cue in comparison to a neutral one. This suggested no impairment in engaging or focusing attention. In contrast, with the invalid cue there was a relative increase in response time in AD patients when compared to controls. This suggests an inability to disengage and switch attention to another location.

Another manipulation by Parasuraman *et al.* (1992) was to place the cue either in the periphery or the centre of the screen. Jonides (1981) has shown that the central cue elicits a more voluntary central resource demanding shift of attention. In addition, the peripheral cue provides a more rapid shift of attention, most effective for very short durations (less than half a second), whilst the central cue needs a longer duration to take effect, but it is a longer lasting effect as well. The performance of AD patients and age-matched controls were compared, and highlighted the specificity of the deficit (see Fig. 4.1). With peripheral cues the difficulty in switching occurs with short intervals showing the impairment is fast acting. With central cues, it becomes apparent with longer durations and is stable over a period. The specificity of this result is indicated by the finding that patients with Parkinson's disease fail to show the normal advantage with valid cues, rather than being penalized more with invalid cues (Wright *et al.* 1990). In their case, the deficit is likely to be the initial focusing of attention. It is not clear why the Freed *et al.* (1989) study produced different results, but Parasuraman *et al.* (1992) speculate that more severely demented patients were investigated and this interacted with the longer intervals used reducing the 'inhibitory' effect.

The above task concerns switching between spatial locations. Other studies have explored switching between stimulus dimensions in the visual domain. Firstly, Filoteo *et al.* (1992) presented subjects with digits visually, which were, in turn, made up from arrays of smaller digits. For example the larger digit 2 might be constructed from 11 smaller digits arranged appropriately. In a control condition the subjects had to indicated whether a '1' or a '2' was seen in terms of the larger digit. In another condition the same judgement had to be made, but judging whether it was seen with either the smaller or larger composite digit. This forces the subject to switch between the 'local' (small digit) or 'global' large digit. This type of switching led to a much greater slowing in response time in the AD patients, suggesting a specific deficit in switching attention.

Similarly, Haxby *et al.* (1991) used a matching-to-sample reaction

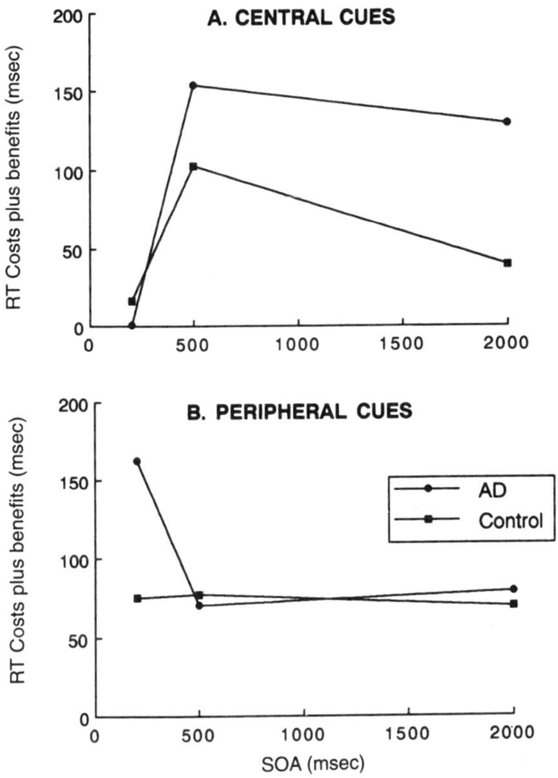

FIG. 4.1 Combined reaction time (RT) costs and benefits on a spatial attention task as a function of cue-target stimulus onset asynchrony (SOA) in Alzheimer's disease patients (AD) and control subjects (from Parasuraman *et al.* 1992).

time task in which one of two choice stimuli shared a visual feature with a sample stimulus. The matching could occur on more than one dimension, for example colour, shape, or number, in a similar fashion to the Wisconsin Card Sorting Task. Different conditions, the main comparison between a simple matching task in which the matching feature was always the same within a series of choice, and a 'divided attention' condition in which the matching feature changed every item. On the control condition, AD patients were only slightly slower than the controls, by an amount easily accounted for by generalized cognitive slowing. The impairment increased markedly on the divided attention condition, suggestive of a substantial impairment in switching attention between dimensions.

Auditory selective attention

In the auditory domain there are parallel deficits in selective attention measured using the dichotic listening task. Here strings of words or digits are presented simultaneously in each ear for remembering. Normally the list presented to the right ear tends to be reported first with an accompanying right-ear advantage in accuracy. The effect is enhanced by instructing the subject to recall the right ear list first and reversed by a left ear instruction. Both effects appear to be impaired in AD. Mohr *et al.* (1990) and Bouma and Van Silfhout (1989) report that the patients fail to show the normal increase in right-ear advantage and also maintain a right-ear advantage when the left-ear first retrieval instruction is given. This can be interpreted as showing that attention is passively driven by the mechanism that determines the right-ear advantage and that the AD patients are unable to switch their attention at will. It is also speculated that damaged right parietal lobe functioning results in an inability to direct attention to the contralateral left ear, and thus enable the patient to overcome the right-ear advantage.

ATTENTION AND REACTION TIME

The visual tasks described above all use reaction time as their principal measure. More generally, reductions in the speed of cognitive processing have been invoked as the cause or consequence or attentional deficits. Certainly, on almost all tasks, a reduction in reaction time (RT) is observed even in early AD (Nebes and Brady 1992). Consistent with this is the association between slowed RT and a reduced amplitude of the Event Related Potential (O'Connor 1980*a*, *b*).

An important issue is whether the slowing is uniform across different mental operations and can account for the pattern of cognitive decline associated with AD. This argument has been used in relation to cognitive changes in the normal elderly (Birren and Birren 1990). The argument is that all cognitive operations are slowed to the same extent. More complex tasks call upon a greater number of stages and so show a greater slowing. Applied to AD, this might explain, for example, the greater differences found on choice rather than simple reaction time tasks. Specifically, Ferris *et al.* (1976) found that AD patients showed a greater increase in RT when required to choose between two response keys according to a particular stimulus, in comparison to responding simply by pressing one key when a stimulus appears. Likewise, when Nebes and Brady (1989) required subjects to search an array of letters for a target letter and varied the number of letters in the array from two, four, to six letters, they found the difference in speed between AD patients and controls increased with the complexity of the task.

A meta-analysis of reaction times by Nebes and Brady (1992) has shown that RTs in AD do indeed appear to conform to a linear function, taking the following form:

$$\text{Control RT} = \text{A} + \text{B} \times \text{Alzheimer-type dementia RT}.$$

They argue against inferring particular types of deficits on the basis of proportionate increases in RTs unless they exceed this particular function. In the case of the Haxby *et al.* (1991) study, cited above, which investigated matching-to-sample with single or multiple dimensional comparisons, this function is exceeded and so supports their conclusion. In other studies, however, the principle produces a more cautious interpretation. Parasuraman and Haxby (1993) have argued that the approach is too stringent and would rule out investigation of information processing which involves very short reaction times (for instance in the millisecond range) where the requirement could not be met. In addition, they question the notion of *task complexity* as an explanation of differential slowing since there are no precise definitions of what this means for a particular task. In the case of the Parasuraman *et al.* (1992) study it is difficult to see why disproportionate slowing should occur with short cue-stimulus intervals with peripheral cues, in contrast to long intervals with central cues (see Parasuraman and Haxby 1993 for a further discussion of this issue).

There is no doubt that RT is increased generally in AD and this is likely to occur at different stages in information processing. By implication, the slowing should have a multiplicative effect with reiterative or more lengthy mental operations involving more sets of cognitive modules. Specifying at what stage the slowing takes place is more difficult. Some hint of this is provided by considering Event Related Potential which can provide an index of the timing of central stages of information processing independent of the response output. In this sense, the P300 latency may provide a purer measure of 'central' processing, and this has indeed been found to be impaired in AD (McCarthy and Donchin 1981). Nevertheless, there is the need to fractionate central processes in a similar fashion to Posner *et al.* (1984*a*), for example the sensory versus executive stage, involving coordinating and executing multiple responses (Nestor *et al.* 1991).

ALZHEIMER-TYPE DEMENTIA AS A DYSEXECUTIVE SYNDROME

The attentional mechanisms considered above, such as switching visual attention to a new location, form just part of an overall executive system controlling cognition. For example the cognitive architecture must be able to deal with several types of processing at once, sequencing activity, timing mental operations, and allocating attentional resources appropriately. This has to take place at different levels within the system, from a low level activation of routine operations as envisaged in contention scheduling models such as that proposed by Shallice and Norman (Shallice 1988), to higher order mechanisms involving acts of the 'will' or metarepresentations (Morris *et al.* 1995; Stuss 1992).

Various cognitive frameworks have been employed to encompass or explain executive functioning phenomena, including the notion of central processing or attentional resources (Kahneman 1973; Norman and Bobrow 1975), in which there is a limited 'multi-purpose' pool of cognitive resources that can be applied to more demanding mental operations. These can be split into different pools of resources, for example for visuospatial or spatial processing, but the central concept is that when several cognitive operations run in parallel these compete for the same resources, leading to decline in individual performance. Applied to AD the most obvious prediction, based on what is known about the physiology of the disease, is that these resources will be more limited, leading to special difficulties with more complex attentionally demanding tasks. Another approach is to postulate specific executive mechanisms and try and parse these into their constituents, an approach used by Baddeley and Hitch's (1974; Baddeley 1992) Working Memory Model or by Norman and Shallice's (1986) model concerning willed and automatic forms of behaviour. The current review presents data within the Working Memory Model, since this has been used most extensively as the framework to explore executive processes in AD (Morris 1994*b*; Morris and Baddeley 1988).

Executive processes and dual tasks performance

According to the Working Memory Model, there is a Central Executive System (CES) which functions to coordinate and schedule mental operations as indicated in Fig. 4.2 (Baddeley 1990). Connected to this system are subsidiary storage mechanisms concerned with maintaining information for short periods for simultaneous processing, termed 'slave systems', including the Articulatory Loop System and Visuospatial Scratchpad. These systems have been fractionated through a combination of cognitive and neuropsychological studies and have been explored individually in AD.

Support for an impairment in executive functioning comes from marked deficits in a variety of dual tasks, which 'stress' the CES. First, there is substantial impairment on tasks such as the Peterson and Peterson (1959) task in which a person is presented with three items,

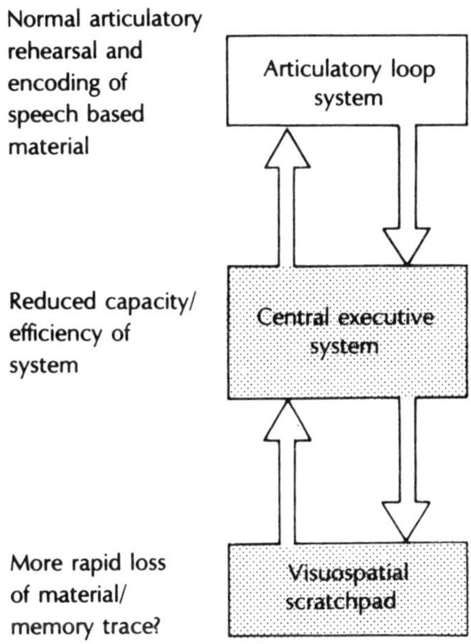

FIG. 4.2 Diagram illustrating areas of deficits in relation to the Baddeley (1992) working memory model (reproduced with permission).

words, or consonants, and distracted by a subsidiary task for varying intervals of up to approximately 30 seconds. This produces significant forgetting in normal subjects and a very substantial impairment in AD (Corkin 1982; Kopelman 1985; Morris 1986; Morris and Kopelman 1990). For example in a study by Kopelman (1985) a marked deficit was seen after a 3-second delay in comparison to no deficit in Korsakoff patients. At the longer 30 second delay the Korsakoff patients were impaired as well, attributable to their long-term memory impairment. In the studies above, demanding distracter tasks were used, such as counting backwards by threes. Morris (1986) found that even simple distracter tasks such as tapping the palm of the right hand on a desk repeatedly was sufficient to cause marked forgetting in AD patients, but no forgetting in controls. Other subsidiary tasks such as saying the word 'the' repeatedly, reversing or additing a series of two single digit numbers, all produced a clear deficit in the patient group.

An issue with respect to this approach is at what level is the dual-task interference operating? If the cognitive operations of the tasks are likely to be similar, for example two tasks requiring verbal material, then there may be structural interference at the level of individual processing systems or modules rather than in the control mechanism (Norman and Bobrow 1975). To focus on a central system it is necessary to make the tasks as dissimilar as possible with respect to modality and processing. Baddeley *et al.* (1986, 1991*b*) used a pursuit tracking task, in which the subject tracked a moving node on a VDU screen with a lightpen, against three different tasks. One involved repeating the digits 1–5 repeatedly (articulation), another detecting tones and responding using a foot switch (tone detection), and another recalling a string of digits (digit span). To control for the possibility of visuoperceptual or motor deficits merely being magnified by combining the tasks, the speed of the moving node was adjusted for each subject to achieve matched levels of accuracy. Similarly, the digit span, the maximum number of digits recalled successfully, was used for the digit-span task.

Baddeley *et al.* (1986) found that the articulation task did not affect tracking performance differentially in AD patients. The remaining tasks, however, had a very significant effect, most salient being digit span since performance on both tasks had been titrated. A potential puzzle is why the articulation task did not produce differential interference. Morris and Baddeley (1988) have argued that it was not sufficiently demanding to disrupt the already titrated tracking task. Of note, on follow-up, Baddeley *et al.* (1991*b*) found that even this task was sufficient to disrupt tracking differentially in AD patients who had progressed to a later stage of their illness.

A potential criticism of inferring a CES impairment specifically is that impairments in perceptual or basic attentional processes might have contributed to the deficit, simply exacerbated by increasing the complexity of mental operations through using two tasks. Against this are results from the titration method used by Baddeley *et al.* (1986, 1991*b*) which effectively should control for this possibility. In addition, attentional mechanisms can be considered as components of the CES, which although having a general purpose capacity become more differentiated as a further understanding of executive processes develops. Another potential difficulty is defining whether a task draws upon the resources of the CES, without resorting to circularity, in other words on the basis of whether dual-task interference is observed. This is perhaps better understood if it is considered that almost all tasks require the action of the CES for their initiation and coordination, but some tasks have much less need for supervisory control. In AD, if the CES is substantially impaired, even a very undemanding task might be sufficient to cause dual-task interference. An example is the tapping task, sufficient to cause substantial forgetting of consonant trigrams in the study conducted by Morris (1986). In relation to this task, Parasuraman *et al.* (1992) have argued that tapping is a relatively automatic task, capable of being performed with little supervisory control. Why then is it capable of producing a deficit in AD? The possibility is that the resources of the CES are so depleted, that even this task can produce a deficit. Clearly, however, it will never be possible to determine precisely how much an individual task draws on the capacity of the CES, and this may vary between individuals and the extent of experience of the task.

Additional studies of divided attention have tended to confirm the results reported by Baddeley *et al.* (1986), but using different approaches. This includes the probe-reaction time dual-task method employed by Nestor *et al.* (1991). As a primary task they used a visual letter and form matching paradigm. When compared to controls AD patients were not substantially impaired on their speed of response on different versions of this task. This task was then combined with a simple auditory reaction time task, to investigate the effect of divided attention. This produced a substantial increase in response latency in the AD patients, but not in the controls (see Fig. 4.3). However, Nestor *et al.* (1991) attribute this deficit to difficulties in coordinating multiple task inputs and responses, rather than the increased attentional 'cost' of performing two tasks. Dual-task impairment has also been found by Grober and Sliwinski (1991). Here the AD patients had to remember short strings of digits and decide simultaneously whether two visually presented letters were the same or different. Specifically, the letters were in lower or upper case and either A or B. A greater divided attention effect in AD was observed in the recall of the digits when order was not specified (free recall). A second condition, which required ordered recall of the digits, did not produce such an effect.

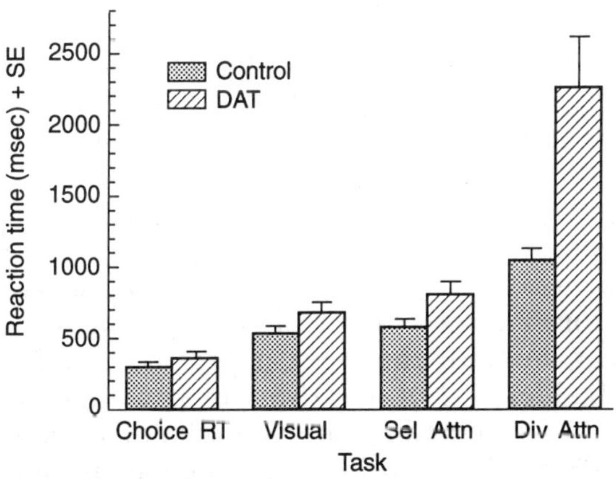

FIG. 4.3 Reaction time (RT) on four visual matching tasks with varying attentional demands for patients with Alzheimer-type dementia (AD) and controls (Sel Attn, selective attention; Div Attn, divided attention).

It is possible, however, that in this latter condition, the AD patients transferred most of their attention away from letter matching, thereby maintaining their relative level of accuracy on digit recall.

A different approach to investigating executive functioning in AD stems from exploring performance on tasks which measure self-initiated activity, rather than divided attention. This relates to the fact that an executive system can be seen more broadly as being involved in purposeful cognitive activity, such as problem solving or monitoring the environment and developing specific strategies for cognitive activity (Baddeley 1986). Under this framework, the coordinating aspects of the CES form just part of the overall executive activity (Shallice 1988).

One task that has been used to tap into this alternative aspect of executive functioning is random generation, in which the subject produces a random string of letters. This task has been found to be attentionally very demanding, with subjects tending to lapse into producing non-random sequences (Baddeley 1986; Shallice 1988). The CES is thought to be 'stressed' by this task, first in the initiation of the retrieval mechanisms, and second, to monitor the retrieved material and inhibit repetition of over-learned sequences. A less rigorous technique, which nevertheless draws on similar processes, is various versions of the word-generation task, known as verbal fluency in the context of investigating dysphasia (Benton and Hamsler 1978). Indeed, combinations of word-generation tasks and other problem-solving tasks such as the Wisconsin Card Storing task are frequently used to investigate the executive impairment associated with frontal lobe impairment (Crawford *et al.* 1992).

This approach has been applied to AD by Becker (1988; Becker *et al.* 1992*a*) using factor analytical techniques deriving a measure of executive impairment using a combination of tests. These include the Wechsler Adult Intelligence Scale (WAIS) Similarities test, the Weigl sorting task (Weigl 1927), letter cancellation (Diller *et al.* 1974) and verbal fluency. An 'executive' factor combines these particular tasks, as established in a preliminary study by Becker (1988). Subsequently, Becker *et al.* (1992*a*) were able to isolate patients with predominately executive impairments using specific cut-off criteria. These could be differentiated from another subset of AD patients who had specific long-term memory impairments (see Chapter 5). A similar analysis was conducted by Baddeley *et al.* (1991*a*), using a slightly different set of psychometric tests, including the Gottschaldt's hidden figure test (Capitani *et al.* 1988). Again, using a specific cut-off they were able to identify patients with specific dysexecutive syndromes.

Focal deficits in AD are not uncommon. Indeed, Becker *et al.* (1992*b*) have found material-specific deficits in long-term memory with patients either having verbal or visuospatial memory impairment.

To what extent does the specificity of these deficits change with time? In a two-year follow-up study, Becker *et al.* (1992*a*) found that all their cases of executive dysfunction became 'non-focal' and that no other case became focal. In addition, the case reported by Baddeley *et al.* (1991*a*) became generalized after approximately six months.

Discussion

In summary, group studies of AD suggest an impairment in divided attention with is relatively consistent. Psychometric studies reveal cases who have specific executive impairments, in other words, those that outstrip the more widespread cognitive degeneration. To what extent can these findings be accommodated within a cognitive framework? Various possibilities emerge and these are well summarized in relation to attention by Parasuraman and Haxby (1993). Executive processes are clearly an amalgam of control mechanisms including, for example, selective attention, scheduling different mental operations, including time sharing, and being able to coordinate mental activity in a manner that facilitates problem-solving activity.

The studies above suggest that, at least in the early stages of dementia, there is some specificity of impairment, rather than a global deficit. For example visual selective attention is impaired at the stage of disengaging from a target. Divided attention appears to be particularly impaired, whilst phasic and tonic arousal appears to be normal and AD patients can be unimpaired on sustained attention.

SUBCOMPONENTS OF WORKING MEMORY

As indicated above, fractionation of executive processes should lead to an increased understanding of AD, in the same way as the differentiation of visual selective attentional processes has shown a specific type of impairment in AD (Parasuraman *et al.* 1992). The peripheral subsystems that enable material to be retained in a temporary fashion have been investigated extensively. These storage mechanisms have been subsumed under the Baddeley and Hitch Working Memory Model (Baddeley 1992). In the verbal domain, the *Articulatory Loop System* (ALS) is proposed to recycle verbal material (for example words, digits) in a relatively automatic fashion. For example when remembering a string of digits, as in digit span, the material is cycled continuously through the ALS to refresh the memory trace (Baddeley 1992; Vallar and Baddeley 1984). An equivalent *Visuospatial Scratchpad* is thought to retain small amounts of visuospatial material in short-term memory. Recent formulations of the model, stress the dynamic interaction between processing and storing information, with both ALS and VSSP having rehearsal and storage mechanisms.

The Articulatory Loop System

Studies of normal subjects have split the ALS into a phonological short-term store (PSS) and an articulatory rehearsal mechanism (ARM) (Baddeley 1992; Vallar and Baddeley 1994) and this distinction has been supported more recently by positron emission tomography (PET) studies (Paulescu *et al.* 1993). The PSS is a more passive repository for phonologically encoded material, whilst the ARM is involved in active rehearsal of this material feeding the PSS. The ALS plays a major part in digit span performance where it is estimated that the equivalent of 2 to 3 items are recycled through the rehearsal mechanism.

A relative preservation of the ALS in AD is indicated by only small deficits in memory span (the maximum number of items a person can recall immediately in serial order) across a range of tasks, including those using digits, words, and letters (e.g. Corkin 1982; Kopelman 1985; Morris 1984; Spinnler *et al.* 1988). Some studies have reported no deficit, including the studies by Martin *et al.* (1985) and Weingartner *et al.* (1983).

There are various methods for investigating the ALS. One is to measure the reduction in memory span when a subject simultaneously mouths an irrelevant word (such as saying 'the' continuously). This technique effectively suppresses the ARM, reducing the contribution to memory span (Baddeley *et al.* 1975). Morris (1984, 1987*a*) has shown equivalent suppression effects in AD and control subjects using both words and digits. The size is also unaltered if the rate of articulating the irrelevant item is paced or unpaced by the experimenter (Morris 1987*a*). The functioning of the ARM is also reflected in the size of what is termed the word length effect (Baddeley *et al.* 1975). This is the finding that memory span for longer words (for instance *university* and *association*) is generally less than that for shorter words (for example *harm* or *wit*). The effect relates to the greater time that longer words take to be recycled and, hence, the increased probability that they will not be retained. Morris (1984) found no diminution of the word length effect in early AD patients. A follow-up study by Morris, Bradley, and Welch (see Morris 1992) replicated this finding using memory for line drawings of objects, whose name differed in length. In this task, the drawings were presented sequentially and the subject had to produce the names in order.

Finally, the *rate* at which patients can rehearse verbal material can be used to explore the functioning of the ALS. If the rate of the ARM is reduced, then less material can be recycled, so reducing memory span. In AD, as indicated in the sections above, slowing is observed on reaction time tasks, so this is a potential cause of reduced short-term verbal memory functioning. To estimate rehearsal rates, Morris (1987*b*) required patients either to read as rapidly as possible strings of digits (reading rate) or to count out loud from one to ten (counting rate). AD patients were found to be impaired on counting but not reading rate. However, Morris (1987*b*) considered the counting rate to be a less reliable estimate of rehearsal rate because of the problems that AD patients have in retrieving the digits from memory. This process is heavily dependent on semantic memory, known to be impaired in AD (see Chapter 8). For example Gewirth *et al.* (1984) have shown that AD patients have considerably longer latencies in producing word associations to cue words. Estimates of rehearsal rate have also been shown to correlate with memory span, on the basis that the faster a person can rehearse material the more material can be recycled (Baddeley *et al.* 1975). Of note, Morris (1987*b*) found a substantial reduction in this correlation between reading rate and memory in AD in comparison to normal controls. This relates to component cognitive processes that make up memory span performance. The latter partially includes a contribution from the ALS, but also that of executive processes to coordinating performance on the task. It is possible that a breakdown in executive processes, for example, which would vary between patients, reduces the association between rehearsal rate and memory span.

A second area of investigation is the PSS. This was investigated by Morris (1984) by comparing memory span for acoustically similar (for example B, C, D, V, and G) or dissimilar (for example E, H, J, R, W, and Y) letters. In normal subjects memory span is reduced when similar sounding verbal material is used, a finding that supports the presence of phonological encoding. If this store is impaired in AD, then the phonological similarity effect should be reduced (Vallar and Shallice 1990). In AD, Morris (1984) found the effect to be undiminished, when comparing elderly AD patients and controls and using both visual and auditory presentation of letters.

In summary, there is reasonably convincing evidence for a preserved ALS in AD, with normal word length and phonological similarity effects and a normal effect of articulatory suppression on memory span performance.

The Visuospatial Scratchpad

In the visual domain, the VSSP is responsible for holding small amounts of information in working memory (Baddeley 1992; Logie and Marchetti 1991). For example if a person is diverted momentarily from viewing a scene, the memory will be retained for a short instance. The VSSP is, in a sense, a counterpart to the ALS and is thought in turn to be split into visual and spatial components.

There is preliminary evidence that the VSSP is impaired in AD, but this is not conclusive. First, AD patients have been shown to be impaired on the Corsi Block Span task. This requires observing an experimenter tapping out a sequence on an array of nine blocks. The same sequence, or locations, are then 'tapped' by the subject. This tests the spatial component of the VSSP. Another test of spatial memory is the Spatial Working Memory task designed originally by Morris (Morris *et al.* 1988; Owen *et al.* 1990). This has a series of 'boxes' which are presented on a visual display unit fitted with a touch-sensitive screen. The subject tries each box in turn to find one which, when touched, will reveal a hidden 'token'. On subsequent searches, the rule is not to go back to the successful boxes. In effect, there is a series of searches in which the subject has to avoid previously successful locations. AD patients were found to be substantially impaired on this task, making significantly more erroneous returns (Sahgal *et al.* 1994).

Other investigations relate to visual, rather than spatial short-term memory. These include investigations using versions of the delayed matching-to-sample task, in which a sample stimulus is shown followed by a short delay and then a choice of other stimuli, one of which matches the sample. Money *et al.* (1992) required subjects to recognize a filled circle of a particular size out of an array of four other circles and found a significant impairment in AD patients. Morris *et al.* (1987) (see also Sahakian *et al.* 1988) used abstract patterns, again with four choice stimuli. Here the deficit was greater with longer delays, which varied between 4 and 16 seconds, indicating a faster forgetting rate.

One of the difficulties in interpreting these results in that none of the tasks specifically test the VSSP. Each are relatively demanding and, for example, have significant executive processing components. For example, in the Spatial Working Memory task there is a specific strategy that can be used, which consists of following a predetermined sequence starting from a particular box and returning to it as soon as a token is found. Sahgal *et al.* (1995) found that this strategy was severely disrupted in AD and may account for the spatial memory deficit, although no covariate analysis was performed to investigate this further. In the Money *et al.* (1992) study the AD patients also had difficulties in discriminating the circles in simultaneous matching conditions, which suggests that perceptual difficulties may have added to the task. In summary, although AD patient show deficits on tasks that are likely to involve use of the VSSP, the specificity of this deficit is unknown. Paradigms used to investigate the VSSP in normal subjects, for example using suppression techniques similar in logic to the

ALS investigations, have proved so far to be too complex for this patient group.

CONCLUSIONS

In conclusion, the studies reviewed above indicate that the attentional and executive deficits associated with AD are nonglobal in nature. Clearly the control processes that guide and direct the flow of information processing are impaired and these have been referred to variously as 'control processes', 'attentional', or 'processing resources' of the functioning of the Central Executive System. (Baddeley 1992; Norman and Bobrow 1975; Shallice 1988). Fractionation of these processes in future studies should provide a more detailed picture and explanation of impairment, although some of this work has been done under the rubric of 'attentional processes'. Some progress has been made in relation to the storage mechanisms that surround the control mechanisms, for example indicating the preserved functioning of the Articulatory Rehearsal Loop (Morris 1984). The underlying neurobiological causes of these dissociations have not been discussed, but will be explored more fully in Chapter 13.

Additional, explanatory frameworks can be used in this context to explain the dysexecutive impairment. One is the concept of limited capacity processing resource, which can be applied to 'service' different cognitive operations. Single 'resource' models hold to the notion that there is a central pool of cognitive processing resources which can be used up by increasing the number of mental operations performed (Gopher 1986; Kahneman 1973; Norman and Bobrow 1975). In AD, it would be proposed that a reduced resource pool would explain a variety of deficits, for example on divided attention tasks (Hartman 1991; Morris and Baddeley 1988). One problem with this approach is the lack of predictive value the framework provides. Since there is no independent measure of processing resources it is not possible to determine whether a particular task, or combination of tasks, is taking up more or fewer resources. Such effects as increased divided attention costs can be shown to be consistent with the framework, but in an *ad hoc* fashion. To some extent, the global notion of a Central Executive System suffers from the same limitations, but at least the framework is concerned with fractionating cognitive mechanisms, and it may be possible in future to determine which components of the CES are impaired in AD.

REFERENCES

Allport, A. (1989). Visual attention. In *Foundations of cognitive science*, (ed. M. I. Posner), pp. 631–82. MIT Press, Cambridge, MA.

Baddeley, A. D. (1986). *Working memory.* Oxford University Press, Oxford.

Baddeley, A. D. (1990). *The psychology of memory.* Basic Books, New York.

Baddeley, A. D. (1992). Working memory. *Science*, **255**, 556–9.

Baddeley, A. D. and Hitch, G. (1974). Working memory. In *Recent advances in learning and motivation, Vol. VIII*, (ed. G. Bower), pp. 47–90. Academic Press, New York.

Baddeley, A. D., Thomson, N., and Buchanan, M. (1975). Word length and the structure of short-term memory. *Journal of Verbal Learning and Verbal Behavior*, **14**, 575–89.

Baddeley, A. D., Logie, R., Bressi, S., Della Sala, S. and Spinnler, H. (1986). Dementia and working memory. *Quarterly Journal of Experimental Psychology*, **38A**, 603–18.

Baddeley, A. D., Bressi, S., Della Sala, S., Logie, R., and Spinnler, H. (1991*a*). The decline of working memory in Alzheimer's disease. *Brain*, **114**, 2521–42.

Baddeley, A. D., Della Sala, S., and Spinnler, H. (1991). The two component hypothesis of memory deficit in Alzheimer's disease. *Journal of Clinical and Experimental Neuropsychology*, **13**, 372–80.

Becker, J. T. (1988). Working memory and secondary memory deficits in Alzheimer's disease. *Journal of Clinical and Experimental Neuropsychology*, **6**, 739–53.

Becker, J. T., Bajulaiye, O., and Smith, C. (1992*a*). Longitudinal analysis of a two-component model of the memory deficit in Alzheimer's disease. *Psychological Medicine*, **22**, 437–45.

Becker, J. T., Lopez, O. L., and Wess, J. (1992*b*). Material-specific memory loss in probable Alzheimer's disease. *Journal of Neurology, Neurosurgery and Psychiatry*, **55**, 1177–81.

Benton, A. L. and Hamsler, K. (1978). *Multilingual aphasia examination.* University of Iowa, Iowa City.

Beradi, A., Gaillard, F., Haxby, J. V., Greenwood, P., and Parasuraman, R. (1992). Sustained attention in dementia of the Alzheimer type. Paper presented at the *Annual Meeting of the Gerontological Society of America*, Washington, DC.

Birren, J. E., and Birren, B. A. (1990). The concepts, models, and history of the psychology of aging. In *Handbook of the psychology of aging*, (ed. J. E. Birren and K. W. Schaie), pp. 3–20. Academic Press, San Diego.

Bouma, A., and Van Silfhout, B. (1989). Dichotic listening in patients with Alzheimer's disease. *Journal of Clinical and Experimental Neuropsychology*, **11**, 369.

Brok, P., Preston, G. C., Traub, M., Poppelton, P., Ward, C., and Stahl, S. M. (1988). Modelling dementia: Effects of scopolamine on memory and attention. *Neuropsychologia*, **26**, 685–700.

Capituni, E., Della Sala, S., and Spinnler, H. (1988). Neuropsychological approach to dementia. In *Neurology* (ed. K. Poeck and B. H. J. Gaensehirt), pp.61–9. Springer-Verlag, Berlin.

Corkin, S. (1982). Some relationships between global amnesias and the memory impairment in Alzheimer's disease. In *Alzheimer's disease: A report of research in progress*, (ed. S. Corkin, K. L. Davis, J. H. Growden, E. Usdin and R. J. Wurtman), pp.192–207. Raven Press, New York.

Crawford, J. R., Parker, D. M., and McKinlay, W. W. (1992). *A handbook of neuropsychological assessment.* Lawrence Erlbaum Associates, Hillsdale.

Diller, L., Ben-Yishay, Y., Gerstman, L. J., Goodkin, R., Gordon, W., and Weinberg, J. (1974). *Studies in cognition and rehabilitation in hemiplegia* (Rehabilitation Monograph No. 50). New York University, New York.

Ferris, S., Crook, T., Sathanathan, G., and Gershon, S. (1976). Reaction time as a diagnostic measure of senility. *Journal of the American Geriatrics Society*, **24**, 529–33.

Filoteo, J. V., Delis, D. C., Massman, P. J., Demadura, T., Butters, N., and Salmon, D. P. (1992). Directed and divided attention in Alzheimer's disease: Impairment in shifting attention to global and local stimuli. *Journal of Clinical and Experimental Neuropsychology*, **14**, 871–83.

Freed, D. M., Corkin, S., Growdon, J. H., and Nissen, M. J. (1989). Selective attention in Alzheimer's disease: characterising cognitive subgroups of Alzheimer's disease. *Neuropsychologia*, **27**, 325–39.

Gewirth, L. R., Shindler, A. G., and Hier, D. B. (1984). Altered patterns of words associations in dementia and aphasia. *Brain and Language*, **21**, 307–17.

Gopher, D. (1986). In defense of resources: On structures, energies, pools and allocation of attention. In *Energetics and human information processing*, (ed. G. R. J. Hockey, A. Gaillard, and M. G. H. Coles), pp. 353–71. Nijhoff, Amsterdam.

Grady, C. L., Grimes, A. M., Partronas, N., Sunderland, T., Foster, N. L., and Rapoport, S. I. (1989). Divided attention, as measured by dichotic speech performance in dementia of the Alzheimer's type. *Archives of Neurology*, **46**, 317–20.

Grober, E. and Sliwinski, M. J. (1991). Dual-task performance in demented and non-demented elderly. *Journal of Clinical and Experimental Neuropsychology*, **13** (5), 667–76.

Hartman, M. (1991). The use of knowledge in Alzheimer's disease: Evidence for impairments of attention. *Neuropsychologia* **29**, 213–28.

Haxby, J. V., Grady, C. L., Koss, E., Horwitz, B., Shapiro, M., Friedland, R. P., *et al.* (1988). Heterogenous anterior – posterior metabolic patterns in dementia of the Alzheimer's type. *Neurology*, **38**, 1853–63.

Haxby, J. V., Parasuraman, R., Gillette, J., and Raffaele, K. (1991). Selective and divided attention to visual features are impaired in patients with early dementia of the Alzheimer-type. *Society for Neuroscience Abstracts*, **17**, 696.

Jonides, J. (1981). Voluntary versus automatic control over the mind's eye movement. In *Attention and performance IX*, (ed. J. Long and A. D. Baddeley), pp. 187–203. Erlbaum, Hillsdale, NJ.

Kahneman, D. (1973). *Attention and effort.* Prentice Hall, Englewood Cliffs, NJ.

Kopelman, M. D. (1985). Rates of forgetting in Alzheimer-type dementia and Korsakoff's syndrome. *Neuropsychologia*, **23**, 623–8.

LaBerge, D. (1990). Thalamic and cortical mechanisms of attention suggested by recent positron emission of tomography experiments. *Journal of Neuroscience*, **2**, 358–72.

Lines, C. R., Dawson, C., Preston, G. C., Reich, S., Foster, C., and Traub, M. (1991). Memory and attention in patients with senile dementia of the Alzheimer type and normal elderly subjects. *Journal of Clinical and Experimental Neuropsychology*, **13**, 691–702.

Logie, R. H. and Marchetti, C. (1991). Visuospatial working memory: Visual, spatial or central executive? In *Mental images in human cognition*, (ed. R. H. Logie and M. Dennis), pp. 105–15. Elsevier Science Publishers, B. V.

McCarthy, G. and Donchin, E. (1981). A metric for thought: A comparison of P300 latency and reaction time. *Science*, **211**, 77–80.

Martin, A., Brouwers, P., Cox., C., and Fedio, P. (1985). On the nature of the verbal memory deficit in Alzheimer's disease. *Brain and Language*, **25**, 323–41.

Mattis, S. (1976). Mental status examination for organic mental syndrome in the elderly patient. In *Geriatric psychiatry*, (ed. L. Bellak and T. B. Karasu), pp. 77–121. Grune and Stratton, New York.

Mohr, E., Cox, C., Williams, J., Chase, T. M., and Fedio, P. (1990). Impairment of central auditory function in Alzheimer's disease. *Journal of Clinical and Experimental Neuropsychology*, **12**, 235–46.

Money, E. A., Kirk, R. C., and McNaughton, N. (1992). Alzheimer's dementia produces a loss of discrimination but no increase in rate of memory decay in delayed matching to sample. *Neuropsychologia*, **30**, 133–43.

Morris, R. G. (1984). Dementia and the functioning of the articulatory loop system. *Cognitive Neuropsychology*, **1**, 143–57.

Morris, R. G. (1986). Short-term forgetting in senile dementia of the Alzheimer's type. *Cognitive Neuropsychology*, **3**, 77–97.

Morris, R. G. (1987*a*). Articulatory rehearsal in Alzheimer-type dementia. *Brain and Language*, **30**, 251–362.

Morris, R. G. (1987*b*). The effect of concurrent articulation on memory span in Alzheimer-type dementia. *British Journal of Clinical Psychology*, **26**, 233–4.

Morris, R. G. (1992). Patterns of short-term memory impairment in Alzheimer's disease. In *Memory functioning in dementia*, (ed. L. Backman), pp. 3–25. Elsevier Science Publishers, Amsterdam.

Morris, R. G. (1994*a*). Recent developments in the neuropsychology of dementia. *International Journal of Psychiatry*, **4**, 85–107.

Morris, R. G. (1994*b*). Working memory in Alzheimer's disease. *Neuropsychology*, **8**, 544–54.

Morris, R. G. and Baddeley, A. D. (1988). Primary and working memory functioning in Alzheimer-type dementia. *Journal of Experimental and Clinical Psychology*, **51**, 757–66.

Morris, R. G. and Kopelman, M. D. (1986). The memory deficits in Alzheimer-type dementia: A review. *Quarterly Journal of Experimental Psychology*, **38**, 575–602.

Morris, R. G., Evenden, J. L., Sahakian, B. J., and Robbins, T. W. (1987). Computer-aided assessment of dementia: comparative studies of Alzheimer-type dementia and Parkinson's disease. In, *Cognitive neurochemistry*, (ed. S. M. Stahl, S. D. Iversen, and E. C. Goodman), pp.21–36. Oxford University Press, Oxford.

Morris, R. G., Downes, J., Sahakian, B., Evenden, J., Heald, A., and Robbins, T. W. (1988). Planning and working memory in Parkinson's disease. *Journal of Neurological, Neurosurgery and Psychiatry*, **51**, 757–66.

Morris, R. G., Swain, S., Fox., N., and Polkey, C. E. (1995). Theory of mind impairment following frontal lobectomy. Annual Meeting of the British Neuropsychological Society, Cambridge, UK.

Nebes, R. D. and Brady, C. B. (1989). Focused and divided attention in Alzheimer's disease. *Cortex*, **25**, 305–15.

Nebes, R. D. and Brady, C. B. (1992). Generalised cognitive showing and severity of dementia in Alzheimer's disease: implications for the interpretation of response-time data. *Journal of Clinical and Experimental Neuropsychology*, **14**, 317–26.

Nebes, R. D. and Brady, C. B. (1993). Phasic and tonic alertness in Alzheimer's disease. *Cortex*, **29**, 77–90.

Nestor, P., Parasuraman, R., Haxby, J. V., and Grady, C. L. (1991). Divided attention and metabolic brain dysfunction in mild dementia of the Alzheimer's type. *Neuropsychologia*, **29**, 379–87.

Norman, D. A. and Bobrow, D. G. (1975). On data-limited and resource-limited processes. *Cognitive Psychology*, **7**, 44–64.

Norman, D. A. and Shallice, T. (1986). Attention to action: Willed and automatic control of behaviour. In *Advances in research and theory*, Vol. 4, *Consciousness and self-regulation* (ed. R. J. Davidson, G. E. Schwartz, and D. Shapiro), pp. 1–18. Plenum Press, New York.

O'Connor, K. P. (1980*a*). Slow potential correlates of attentional dysfunction in senile dementia: I. *Biological Psychology*, **11**, 193–202.

O'Connor, K. P. (1980*b*). Slow potential correlates of attentional dysfunction in senile dementia: II. *Biological Psychology*, **11**, 203–16.

Owen, A. M., Downes, J.J., Sahakian, B. J., Polkey, C. E., and Robbins, T. W. (1990). Planning and spatial working memory following frontal lobe lesions in man. *Neuropsychologia* **28**, 1021–34.

Parasuraman, R., and Giambra, L. (1991). Skill development in vigilance: effects of event rate and age. *Psychology and Aging*, **6**, 155–69.

Parasuraman, R., and Haxby, J. V. (1993). Attention and brain function in Alzheimer's disease: A review. *Neuropsychology*, **7**, 242–72.

Parasuraman, R., Mutter, S. A., and Molloy, R. (1991). Sustained attention following mild closed head injury. *Journal of Clinical and Experimental Neuropsychology*, **13**, 789–811.

Parasuraman, R., Greenwood, P. M., Haxby, J. V., and Grady, C. L. (1992). Visuospatial attention in dementia of the Alzheimer's type. *Brain*, **115**, 711–33.

Paulescu, E., Frith, C. D., and Frackowiak, R. S. J. (1993). The neural correlates of the verbal components of working memory. *Nature*, **362**, 342–5.

Peterson, L. R. and Peterson, M. J. (1959). Short-term retention of individual verbal items. *Journal of Experimental Psychology*, **58**, 193–8.

Posner, M. I. (1980). Orienting of attention. *Quarterly Journal of Experimental Psychology*, **32**, 3–25.

Posner, M. I., Cohen, Y., Choate, L. S., Hockey, R., and Maylor, E. (1984*a*). Sustained concentration: passive filtering or active orienting? In *Preparatory states and processes*, (ed. S. Kornblum and J. Requin), pp. 49–65. Lawrence Erlbaum, Hillsdale, NJ.

Posner, M. M., Walker, J. A., Friedrich, F. J., and Rafal, R. D. (1984*b*). Effects of parietal injury on covert orienting of attention. *Journal of Neuroscience*, **4**, 1863–74.

Sahakian, B. J., Morris, R. G., Evenden, J. L., Heald, A., Levy, R., Philpot, M., *et al.* (1988). A comparative study of visuo-spatial memory and learning in Alzheimer-type dementia and Parkinson's disease. *Brain*, **111**, 695–718.

Sahgal, A., McKeith, I. G., Galloway, P. H., Tasker, N., and Steckler, T. (1995). Do differences in visuospatial ability between senile dementias of the Alzheimer and Lewy body types reflect differences solely in mnemonic function. *Journal of Clinical and Experimental Neuropsychology*, **17**, 35–43.

Shallice, T. (1988). *From neuropsychology to mental structure*. Cambridge University Press, New York.

Spinnler, H., Della Sala, S., Bandera, R., and Baddeley, A. D. (1988). Dementia, ageing and the structure of human memory. *Cognitive Neuropsychology*, **5**, 193–211.

Stuss, D. T. (1992). Biological and psychological development of executive functions. *Brain and Cognition*, **20**, 8–23.

Vallar, G., and Baddeley, A. D. (1984). Fractionation of working memory: Neuropsychological evidence for a phonological short-term store. *Journal of Verbal Learning and Verbal Behaviour*, **34**, 53–60.

Vallar, G., and Shallice, T. (ed.) (1990). *Neuropsychological impairments of short-term memory*. Cambridge University Press, Cambridge.

Weigl, E. (1927). On the psychology of so-called processes of abstraction. *Journal of Abnormal and Social Psychology*, **36**, 3–33.

Weingartner, H., Grafman, J., Boutelle, W., Kaye, W., and Martin, P. R. (1983). Forms of memory failure. *Science*, **221**, 380–2.

Wright, M. J., Burns, R. J., Geffen, G. M., and Geffen, L. B. (1990). Covert orientation of visual attention in Parkinson's disease: an impairment in the maintenance of attention. *Neuropsychologia*, **28**, 151–9.

FIVE

Episodic memory: differential patterns of breakdown

James T. Becker, Oscar L. Lopez, and Meryl A. Butters

BACKGROUND

A diagnosis of Alzheimer-type dementia (AD) can only be made in the presence of significant impairments in at least two areas of cognitive function (APA 1987; McKhann *et al.* 1984), and memory loss is the most common presenting symptom. Analyses of groups of AD patients have revealed the existence of subgroups (Jorm 1985; Martin 1990), characterized on the basis of the pattern of their neuropsychological deficits. Some patients may have pronounced defects in visuospatial functions, whilst others may have focal lexical/semantic impairments, and still others may have profound dysexecutive syndromes; all of these patients nevertheless meet the criteria for Probable AD (Baddeley *et al.* 1991; Becker 1988; Martin *et al.* 1986). Analysis of the cognitive functions of these patients has revealed important features of their neuropsychological impairments (Martin *et al.* 1985*b*), as well as correlations with regional cerebral glucose metabolism (Martin *et al.* 1985*a*). Further, follow-up of these patients has revealed differential rates of decline among some of the subgroups (Becker *et al.* 1992*a*).

At some point during the course of AD, it is likely that individual patients will show relative sparing of certain cognitive functions. In some cases, as noted above, these dissociations are striking, and the patient can be included in a subgroup of AD. These different patterns of impairment severity may reflect the relative distribution of neuropathological changes, which typically disrupt cortical–cortical connections (see Chapter 13). However, membership in any of the subgroups described to date cannot be predicted by predispositional factors such as age or education and appear not to alter prognosis. This chapter describes the nature of the episodic memory breakdown in AD, with specific reference to the nature of the patient subgroups that have been identified along this dimension. We will also discuss the nature of the CNS functional abnormality associated with verbal memory, as visualized with [^{15}O] water positron emission tomography (PET). We will focus on a dichotomy between long-term memory and working memory function, in part because it provides a reasonable conceptual framework. However, we will also describe new data which suggest the existence of one patient subgroup that does have a significant prognostic value.

EPISODIC MEMORY

To begin at the beginning, it is important to understand the context in which memory loss became the principal symptom of dementia. Berrios and Freeman (1991) point out that the recognition that dementia could arise in the presence of a specific neuropathological abnormality (for example senile plaques), occurred in the late 1800s when the *quantitative* study of memory and memory function was gaining in importance; quantification of other cognitive functions (such as language, perception) was somewhat less advanced. Thus, both memory *function* and *loss* could be relatively easily measured, whereas other functions (such as language or constructional skills) were not as easily measured. Thus, memory loss became *de facto* the prime symptom of AD, and this was later codified in the various diagnostic schema (see also Becker *et al.* 1994*b*).

Memory complaints and mild deficits in episodic memory are common in elderly non-demented individuals. Studies on normal age-related changes in episodic memory find a decrement in the availability of processing resources at the time of encoding and retrieval, but recall of previously learned information is relatively preserved (Petersen *et al.* 1992). Although normal individuals complain of subtle memory problems with advancing age, these changes are not of the magnitude observed in AD (Welsh *et al.* 1991; Welsh *et al.* 1992). The memory impairment in AD is not only quantitatively different from normal ageing, but qualitatively different as well, involving aspects of memory that are preserved in normal ageing (Petersen *et al.* 1994).

The memory impairment exhibited by AD patients has been the focus of substantial research, as it is the most distinguishing feature of the disease. Both episodic and semantic memory are affected early in the course of the disease, while procedural memory is unimpaired until the very late stages (see Chapter 7). The episodic memory impairment is a genuine amnesia, in that patients are unable to learn and remember new information. This aspect of the memory defect, best characterized as a lack of storage, or consolidation of new information, has been demonstrated in numerous studies by a variety of methods.

The episodic memory loss has often been characterized as an extremely rapid rate of forgetting, and this differentiates AD from other forms of dementia and has proven to be the single best indicator of early AD (Butters *et al.* 1988; Hart *et al.* 1988; Knopman and Ryberg 1989; Kramer *et al.* 1989; Troster *et al.* 1993). For example when the performance of AD patients was compared with that of patients with Huntington's disease (HD) (a subcortical dementia) or alcoholic Korsakoff's syndrome on word list recall, all three patient groups were equally impaired relative to the controls after a brief delay (15 seconds). However, after 2 minutes, the AD patients recalled significantly fewer words than either the HD or Korsakoff groups. Moreover, when the rate of forgetting (the number of words recalled at the longer delay expressed as a percentage of the number of words recalled at the shorter delay) was assessed, the AD patients showed a significantly greater loss of information than did any of the other groups. The abnormally rapid rate of forgetting appears to be related to the transfer of information or consolidation of information into a longer-term store, and has its greatest impact within (approximately) 2 minutes of retention (Kopelman 1992). An analysis of the performance of AD patients on various memory measures derived from a ten-word list learning task in the 'Consortium to Establish a Registry for Alzheimer's Disease test battery', found that even very mildly impaired AD patients performed poorly relative to normal controls on all of the measures (Welsh *et al.* 1991; Welsh *et al.* 1992). However, the clinical sensitivity and specificity was not equivalent across the measures; delayed recall and forgetting rate were best at discriminating very early AD patients from normal controls.

The inability to transfer new information from short-term to long-term storage exhibited by AD patients is also evident in the reduction of the primacy effect in verbal-free recall tasks (the tendency to recall more of the first few items of a list of words) (Delis *et al.* 1991*a*; Miller 1971; Wilson *et al.* 1983), in their poor recognition memory (Delis *et al.* 1991*b*), and their inability to acquire additional information over repeated trials (Buschke and Fuld 1974; Masur *et al.* 1989; Wilson *et al.* 1983). When the performance of AD and Korsakoff patients was compared on the California Verbal Learning Test (CVLT) (Delis *et al.* 1987), both groups had severely impaired recognition discriminability and did not perform better on recognition testing than they did on free recall, unlike patients with Huntington's disease. This suggests that the AD patients had impairments in *both* encoding and storage of new information, rather than the more pronounced retrieval deficit seen in the HD patients (Butters *et al.* 1985; Heindel *et al.* 1989). Moreover, the AD and Korsakoff patients exhibited a tendency to recall words passively from the recency region of the list.

THE CASE FOR SUBGROUPS

Although the argument for the existence of subgroups of AD patients determined *between* cognitive domains has been made earlier, we expanded the analogy to work *within* a single domain, specifically episodic memory. Our initial analysis included 191 AD patients (Becker *et al.* 1992*b*), and found that 13% of the cases had a material-specific deficit; in this case comparing verbal versus non-verbal memory loss. We have reanalysed these data based on the more recent dataset of 181 probable or definite AD cases (Becker *et al.* 1994*a*), and the results are virtually the same; 8 of the patients (4.5%) had focal verbal memory loss and 11 (6.3%) had focal non-verbal memory loss (Becker *et al.* 1992*b*). As shown in Fig. 5.1, those AD patients with verbal memory loss ('story impaired') performed poorly at immediate recall of a short story, but normally at recall of a modified Rey figure. By contrast, those patients with non-verbal memory loss ('figure impaired') recalled the story well, but had a significant deficit in figure recall. These material-specific deficits could not be attributed to perceptual or pre-processing defects and appeared specifically related to episodic memory dysfunction. The finding that some AD patients could be normal in one aspect of episodic memory, while being profoundly impaired in another, led us

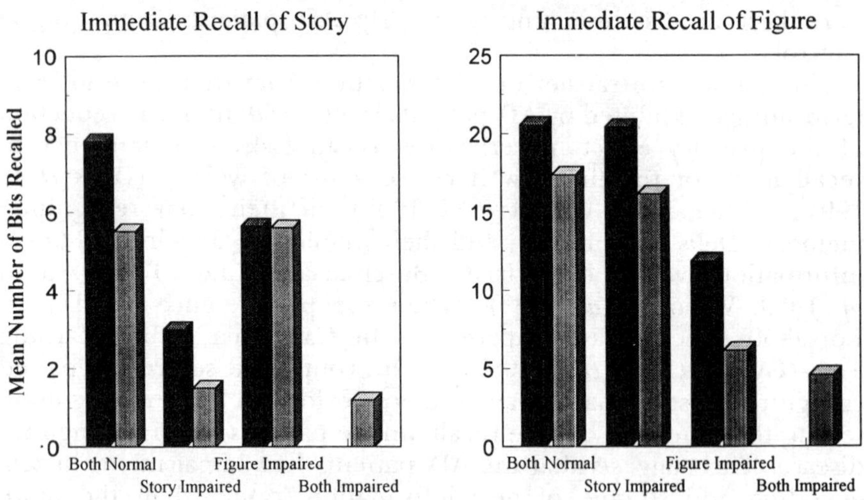

FIG. 5.1 Performance by AD patients (dark bars) and normal control subjects (light bars) on the immediate recall of a story and a figure. Subjects are classified relative to the 5% tile of normals, and were grouped according to the pattern of impairment.

to our study of what were perhaps more subtle processing dissociations (Becker 1988).

The beginning of the study of the multiple processing deficits responsible for the memory loss in AD can probably be traced to the work of Edgar Miller in the 1970s (Miller 1971, 1973) when he noted that there was a difference in the breakdown of primary memory and secondary memory. Using an auditory—verbal free recall task (Glanzer and Cunitz 1966), he demonstrated that AD patients have impairments in recall for both the short-term (recency effect) and long-term (primacy effect) memory components of the serial position curve (Miller 1971) unlike amnesic patients, who have impairments restricted to the long-term memory component of the task (Baddeley and Warrington 1970). However, the patients also failed to show a normal response (that is an increase in the primacy effect) to a slower rate of word presentation, leading Miller to conclude that the memory loss had at least two components—one related to short-term or working memory, and one related to long-term memory. This hypothesis was supported by further data (Miller 1973) demonstrating that not only were AD patients impaired at immediate recall of short word lists, but were also impaired at learning lists that exceeded their word span by one, two, or three words—even with repeated exposure.

Morris and Kopelman (1986) followed on this tradition, arguing that the memory loss in AD was due to a profound amnesic syndrome similar to that seen in patients with focal amnesic disorders (accounting for the secondary memory loss), with an additional information processing defect which had an impact on their short-term memory. Our own data suggested that this additional deficit might reflect a dysexecutive syndrome (Becker 1988), based on a model of Working Memory developed by Baddeley and Hitch (1974). A cross-sectional analysis of the neuropsychological data demonstrated the existence of two subgroups of AD patients based on this model—one with a profound amnesic syndrome and normal executive functions, and the other with a significant dysexecutive syndrome and normal secondary memory. A subsequent longitudinal analysis (Becker *et al.* 1992) revealed that the pattern of decline in these two subgroups of patients differed, with the dysexecutive patients demonstrating a dramatic loss of secondary memory functions over a one-year period. Baddeley and colleagues from Milan (Baddeley *et al.* 1991) examined a separate database consisting of AD patients who had completed a comprehensive battery of neuropsychological tests (Spinnler and Tognoni 1987). By analysing the patterns of performance of these patients, this group was also able to identify 'amnesic' and 'dysexecutive' AD patients (see also Morris, Chapter 4).

All of the patient data that will be described below were gathered as part of the Alzheimer Research Program (ARP) at the University of Pittsburgh (program director: F. Boller, MD, PhD). Details of the recruitment and assessment procedures have been published previously (Becker *et al.* 1994). All subjects, patients, and controls alike completed an extensive battery of neuropsychological tests that evaluated a wide range of cognitive functions and evaluations were completed on an annual basis.

Of critical importance for this report was our method of reducing the extensive neuropsychological data into manageable units. We have used factor analytic strategies (Becker 1988; Becker *et al.* 1988, 1992) to compile the data into summary variables with both face and construct validity. First, the individual test scores were transformed into standard scores using the mean and standard deviations of the control group. In the event that a subject was missing a particular test score, the mean value for the study group, was substituted. In the event that a subject (usually a patient) was unable to complete a particular test due to the severity of their dementia, then the maximum error score was substituted. The total number of data substitutions comprised less than 1% of the total dataset.

These standard scores were then averaged, using the appropriate sign, to create a score reflecting the subject's observed performance on the tasks. The data from the control group were then entered into a multiple regression analysis to evaluate the effects of age, education, and sex on the particular summary score. We then used these regression equations to *predict* individual performance based on age, education, and sex. The arithmetic difference between the observed and predicted scores constituted the composite variable. Thus, the composite scores can be interpreted as reflecting the deviation of an individual's performance from that expected based on their age, education, and sex. The mean value of these composite scores among the controls subjects varies about zero, while those of the patients were in the negative range, indicating performance worse than that expected (Becker *et al.* 1994).

Memory and executive functions:

In our initial cross-sectional (Becker 1988) and longitudinal (Becker *et al.* 1992) analysis of these data, we classified each subject with respect to their scores on the memory and executive composite variables. In order to be classified into one of the patient subgroups, a patient had to have scored within normal limits on one of the composite variables (such as memory)—defined as a score >–2.00, and significantly worse on the other variable (such as executive)—defined as >–2.00 standard units. Patients could thus be classified as either 'amnesic', 'dysexecutive', or 'non-focal' based on their pattern of performance. Each of the patients who were classified as belonging to one of the focal impairment groups otherwise met the NINCDS–ADRDA criteria for probable or definite AD (Khachaturian 1985; McKhann *et al.* 1984); they simply had an aspect of their cognitive functions which suggested a more focal pattern of impairment.

We next addressed the question of whether the subgroups of patients that we had identified had different patterns of progression than the non-focal AD patients. Patients with focal visuospatial or language dysfunction appear to progress towards a 'non-focal' pattern of impairment (Becker *et al.* 1988), suggesting that although the disease distinguished itself in different domains initially, by the 'middle' stages, the subgroups were equivalent, and we had simply captured our patients at different points in the progression of their disease. Longitudinal analysis of the performance of AD patients classified relative to their memory and executive functions, however, revealed a similar lack of differentiation from the non-focal patients, but with an interesting interaction. Specifically, of the patients classified as 'amnesic' at study entry, 5/24 (20.8%) progressed into the non-focal group while 79.2% were still classified as amnesic one year later. However, 18 patients who had been mildly, but non-focally, impaired at study entry, were now classified as amnesic at the follow-up visit. This provided support for the idea that we were observing our patients at different stages of the development of their dementia, and that they would progress to the more typical non-focal presentation. By contrast, of the patients classified as dysexecutive at study entry, *all* were classified as non-focal at the second visit. Although the rate of progression of their executive dysfunction was close to that of the group overall (visit 1 = –3.69, visit 2 = –3.80), their memory functions declined significantly faster than the other patient groups (visit 1 = –0.92, visit 2 = –5.06). Furthermore, there were *no* incident classifications of dysexecutive syndromes at the second visit. These latter data have led us to speculate that the dysexecutive syndrome can actually occur as the earliest symptom of AD (Becker *et al.* 1992). It can be of sufficient severity to disrupt activities of daily living, alter work habits, and interfere with normal functioning. At this stage of the disease, memory retrieval is most likely affected, and thus the patient appears 'forgetful'. Memory storage is only affected later, and this symptom most likely stimulates the clinical evaluation.

These initial studies of amnesic and dysexecutive AD patients utilized a subsample of the final study sample. More recently, we replicated these studies using the entire study group (n = 181) and utilizing more sophisticated statistical analyses (Butters 1996). Accordingly, we examined the structure of the data using a K-Means cluster analysis

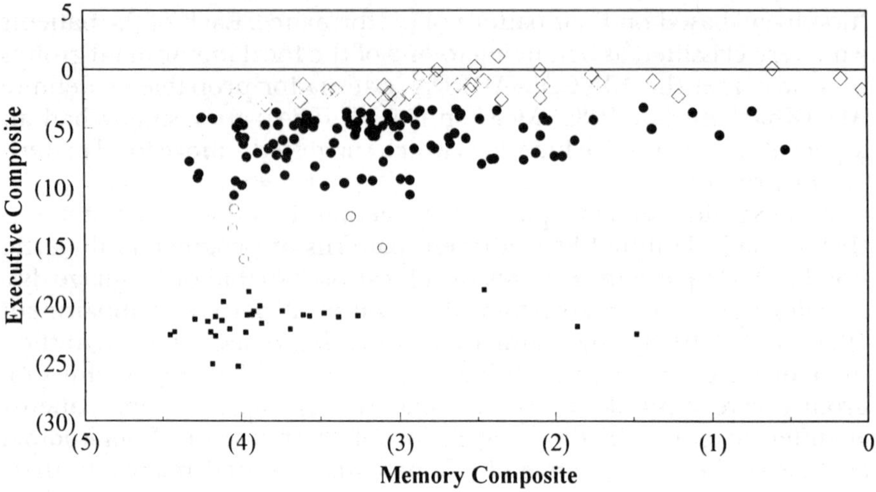

FIG. 5.2 A scatterplot of the performance of 181 probable AD patients on the Memory and Executive Composite scores. The symbols corresponding to the three non-focal groups are: mild (closed circles), moderate (open circles), and severe (closed squares) impairments. The temporal lobe subgroup is shown in open diamonds.

which identified four different clusters of AD patients based on their scores on the memory and executive composite scores. Three of the groups of AD patients appeared to be related to increasing severity of the dysexecutive syndrome with a relatively constant score on the memory composite. These groups are described as mild, moderate, and severely impaired on the degree of executive systems dysfunction (see Fig. 5.2). The fourth group of patients was impaired in only two areas of cognitive function, those related to episodic (both verbal and non-verbal) and semantic memory. There were no significant impairments in perception, construction, or attention. Thus, these patients are described as having 'temporal lobe' impairments—verbal and non-verbal memory are impaired, as are naming, fluency, and the ability to associate highly related words (i.e. easy paired associates).

The performance of these groups of patients on a global measure of dementia the Mini-Mental State (MMS) examination showed that the rate of decline among the patients in the temporal lobe group is significantly slower than that of the other three groups of patients. After two years of evaluation, the mean MMS score remains in the mildly impaired range (mean = 20.44, s.d. = 5.49), and is significantly different from that of the patients in the mild group (mean = 10.77, s.d. = 6.37).

FUNCTIONAL NEUROIMAGING OF EPISODIC MEMORY FUNCTION IN AD

Functional neuroimaging studies of regional cerebral blood flow (rCBF) and cerebral glucose metabolism of AD patients have demonstrated decreased functioning of the parietal and temporal cortices when patients are at rest, consistent with the pattern of neurodegenerative changes in these regions (Haxby *et al.* 1985, 1986, 1990; Jagust *et al.* 1990; Johnson *et al.* 1990; Smith *et al.* 1992; Stern *et al.* 1992) (see also Chapter 13). More recent studies of young, healthy normal volunteers have revealed distinct patterns of functional activity as the subjects engage in tasks related to auditory verbal short-term memory (Becker *et al.* 1994; Grasby *et al.* 1993; Kapur *et al.* 1994; Paulescu *et al.* 1993; Shallice *et al.* 1994; Tulving *et al.* 1994). These studies are of particular relevance because the procedures have the potential for revealing specific functional defects related to specific information processing deficits, prior to any observable structural abnormalities. We utilized these procedures to study the changes in rCBF of AD patients during the performance of verbal memory tasks that place differential demands on cognition, and presumably different functional processing systems (Becker *et al.* 1996).

Five women and two men meeting the NINCDS–ADRDA criteria for probable AD (McKhann *et al.* 1984) participated in the study (Becker *et al.* under editorial review). Their overall level of cognition was mildly impaired (mean MMS score = 21.7 ± 3.4). These patients were compared with seven age-, education-, and sex-matched controls who all completed the same PET procedures. Each subject was scanned eight times measuring rCBF using ^{15}O [water] with standard laboratory procedures (Becker *et al.* 1994). During the first and last scans, the subjects were instructed to lie still and fix their gaze on a cross-hair target on a video screen suspended over their head and perpendicular to their line of vision ('Rest' condition). During the remaining six scans, the subjects were tested on single word repetition one (1WR), three word repetition (3WR), and eight word free recall (8WR). The scan order was counterbalanced and fixed for all subjects: Rest, 1WR, 3WR, 8WR, 3WR, 1WR, and Rest.

Contrasting 3WR with Rest among the control subjects revealed those brain regions more active during auditory processing, working memory, and speech output than at rest. Fig. 5.3 shows the statistical parametric map (SPM) (Friston *et al.* 1991) of the 3WR—Rest contrast for the seven elderly control subjects. Previous studies from this and other laboratories have identified those brain regions activated during relatively lower-level, automatic processes associated with working memory in healthy young subjects (Becker *et al.* 1994; Grasby *et al.* 1993; Paulescu

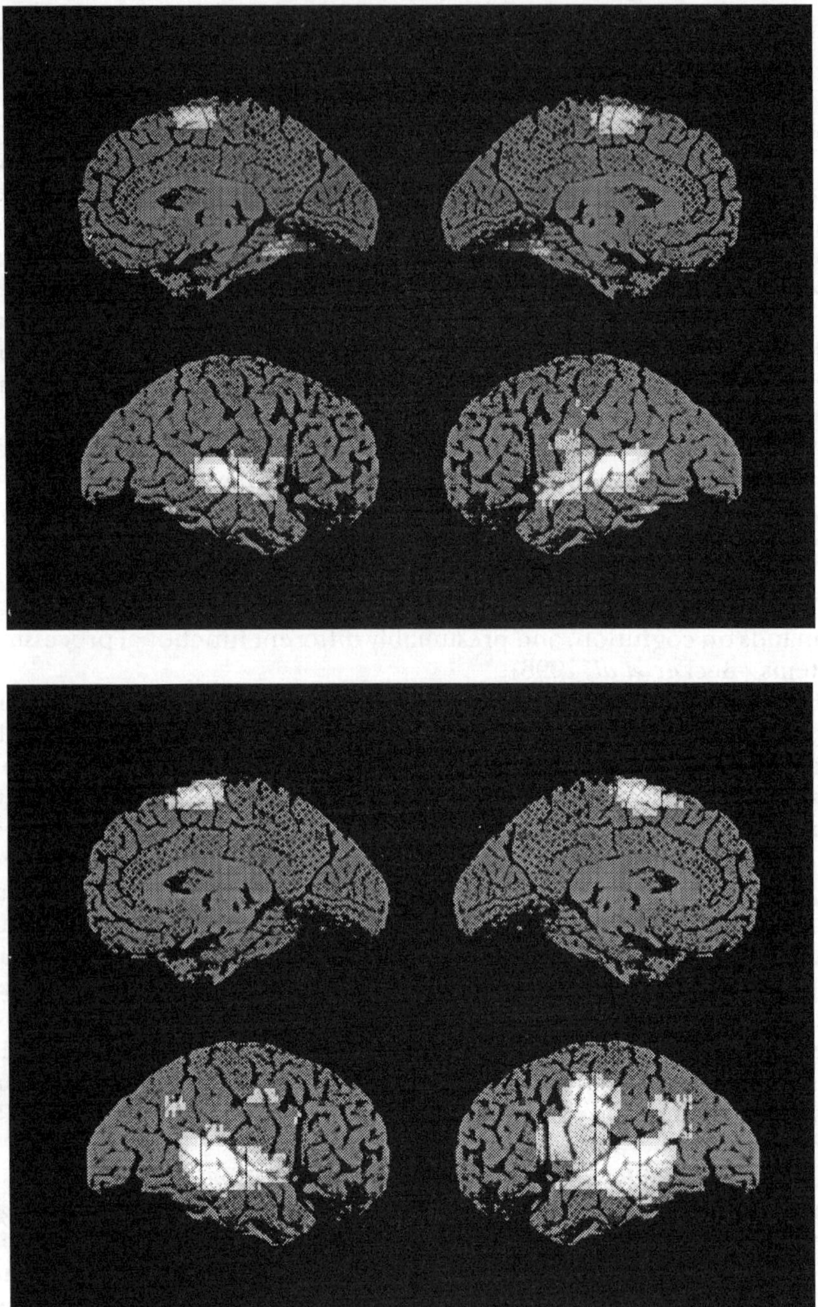

FIG. 5.3 Statistical parametric map of the comparison between three word recall and rest. Data from the control subjects are in the top panel, and those from the AD patients are in the lower panel.

et al. 1993). The healthy elderly subjects showed a similar pattern of functional anatomical relationships, with significant increases in rCBF in brain regions responsible for auditory perception, phonological storage, and articulatory rehearsal and articulated speech.

All seven AD subjects were able to complete the 3WR task accurately and, like the normal control subjects, the AD patients showed significant activations in brain regions associated with speech and language function, and with phonological storage (Fig. 5.3, bottom). By contrast, there was no significant activation in the hippocampal formation, a brain region implicated in long-term, but not short-term memory function (Kopelman and Corn 1988; Smith 1989). Of particular note, however, is that of the regions that showed significant activation, there was an apparent increase in their spatial extent. In all regions examined, the field of activity observed in the AD patients was greater than the activation in the same region in the normal controls. However, for the 3WR—Rest comparison there were no brain regions activated in the AD patients that were not also activated by the control subjects.

By comparing the pattern of rCBF seen in the 8WR condition with that seen in the 3WR condition, it is possible to isolate those brain mechanisms responsible for the encoding and retrieval of information from secondary episodic memory. That is, while the input and output demands of the two tasks were similar, and the demands on working memory were similar, the 8WR task required encoding of information into, and retrieval of information from, secondary memory. The control subjects showed significant activation primarily in BA10 of the middle frontal gyrus, bilaterally (Fig. 5.4, top).

By contrast, the SPM for the 8WR—3WR comparison in the AD patients showed significant activity in the dorsolateral prefrontal cortex across the convexity, bilaterally. Brodmann's Area 8, BA9, and BA10 all showed significant activation, extending down to a level approximately 12 cm above the inter-commissural line. Posteriorly, the AD patients had regional activation in the supramarginal gyrus on the left (BA40), in the angular gyrus (BA39), and in the cuneate (BA31).

The finding that the spatial extent of activation seen in the AD patients is greater than that seen in the control subjects suggests that there is a broadening of the cortical field in response to the altered cortical connections due to the neuropathological changes. Although the focus, or specific locus of activity remains the same, the area around these foci has changed. This view is consistent with the observation that areas of cortical representation of information can be altered by changes in the input to those brain regions (Merzenich and Sameshima 1993). Further, one aspect of the dysfunction in *semantic* memory in AD may be a 'loss of constraints ... needed to push the network towards a stable pattern of activation' (Tippett and Farah

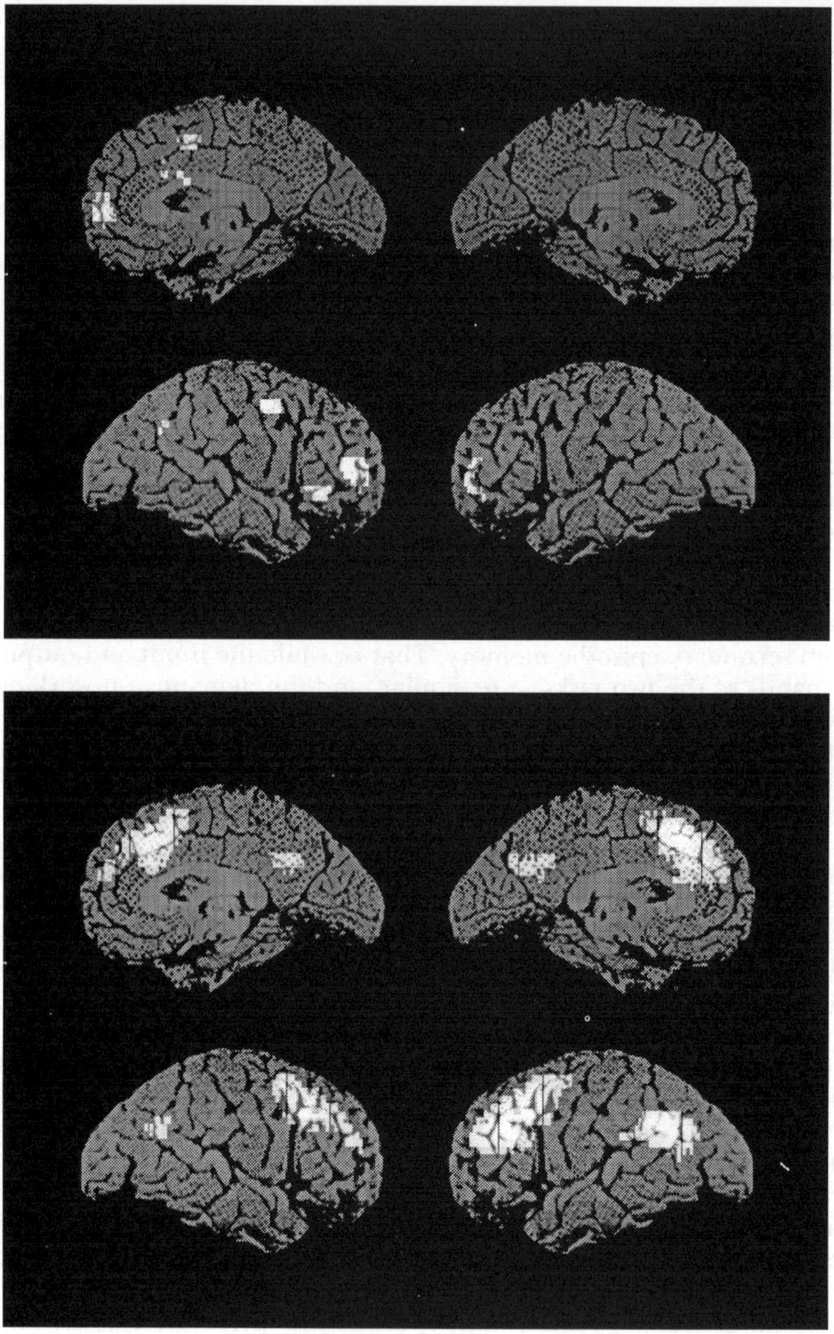

FIG. 5.4 SPM comparison of 8WR—3WR.

1994), which might be represented here as a broadening of the spatial extent of activity.

CONCLUSIONS

The data described in this chapter make several points relevant to our understanding of Alzheimer's disease. They reinforce the finding that Alzheimer's disease can present with relative sparing and impairment of specific cognitive functions, even as it relates to a single sphere of cognition, and the breakdown conforms to known structure–function relationships. We identified a group of patients with impaired episodic and semantic memory, with few additional cognitive impairments, who had a slower rate of intellectual decline than other AD patients. These patients are felt to have a focal impairment in the functions of the temporal lobes, bilaterally, in the context of probable AD. Further, the pattern of rCBF during verbal memory tasks suggests an alteration in the extent of the cortical fields supporting memory-related processes.

It seems clear that while the most common pattern of impairment includes loss of episodic memory function early in the course of AD, this may be accompanied by differential sparing and impairments of function. These patterns of impairment correspond to the altered regional CNS function as revealed by positron emission tomography (Haxby *et al.* 1985, 1990), demonstrating a close link between loss of brain function and abnormal cognition. The specific pattern of impairment is important. Thus, the identification of a 'temporal lobe' pattern of dysfunction appears to have significance for predicting a slower rate of decline in function, while the presence of a language or construction deficit does not have the same predictive value. This suggests that when the cognitive dysfunction associated with AD begins with processes ascribed to the temporal lobes, and not, for example, the parietal lobes, then the rate of spread of these abnormalities may be different. This observation may have implications for understanding the nature of the progression of AD-related neuropathological changes throughout the brain.

These data make an important point about clinical pharmacological trials in AD. We take the view that the assessment of *cognitive* function is the most sensitive and specific index of *cortical* function (Goldstein *et al.* 1973). As such, it seems important to view such functions as an important indicator variable in clinical trials. However, at the present time there are no criteria for entry into studies based on the *pattern* of impairment. The assumption appears to be that in a large study, random assignment of patients to treatment or placebo conditions should eliminate any potential problems related to subgroup classification. This is probably true in terms of determining efficacy provided that the samples are large enough. However, in small studies (for instance < 20 per group), a bias in terms of patient characteristics could have important effects. Perhaps more important is the fact that these characteristics are not considered in the design of these studies. The scientific and clinical merits of these pharmacological trials would be increased dramatically if these sorts of patient characteristics were used as blocking variables and as outcome measures (see, for example, Bilder *et al.* 1992). It may be the case, for example, that while a particular compound has only a marginal effect on cognition when measured by summary variables, specific aspects of cognition are affected more than others, and certain subgroups of patients may show marked improvement relative to other subgroups. This kind of interaction between neuropsychology and psychopharmacology in the context of treating dementia syndromes is an important source of information on brain mechanisms in cognition.

As our understanding of the biology of AD advances, it seems that it would be advantageous for this progress to be made in the context of our long-standing understanding of the nature and patterns of cognitive loss. While the analysis of patient subgroups is but one method for such cross-fertilization, we feel that in the long run it will be an extremely fruitful interaction.

ACKNOWLEDGEMENTS

The preparation of this chapter was supported, in part, by funds from the National Institute on Aging (AGO5133). J.T.B. is the recipient of a Research Scientist Development Award—Level II (K02–MH0177).

REFERENCES

APA. (1987). *Diagnostic and statistical manual on mental disorders—Revised (DSM-III-R)*, (3rd edn, revised) American Psychiatric Press, Washington, DC.

Baddeley, A. D. and Hitch, G. (1974). Working memory. In *The psychology of learning and motivation* (ed. G. H. Bower), pp. 47–90. Academic Press, San Diego.

Baddeley, A. D., and Warrington, E. K. (1970). Amnesia and the distinction between long-and short-term memory. *Journal of Verbal Learning and Verbal Behavior*, **9**, 176–89.

Baddeley, A. D., Della Salla, S., and Spinnler, H. (1991). The two-component hypothesis of memory deficit in Alzheimer's disease. *Journal of Clinical and Experimental Neuropsychology*, **13**, 372–80.

Becker, J. T. (1988). Primary memory and secondary memory deficits in Alzheimer's disease. *Journal of Clinical and Experimental Neuropsychology*, **10** 739–53.

Becker, J. T., Huff, F. J., Nebes, R. D., Holland, A., and Boller, F. (1988). Neuropsychological functioning in Alzheimer's disease: Pattern of impairment and rates of progression. *Archives of Neurology*, **45**, 263–8.

Becker, J. T., Bajulaiye, O., and Smith, C. (1992*a*). Longitudinal analysis of a two-component model of the memory deficits in Alzheimer's disease. *Psychological Medicine*, **22**, 437–46.

Becker, J. T., Lopez, O. L., and Wess, J. (1992*b*). Material specific memory loss in probable Alzheimer's disease. *Journal of Neurology, Neurosurgery and Psychology*, **55**, 1177–81.

Becker, J. T., Boller, F., Lopez, O. L., Saxton, J., and McGonigle, K. (1994*a*). The natural history of Alzheimer's disease: Description of study cohort and accuracy of diagnosis. *Archives of Neurology*, **51** 585–94.

Becker, J. T., Martin, A., and Lopez, O. L. (1994*b*). The dementias and AIDS. In *Neuropsychology of HIV infection*, (ed. I. Grant and A. Martin), pp. 133–45. Oxford University Press, New York.

Becker, J. T., Mintun, M. A., Diehl, D. J., Dobkin, J., Martidis, A., Madoff, D. C., *et al.* (1994*c*). Functional neuroanatomy of verbal free recall: A replication study. *Human Brain Mapping*, **1**, 284–92.

Becker, J. T., Mintun, M. A., Aleva, K., Wiseman, M. B., Nichols, T., and DeKosky, S. T. (1996). Compensatory reallocation of brain resources supporting verbal episodic memory in Alzheimer's disease. *Neurology*, **46**, 692–700.

Berrios, G. E., and Freeman, H. L. (1991). *Alzheimer and the dementias (eponymists in medicine)*. Royal Society of Medicine Services, London.

Bilder, R. M., Turkel, E., Lipschitz-Broch, L., and Lieberman, J. A. (1992). Antipsychotic medication effects on neuropsychological functions. *Psychopharmacology Bulletin*, **28**, 353–66.

Buschke, H., and Fuld, P. A. (1974). Evaluating storage, retention, and retrieval in disoriented memory and learning. *Neurology*, **24**, 1019–25.

Butters, N., Wolfe, J., Martone, M., Granholm, E., and Cermak, L. S. (1985). Memory disorders associated with Huntington's disease: Verbal recall, verbal recognition and procedural memory. *Neuropsychologia*, **23**, 729–43.

Butters, N., Salmon, D. P., Heindel, W., and Granholm, E. (1988). Episodic, semantic and procedural memory: Some comparisons of Alzheimer and Huntington disease patients. In *Aging and the brain*, (ed. R. D. Terry), Raven Press, pp. 63–87. New York.

Butters, M. A., Lopez, O. L., and Becker, J. T. (1996). Focal temporal lobe dysfunction in Probable Alzheimer's disease predicts a slow rate of decline. *Neurology*, **46**, 687–92.

Delis, D. C., Kramer, J. H., Kaplan, E., and Ober, B. A. (1987). *The California Verbal Learning Test.* Psychological Corporation, New York.

Delis, D. C., Massman, P. J., Butters, N., Salmon, D. P., Cermak, L. S., and Kramer, J. H. (1991 *a*). Profiles of demented and amnesic patients on the California Verbal Learning Test: Implications for the assessment of memory disorders. *Psychological Assessment*, **3**, 16–19.

Delis, D. C., Massman, P. J., Butters, N., Salmon, D. P., Kramer, J. H., and Cermak, L. (1991 *b*). Profiles of demented and amnesic patients on the California Verbal

Learning Test: Implications for the assessment of memory disorders. *Psychological Assessment: A Journal of Consulting and Clinical Psychology*, **3**, 19–26.

Friston, K. J., Frith, C. D., Liddle, P. F., and Frackowiak, R. S. J. (1991). Comparing functional (PET) images: The assessment of significant change. *Journal of Cerebral Blood Flow Metabolism*, **10**, 458–66.

Glanzer, M., and Cunitz, A. R. (1966). Two storage mechanisms in free recall. *Journal of Verbal Learning and Verbal Behavior*, **5**, 351–360.

Goldstein, S., Deysach, R., and Kleinknecht, R. (1973). Effect of experience and amount of information on the identification of cerebral impairment. *Journal of Consulting and Clinical Psychology*, **41**, 30–4.

Grasby, P. M., Frith, C. D., Friston, K. J., Bench, C., Frackowiak, R. S. J., and Dolan, R. J. (1993). Functional mapping of brain areas implicated in auditory–verbal memory function. *Brain*, **116**, 1–20.

Hart, R. P., Kwentus, J. A., and Harkins, S. W. (1988). Rate of forgetting in mild Alzheimer-type dementia. *Brain Cognition*, **7**, 31–8.

Haxby, J. V., Duara, R., and Grady, C. L. (1985). Relations between neuropsychological and cerebral metabolic asymmetries in early Alzheimer's disease. *Journal of Cerebral Blood Flow Metabolism*, **5**, 193–200.

Haxby, J. V., Grady, C. L., Duara, R., Schlageter, N., Berg, G., and Rapoport, S. I. (1986). Neocortical metabolic abnormalities precede nonmemory cognitive deficits in early Alzheimer's-type dementia. *Archives of Neurology*, **43**, 882–5.

Haxby, J. V., Grady, C. L., Koss, E., Horwitz, B., Hexton, L., Schapiro, M. *et al.* (1990). Longitudinal study of cerebral metabolic asymmetries and associated neuropsychological patterns in early dementia of the Alzheimer type. *Archives of Neurology*, **47**, 753–60.

Heindel, W. C., Salmon, D. P., Shults, C. W., Walicke, P. A., and Butters, N. (1989). Neuropsychological evidence for multiple implicit memory systems: A comparison of Alzheimer's, Huntington's, and Parkinson's disease patients. *Journal of Neuroscience*, **9**, 582–7.

Jagust, W. J., Reed, B. R., Seab, J. P., and Budinger, T. F. (1990). Alzheimer's disease: Age at onset and single-photon emission computed tomographic patterns of regional cerebral blood flow. *Archives of Neurology*, **47**, 628–33.

Johnson, K. A., Holman, B. L., Rosen, T. J., Nagel, J. S., English, R. J., and Growdon, J. H. (1990). Iofetamine I^{133} single photon emission computed tomography is accurate in the diagnosis of Alzheimer's disease. *Archives of Internal Medicine*, **150**, 752–6.

Jorm, A. F. (1985). Subtypes of Alzheimer's dementia: A conceptual analysis and critical review. *Psychological Medicine*, **15**, 543–53.

Kapur, S., Craik, F. I. M., Tulving, E., Wilson, A. A., Houle, S., and Brown, G. M. (1994). Neuroanatomical correlates of encoding in episodic memory: Levels of processing effect. *Proceeding of the National Academy of Sciences, USA*, **91**, 2008–11.

Khachaturian, Z. (1985). Diagnosis of Alzheimer's disease. *Archives of Neurology*, **42**, 1097–105.

Knopman, D. S. and Ryberg, S. (1989). A verbal memory test with high predictive accuracy for dementia of the Alzheimer type. *Archives of Neurology*, **46**, 141–6.

Kopelman, M. D. (1992). Storage, forgetting, and retrieval in the anterograde and retrograde amnesia of Alzheimer dementia. In *Memory functioning in dementia*, (ed. L. Backman), pp. 45–72). North-Holland, Amsterdam.

Kopelman, M. D., and Corn, T. H. (1988). Cholinergic 'blockade' as a model for cholinergic depletion: A comparison of the memory deficits with those of Alzheimer-type dementia and the alcoholic Korsakoff syndrome. *Brain*, **111**, 1079–110.

Kramer, J. H., Levion, B. E., Brandt, J., and Delis, D. C. (1989). Differentiation of Alzheimer's, Huntington's, and Parkinson's disease patients on the basis of verbal learning characteristics. *Neuropsychology*, **3**, 111–12.

McKhann, G., Drachman, D. A., Folstein, M. F., Katzman, R., Price, D. L., and Stadlan, E. (1984). Clinical diagnosis of Alzheimer's disease: Report of the NINCDS—ADRDA Work Group under the auspices of the Department of Health and Human Services Task Force on Alzheimer's disease. *Neurology*, **34**, 939–44.

Martin, A. (1990). Neuropsychology of Alzheimer's disease: The case for subgroups. In *Modular deficits in Alzheimer's-type dementia*, (ed. M. Schwartz), pp. 143–76. Bradford/MIT, Cambridge, MA.

Martin, A., Brouwers, P., Cox, C., and Fedio, P. (1985*a*). On the nature of the verbal memory deficit in Alzheimer's disease. *Brain and Language*, **25**, 323–41.

Martin, A., Cox, C., Brouwers, P., and Fedio, P. (1985*b*). A note on the different patterns of impaired and preserved cognitive abilities and their relation to episodic memory deficits in Alzheimer's patients. *Brain and Language*, **25**, 323–41.

Martin, A., Brouwers, P., Lalonde, F., Cox, C., Teleska, P., Fedio, P., *et al.* (1986). Towards a behavioral typology of Alzheimer's patients. *Journal of Clinical and Experimental Neuropsychology*, **8**, 594–610.

Masur, D. M., Fuld, P. A., Blau, A. D., Thal, L. J., Levin, H. S., and Aronson, M. K. (1989). Distinguishing normal and demented elderly with the Selective Reminding Test. *Journal of Clinical and Experimental Neuropsychology*, **11**, 615–30.

Merzenich, M. M. and Sameshima, K. (1993). Cortical plasticity and memory. *Current Opinion in Neurobiology*, **3**, 187–96.

Miller, E. (1971). On the nature of the memory disorder in presenile dementia. *Neuropsychologia*, **9**, 75–81.

Miller, E. (1973). Short-and long-term memory in presenile dementia (Alzheimer's Disease). *Psychological Medicine*, **3**, 221–4.

Morris, R. G. and Kopelman, M. D. (1986). The memory deficits in Alzheimer-type dementia: A review. *Quarterly Journal of Experimental Psychology*, **38**, 575–602.

Paulescu, E., Frith, C. D., and Frackowiak, R. S. J. (1993). The neural correlates of the verbal component of Working Memory. *Nature*, **362**, 342–5.

Petersen, R. C., Smith, G., Kokmen, E., Ivnik, R. J., and Tangalos, E. G. (1992). Memory function in normal aging. *Neurology*, **42**, 396–401.

Petersen, R. C., Smith, G. E., Ivnik, R. J., Kokmen, E., and Tangalos, E. G. (1994). Memory function in very early Alzheimer's disease. *Neurology*, **44**, 867–72.

Shallice, T., Fletcher, P., Frith, C. D., Grasby, P., Frackowiak, R. S. J., and Dolan, R. J. (1994). Brain regions associated with acquisition and retrieval of verbal episodic memory. *Nature*, **368**, 633–5.

Smith, G. S., DeLeon, M. J., George, A. E., Kluger, A., Volkow, N., McRae, T., *et al.* (1992). Topography of cross-sectional and longitudinal glucose metabolic deficit in Alzheimer's disease. *Archives of Neurology*, **49**, 1142–50.

Smith, M. L. (1989). Memory disorders associated with temporal-lobe lesions. In *Handbook of neuropsychology*, (ed. F. Boller and J. Grafman), pp. 91–8. Elsevier Science, New York.

Spinnler, H. and Tognoni, G. (ed.). (1987). *Standardizzazione e taratura Itialiana di test neuropsicologici.* Masson Italia Periodici, Milano, Italy.

Stern, Y., Alexander, G. E., Prohovnik, I., and Mayeux, R. (1992). Inverse relationship between education and parietotemporal perfusion deficit in Alzheimer's disease. *Annals of Neurology*, **32** (3), 371–5.

Tippett, L. J. and Farah, M. J. (1994). A computation model of naming in Alzheimer's disease: Unitary or multiple impairments? *Neuropsychology*, **8**, 3–13.

Troster, A. I., Butters, N., Salmon, D. P., Cullum, C. M., Jacobs, D., Brandt, J., *et al.* (1993). The diagnostic utility of savings scores: differentiating Alzheimer's and Huntington's diseases with the Logical Memory and Visual Reproduction tests. *Journal of Clinical and Experimental Neuropsychology*, **15**, 773–88.

Tulving, E., Kapur, S., Craik, F. M. I., Moscovitch, M., and Houle, S. (1994). Hemispheric encoding/retrieval asymmetry in episodic memory: Positron emission tomography findings. *Proceedings of the National Accademy of Sciences, USA*, **91**, 2016–20.

Welsh, K., Butters, N., Hughes, J., Mohs, R., and Heyman, A. (1991). Detection of abnormal memory decline in mild cases of Alzheimer's disease using CERAD neuropsychological measures. *Archives of Neurology*, **48**, 278–81.

Welsh, K. A., Butters, N., Hughes, J. P., Mohs, R. C., and Heyman, A. (1992). Detection and staging of dementia in Alzheimer's disease: Use of neuropsychological measures developed for the consortium to establish a registry for Alzheimer's disease. *Archives of Neurology*, **49**, 448–52.

Wilson, R. S., Bacon, L. D., and Fox, J. H. (1983). Primary memory and secondary memory in dementia of the Alzheimer type. *Journal of Clinical and Experimental Neuropsychology*, **5**, 337–44.

SIX

Knowledge and memory in Alzheimer's disease: a relationship that exists

Lars Bäckman and Agneta Herlitz

INTRODUCTION

It is widely accepted that a deficit in episodic memory functioning (namely the ability to encode, store, and retrieve temporally and spatially bound information) constitutes a cardinal symptom of Alzheimer's disease (AD) that is seen early in the pathogenesis (see Morris and Kopelman 1986; Nebes 1992, for overviews). Markers of episodic memory (for example, tests of recall or recognition) have been found to discriminate particularly well between early AD patients and age-matched controls (e.g. Branconnier *et al.* 1982; Herlitz *et al.* 1995; Storandt and Hill 1989; Welsh *et al.* 1992), and there is even evidence to suggest that episodic memory may start declining in patients who will later develop AD several years prior to diagnostically significant cognitive and social change (e.g. Almkvist and Bäckman 1993; Fuld *et al.* 1990; Masur *et al.* 1990).

However, unlike other groups of individuals suffering from episodic memory impairments (for example normal old persons, anterograde amnesics, depressed patients), AD patients also exhibit marked deficits in other varieties of memory, including semantic memory (that is, general knowledge about words, concepts, and symbols, their meanings and associations, as well as rules for manipulating these concepts and symbols) (see, for example, Butters *et al.* 1987; Hodges *et al.* 1991; Martin and Fedio 1983; Nebes 1989) and some forms of implicit memory retrieval without conscious recollection (see, for example, Brandt *et al.* 1988; Randolph 1991; Shimamura *et al.* 1987) (see also Chapter 7).

In research on episodic memory in AD, considerable attention has been directed at whether AD patients, like their healthy aged counterparts, are able to benefit from various forms of cognitive support for improving memory. In these studies, memory performance in a condition involving little cognitive support at encoding or retrieval is typically contrasted with a condition which involves more support (such as recognition of words versus recognition of objects; free recall of organizable words versus cued recall of organizable words).

Much of the early work addressing this issue revealed failures to utilize or benefit from cognitive support in AD (see Bäckman *et al.* 1990, for an overview). Thus, when support was provided in the form of organizational instructions (Diesfeldt 1984), verbal mediators (Butters *et al.* 1983), more study time (Strauss *et al.* 1985), a rich stimulus input (Rissenberg and Glanzer 1986), an inherent organizational task structure (Weingartner *et al.* 1981), or self-generation activity (Dick *et al.* 1989*a*; Mitchell *et al.* 1986), AD patients tended to perform at the same level as in control conditions in which these forms of support were lacking. In a related vein, there is evidence that support at retrieval in terms of category cues may not boost the level of recall in AD (Davis and Mumford 1984; Diesfeldt 1984).

Successful attempts to benefit from cognitive support in memory tasks may be viewed as illustrations of how the individual's knowledge structures aid the encoding and retrieval of episodic information. In other words, in many instances the degree to which cognitive support increases episodic memory performance may relate to successful use of semantic memory skills. Conversely, dementia-related deficits with regard to the structure of semantic memory (e.g. Chertkow and Bub 1990; Hodges *et al.* 1992; Martin 1987) as well as impaired access to information stored in semantic memory (e.g. Hartman 1991; Nebes 1989), may contribute to failures in utilizing cognitive support efficiently. From a somewhat different perspective, several researchers have argued that the potential for memory improvement in AD is negligible, because the basic neurobiological memory system is so impaired it cannot be ameliorated (e.g. Dick *et al.* 1989*b*; Martin *et al.* 1985).

However, it is important to note that the early research demonstrating failures to utilize cognitive support in AD rarely involved patients in an early phase of the disease. There are reasons to believe that performance gains following the provision of cognitive support are most likely to occur for AD patients who are relatively early in the pathogenesis. As well, in most of these studies, cognitive support was provided at either encoding or retrieval. Given the gross deterioration of episodic memory skills in AD, it may be necessary to provide cognitive support at both encoding and retrieval of information in order to demonstrate memory improvement in these patients.

KNOWLEDGE AND MEMORY IN AGEING AND DEMENTIA: A CONTINUITY VIEW

The purpose of this chapter is to provide an overview of recent work regarding the effects of cognitive support on episodic memory in AD. In particular, we are interested in exploring whether it is possible to entertain a continuity view of the potential for memory improvement in normal ageing and AD. An important prerequisite for adopting such a perspective is that relevant empirical results should indicate that differences between normal old adults and patients with AD regarding beneficial effects of cognitive support on memory could be viewed as differences in degree rather than as qualitative differences.

The studies pertaining to this issue are organized into three main categories: (1) richness of materials, (2) encoding–retrieval compatibility, and (3) prior knowledge; concepts that are explained below. Unless otherwise noted, the research reviewed focuses on patients in a mild to moderate stage of AD. In addition, in all studies selected for review, the AD patients are compared with normal old adults matched on relevant background characteristics (for instance, age and education).

Richness of materials

A basic premise behind memory research in which the richness of materials is varied, is that a *richer* stimulus will lead to a more elaborated memory representation and, ultimately, to better memory performance. Perhaps the most well-known demonstration of the importance of a rich stimulus input for episodic memory proficiency is the so-called picture superiority effect (e.g. Nelson *et al.* 1974; Paivio and Caspo 1973), which denotes the recall advantage of pictures over words. Other examples include the greater memorability of real-life objects compared with words (e.g. Gollin and Sharps 1988; Spoehr and Lehmkuhle 1982), and the superiority in recall of self-performed actions (so-called subject-performed tasks or SPTs) over words or sentences (e.g. Bäckman *et al.* 1986; Cohen 1981).

In an initial study examining the effects of richness of materials on memory, we compared memory for categorizable sentences (for instance, lift the spoon, roll the marble) encoded in the form of a motor act (SPTs) with memory for the same verbal information encoded without requirement of motor activity (Karlsson *et al.* 1989). Memory was tested with free and cued (taxonomic category names) recall, and there were five goups of subjects: 73-year-old and 82-year-old normal adults, and mildly, moderately, and severely demented AD patients.

The encoding situation in the SPT condition differed from that in the verbal control condition in several important respects. First, whereas the verbal task was presented bimodally (that is, visually and auditorily), the presentation format for SPTs was multimodal in the sense that several sensory systems may be activated at encoding. In addition to the visual and auditory modes, the tactual mode is activated because subjects are instructed to handle various objects, and some SPTs (for example, 'eat the raisin', or 'smell the flower') also result in activity in the gustatory and olfactory modalities.

Second, within each modality, SPTs comprise a variety of features on which the encoding may be based. The instructions read by the experimenter involve verbal features, but features of colour, shape, weight, texture, and sound related to the specific objects involved are also available during SPT encoding. By contrast, the features that are nominally present during encoding of verbal materials are typically limited to semantic, phonemic, and orthographic characteristics of the information to be remembered.

An important assumption in the Karlsson *et al.* (1989) study was that the rich encoding situation in the SPT task, and the requirement of execution of highly overlearned motor programmes, may activate otherwise inaccessible information in semantic memory, which should facilitate an elaborate encoding and subsequent recall in AD. The latter assumption was supported by earlier data showing that object naming may be improved in AD when patients are allowed to demonstrate the use of objects prior to their naming (Lawson and Barker 1968)

Several findings from the Karlsson *et al.* (1989) study should be highlighted. First, replicating earlier studies (e.g. Bäckman and Nilsson 1984, 1985), both groups of normal old adults showed a clear performance advantage for SPTs over sentences in free and cued recall alike; their performance level was approximately twice as high in the SPT conditions compared with the corresponding verbal conditions. Second, all three groups of AD patients performed at the same level for both types of materials when memory was tested with free recall, thus conforming to the pattern that the ability to benefit from cognitive support is impaired in AD. These two results were also reported in a related study by Dick *et al.* (1989*b*). Third, and perhaps most important, Karlsson *et al.* (1989) found that when memory was tested with cued recall, all patient groups showed a superiority in recall of SPTs over recall of verbally presented sentences.

This pattern of results indicates that AD patients may require support at both encoding (in the form of a rich and multimodal input) and retrieval (taxonomic cues) in order to exhibit memory improvement. Phrased somewhat differently, in order to detect effects of encoding manipulations in AD, it may be necessary also to provide support at retrieval.

In a follow-up study by Herlitz *et al.* (1991) mildly, moderately, and severely demented AD patients were compared with a group of normal old adults in free and cued recall of five different types of categorizable materials: words, objects, objects with a semantic orienting task, objects with a semantic/motoric orienting task, and SPTs.

Replicating and extending the Karlsson *et al.* data, this study demonstrated that (1) the normal old adults showed beneficial effects from the provision of category cues in all conditions, (2) the mildly and moderately demented patients showed cue benefits not only in the SPT task, but also for the other conditions involving the presentation of objects at encoding, and (3) the severely demented patients showed memory improvement only when SPT encoding was combined with category cues at retrieval. The latter finding indicates that the ability to use motor activity at encoding may be preserved later in the disease process than the ability to benefit from other forms of encoding support.

A common theme from these two studies is that providing cognitive support at both encoding and retrieval appears to be important in order to obtain memory facilitation in AD. This point will be further demonstrated in the next subsection.

Encoding–retrieval compatibility

The *encoding specificity* principle (Tulving and Thomson 1973) states that the amount of informational overlap between a cue presented at the time of retrieval and the memory representation laid down at encoding is critical to episodic memory proficiency. Thus, the more congruent a cue is with the context prevailing during encoding, or with the cognitive operations carried out during encoding, the more effective it will be at retrieval. Several recent studies have addressed whether compatible conditions at encoding and retrieval boost memory performance in AD. In an early study, Diesfeldt (1984) examined normal old adults and AD patients in free and taxonomic cued recall following presentation of an organizable word list that was acquired under two encoding conditions: standard instructions versus instructions to cluster the words into categories during learning.

Results indicated that whereas the normal old were able to benefit from directed organizational instructions in both free and cued recall, the AD patients showed such an effect only when memory was assessed with cued recall. Thus, in order to use the organizational structure established at encoding, the AD patients required that these structures were reactivated at test through the provision of categorical cues.

The pattern of results observed by Diesfeldt (1984) was replicated and extended in a subsequent study by Herlitz and Viitanen (1991). In this study, normal old adults and mildly and moderately demented AD patients were examined in free recall of random (that is, semantically unrelated) and categorizable (on the basis of taxonomic membership) words. The categorizable words were presented either in an unclustered fashion (organizable), or clustered into categorical blocks (blocked). For the two types of categorizable words, memory was also assessed with taxonomic cued recall.

The results for the normal old revealed a systematic increase of free recall performance as a function of increasing organizational support at encoding. In this group, free recall was better for blocked words than for organizable words which, in turn, were better recalled than random words. In addition, cue benefits at retrieval were observed in both categorizable lists. In contrast, none of the AD groups showed an effect of item organizability in free recall. However, in cued recall the mildly demented patients demonstrated a performance increment for both organizable and blocked words. For the moderately demented, this facilitative effect was seen for blocked words only; that is, when the level of organizational support at encoding was maximal.

These data provide further support for the view that AD patients may show performance gains in memory tasks when the products of the cognitive activity undertaken at encoding are reactivated when memory is tested. Furthermore, the results suggest that it is necessary to provide cognitive support at both encoding (organizability) and retrieval (cues) to demonstrate memory improvement in AD. Finally, it appears that the level of support required at encoding for cue benefits to occur may increase with increasing severity of dementia.

A somewhat different approach to the issue of encoding–retrieval compatibility and episodic memory in AD was taken in two studies by Bird and Luszcz (1991, 1993). Bird and Luszcz (1991) compared normal old adults and AD patients in free and taxonomic cued recall of pictures encoded either with a semantic orienting task or under standard conditions. The important finding from this study was that although the normal old benefited from a semantic encoding in both free recall and cued recall, the AD patients showed an effect of the encoding manipulation only when retrieval was assisted through the provision of category cues. Thus, these results conform to the pattern that support has to be present at both ends of the processing continuum to be beneficial in AD.

In a follow-up study using the same materials, Bird and Luszcz (1993) examined a group of AD patients in free recall, alphabetical cued recall, and category cued recall, following either an alphabetical orienting task or a categorical orienting task. The results showed that both cued recall tasks were superior to the free recall task, irrespective of encoding condition. In addition, the condition in which categorical cues at encoding was combined with alphabetical cues at retrieval was inferior to the remaining three cued recall conditions.

This pattern of data indicates that the provision of categorical cues at test carried the greatest weight with regard to facilitative effects on memory as long as encoding was supported either by alphabetical cues or category cues. In addition, there were effects of encoding–retrieval compatibility such that for both cueing conditions, performance was optimized when retrieval cues were congruent with encoding cues.

It is noteworthy that the results of the Bird and Luszcz (1991, 1993) studies are at odds with an earlier study of Granholm and Butters (1988). These investigators failed to find encoding–specificity effects in AD in a paradigm in which cue–target associations provided at encoding and retrieval were identical (weak–weak, strong–strong) or different (weak–strong, strong–weak). A possible reason for the discrepant findings may be that the requirements of elaborative activity at encoding were greater in the Bird and Luszcz (1991, 1993) studies than in the Granholm and Butters (1988) study. Given that AD patients have difficulties in spontaneously focusing on distinctive properties of stimuli during encoding (Chertkow *et al.* 1989; Martin *et al.* 1985), task-induced control of item elaboration may be particularly critical in order to optimize memory performance in this group of patients.

As alluded to earlier, there is research suggesting that the so-called generation effect (Slamecka and Graf 1978), which denotes the superiority in memory performance of self-generated over experimenter-provided items, may be non-existent (Mitchell *et al.* 1986) or reduced in AD relative to normal ageing (Dick *et al.* 1989*a*). It may be noted, however, that in these two studies subjects were required to generate and remember words in the context of sentences. Thus, they were relatively restricted in their generation activity, and had to form associations between the target words and the whole surrounding sentence context.

Lipinska *et al.* (1994) approached the relationship between self-generation activity and memory in AD from a different perspective, following a procedure devised by Mäntylä and colleagues (Mäntylä 1986; Mäntylä and Nilsson 1983). In two experiments, the effects of self generated cues on memory for words were examined in normal old and mildly demented AD patients. The reasoning was that providing AD patients with self-generated and compatible cues at retrieval may circumvent some of the semantic memory problems that hinder AD patients in utilizing cues in an efficient manner.

In the first experiment, subjects generated properties to target words at study. Following free recall, they were either presented with their self-generated properties, or with taxonomic cues as retrieval support. The results from this experiment showed that normal old adults and AD patients alike performed better with self-generated cues than with taxonomic cues, although there was a clear superiority of taxonomic cued recall over free recall. In the second experiment, encoding–retrieval compatibility was held constant and self-generation activity at encoding was varied. Again, both normal old adults and AD patients showed higher performance with self-generated than with categorical cues which, in turn, resulted in performance gains relative to free recall.

The overall data pattern from this study indicates that the factors that promote an optimal utilization of cues in this task situation (that is, self-generation activity at encoding and encoding–retrieval compatibility) are similar in normal ageing and early AD. Thus, as with the bulk of studies reviewed hitherto, this research suggests no qualitative differences between normal old adults and AD patients with regard to utilization of cognitive support for episodic memory.

Prior knowledge

It is well known that both normal old adults' and AD patients possess more knowledge of dated than of contemporary public events and famous figures (Beatty *et al.* 1988; Kopelman 1989; Sagar *et al.* 1988). One interpretation of these findings is that there are specific periods in a person's lifespan during which general knowledge regarding such domains as music, film, sports, and literature are most likely to be encoded elaboratively. There is also evidence that normal old adults are able to utilize prior knowledge to enhance episodic memory. Specifically, research shows that normal old people perform better with dated than with contemporary materials in word recall (Barrett and Wright 1981; Worden and Sherman-Brown 1983), text recall (Hultsch and Dixon 1983), name recall (Bäckman *et al.* 1987; Hanley-Dunn and McIntosh 1984), and face recognition (Bäckman 1991; Wahlin *et al.* 1993).

In two studies (Bäckman and Herlitz 1990; Lipinska *et al.* 1992), we explored whether AD patients, like their healthy aged counterparts, could use their knowledge advantage of dated over contemporary general information to improve episodic face recognition. Bäckman and Herlitz (1990) presented a series of dated (from the 1940s) and contemporary (from the 1980s) famous faces to test episodic recognition in groups of normal old adults and mildly demented AD patients. In conjunction with the episodic recognition test, subjects level of prior knowledge for the two types of faces was assessed by asking subjects to (1) rate the faces in terms of perceived familiarity, and (2) select the correct name for each of the faces presented in a four-alternative multiple-choice test. It was found that although the normal old had better pre-experimental knowledge for the famous faces than the AD patients, both groups were more knowledgeable of the dated than of the contemporary faces.

In the episodic recognition test, the normal old showed better performance for the dated compared with the contemporary faces, indicating proficient use of prior knowledge in episodic memory. However, in contrast to what was true in the tests of prior knowledge, the AD patients performed equally well for both types of faces in the episodic recognition test. These results indicate that AD may be associated with a deficit in the ability to utilize prior knowledge to enhance face recognition.

However, the support provided at encoding was rather poor in this study; there were no requirements of elaborative cognitive activity during the presentation of faces. In a subsequent study, Lipinska *et al.* (1992) investigated whether an increase in the level of semantic activation would also result in AD patients being able to benefit from prior knowledge in this task situation. The increase of semantic activation was accomplished by (1) having subjects generate statements concerning the famous figures at encoding, and (2) providing the names of the characters along with the faces at both encoding and retrieval. The underlying assumption was that the generation of statements and the provision of names should increase the activation of relevant knowledge structures, thus facilitating an elaborate encoding of the faces to be remembered.

The results indicated that both the normal old and the AD patients generated more correct statements concerning the dated compared with the contemporary characters, indicating better prior knowledge of the dated persons. Interestingly, separate analyses revealed that both groups of subjects generated statements from more domains (for example, professsion, family life, hobbies) for the dated relative to the contemporary faces; in contrast, there was no difference between the two types of faces with regard to the number of correct statements per domain. This suggests that the knowledge advantage for dated over contemporary general knowledge in normal ageing and AD may reflect a greater breadth rather than depth of the knowledge possessed.

The interesting issue, then, was whether the increase in semantic activation in Lipinska *et al.* (1992) would result in positive effects of prior knowledge on face recognition for the AD patients. The answer to this question is yes: both groups of subjects in this study performed better with the dated than with the contemporary faces in the episodic recognition test. Thus, the results from this research indicate that early AD patients are able to utilize prior knowledge in the context of face recognition, although they require more cognitive support than normal old adults to exhibit such effects.

In general, then, the research reviewed in this chapter provides little evidence for the position that there are qualitative differences between normal old adults and AD patients in the effects of cognitive support on episodic memory. On the contrary, using rather different experimental paradigms this research indicates that differences between normal ageing and AD in this regard may be conceptualized as differences in degree. To this end, it may be noted that there is a growing body of research suggesting that most, if not all, differences in patterns of memory performance between normal old adults and mildly to moderately demented AD patients are quantitative in nature (Becker and Lopez 1992; Herlitz *et al.* 1992; Huppert 1994; Kopelman 1992; Nebes 1992). The proposed continuity view of the relationship between knowledge and memory in normal ageing and dementia is elaborated in the next and final section.

CONCLUDING REMARKS

On the basis of the current review, the following conclusions concerning the relationship between semantic knowledge and episodic memory in AD are offered. First, AD results in a deficit in utilizing cognitive support to utilize episodic memory. Second, AD patients are nevertheless able to use cognitive support in episodic memory tasks; however, they need more support (for example, in terms of a rich input, item organizability, cues, prior knowledge) than their healthy aged counterparts, to show memory facilitation. Third, in order to show effects on episodic memory performance of various encoding manipulations in AD, it is also critical to provide support at retrieval. Fourth, proficient use of retrieval support is most likely to be seen in AD when the encoding demands force the subject to engage in elaborative cognitive activity. Fifth, with increasing severity of dementia, there is an increase in the level of support required to improve memory. Finally, the ability to use motor activity at encoding may be preserved later in the disease process than the ability to use other forms of encoding support.

A continuity view of cognitive support and episodic memory in normal ageing and dementia would be supported by findings indicating quantitative variations in the level of support required to show memory improvement also among non-demented older adults. Recent research indicates that this is indeed the case. For example, there is evidence that older adults with major depression have problems in using visual imagery (Hart *et al.* 1987) as well as an inherent organizational structure in the materials (Watts *et al.* 1990; Weingartner and Silberman 1982). In a recent study, Bäckman and Forsell (1994) showed that old age depression resulted in deficits in the ability to use study time and item organizability in free recall, although depressed patients profited from taxonomic cues to the same extent as normal old adults. Interestingly, when memory was assessed with recognition, depressed patients showed similar gains as the normal old from more study time.

In a follow-up study, Bäckman *et al.* (1996) demonstrated that variations in depressive symptomatology among non-depressed older adults may also affect the extent to which supportive task conditions can be utilized in memory tasks. This study showed that performance gains from more study time in free recall decreased as the number of motivation-related depressive symptoms (such as concentration difficulties, lack of interest) increased.

Using a paradigm in which the presence of cues was manipulated at encoding and retrieval, Craik *et al.* (1987) showed that the level of cognitive support required to demonstrate memory facilitation was greater for socially inactive and less well-educated older adults than for similar-aged active persons with more schooling. These data were replicated and extended in a recent study with very old adults by Hill *et al.* (1995). These investigators found that educational level was positively related to the magnitude of gains from more study time and organizability in free recall. In addition, level of social activity was positively related to the size of performance increments from the provision of retrieval cues.

As a final example, several studies have demonstrated that the degree of cognitive support required to improve memory in normal ageing may increase from early to later portions of the late adult lifespan. Such results have been demonstrated in a variety of task situations, including free recall of words (Hill *et al.* 1995), free and cued recall of words and objects (Bäckman and Larsson 1992), and face recognition (Bäckman 1991).

Thus, in drawing together the reviewed work on normal ageing and dementia with the research on cognitive support and memory in non-demented older adults discussed above, a continuity view of the modifiability of episodic memory in old age is emerging. Specifically, one might think of a continuum where the anchor points are represented by young old, highly educated, and socially active adults versus severely demented patients, and where intermediate positions are occupied by, for example, very old sedentary normal persons, depressed older adults, and demented patients in an early phase of the disease. As one progresses along this continuum, there is, of course, a gradual decrease in episodic memory functioning. But there is also a decrease in the ability to utilize cognitive support for improving episodic memory, and a concomitant increase in the degree of support required to show memory improvement.

ACKNOWLEDGEMENT

Preparation of this chapter was supported by grants from the Swedish Council for Research in the Humanities and the Social Sciences, and the Swedish Council for Social Research.

REFERENCES

Almkvist, O. and Bäckman, L. (1993). Progression in Alzheimer's disease: Sequencing of neuropsychological decline. *International Journal of Geriatric Psychiatry*, **8**, 755–63.

Bäckman, L. (1991). Recognition memory across the adult life span: The role of prior knowledge. *Memory and Cognition*, **19**, 63–71.

Bäckman, L. and Forsell, Y. (1994). Episodic memory functioning in a community-based sample of old adults with major depression: Utilization of cognitive support. *Journal of Abnormal Psychology*, **103**, 361–70.

Bäckman, L. and Herlitz, A. (1990). The relationship between prior knowledge and face recognition memory in normal aging and Alzheimer's disease. *Journal of Gerontology: Psychological Sciences*, **45**, 94–100.

Bäckman, L. and Larsson, M. (1992). Recall of organizable words and objects in adulthood: Influences of instructions, retention interval, and retrieval cues. *Journal of Gerontology: Psychological Sciences*, **47**, 273–8.

Bäckman, L. and Nilsson, L.-G. (1984). Aging effects in free recall: An exception to the rule. *Human Learning*, **3**, 53–69.

Bäckman, L. and Nilsson, L.-G. (1985). Prerequisites for lack of age differences in memory performance. *Experimental Aging Research*, **11**, 67–73.

Bäckman, L., Nilsson, L.-G., and Chalom, D. (1986). New evidence on the nature of the encoding of action events. *Memory and Cognition*, **14**, 339–46.

Bäckman, L., Herlitz, A., and Karlsson, T. (1987). Pre-experimental knowledge facilitates episodic recall in young, young-old, and old-old adults. *Experimental Aging Research*, **13**, 89–91.

Bäckman, L., Mäntylä, T., and Herlitz, A. (1990). The optimization of episodic remembering in old age. In *Successful aging: Perspectives from the behavioral sciences* (ed. P. B. Baltes and M. M. Baltes), pp. 118–63. Cambridge University Press, Cambridge.

Bäckman, L., Hill, R. D., and Forsell, Y. (1996). The influence of depressive symptomatology on episodic memory functioning among nondepressed older adults. *Journal of Abnormal Psychology*, **105**, 97–105.

Barrett, T. R. and Wright, M. (1981). Age-related facilitation in recall following semantic processing. *Journal of Gerontology*, **36**, 194–9.

Beatty, W. W., Salmon, D. P., Butters, N., Heindel, W. C., and Granholm, E. L. (1988). Retrograde amnesia in patients with Alzheimer's disease or Huntington's disease. *Neurobiology of Aging*, **9**, 181–6.

Becker, J. T. and Lopez, O. L. (1992). Episodic memory in Alzheimer's disease: Breakdown of multiple memory processes. In *Memory functioning in dementia* (ed. L. Bäckman), pp. 27–43. North-Holland, Amsterdam.

Bird, M. and Luszcz, M. (1991). Encoding specificity, depth of processing, and cued recall in Alzheimer's disease. *Journal of Clinical and Experimental Neuropsychology*, **13**, 508–20.

Bird, M. and Luszcz, M. (1993). Enhancing memory performance in Alzheimer's disease: Acquisition assistance and cue effectiveness. *Journal of Clinical and Experimental Neuropsychology*, **15**, 921–32.

Branconnier, R. J., Cole, J. O., Pera, K. F., and DeVitt, D. R. (1982). Recall and recognition as diagnostic indices of malignant memory loss in senile dementia: A Bayesian analysis. *Experimental Aging Research*, **8**, 189–93.

Brandt, J., Spencer, M., McSorley, P., and Folstein, M. F. (1988). Semantic activation and implicit memory in Alzheimer's disease. *Alzheimer's Disease and Related Disorders*, **2**, 112–19.

Butters, N., Albert, M. S., Sax, D. S., Miliotis, P., Nagode, J., and Sterste, A. (1983). The effect of verbal mediators on the pictorial memory of brain-damaged patients. *Neuropsychologia*, **21**, 307–23.

Butters, N., Granholm, E. L., Salmon, D. P., Grant, I., and Wolfe, J. (1987). Episodic and semantic memory: A comparison of amnesic and demented patients. *Journal of Clinical and Experimental Neuropsychology*, **9**, 479–97.

Chertkow, H. and Bub, D. (1990). Semantic memory in dementia of Alzheimer's type: What do various measures measure? *Brain*, **113**, 397–417.

Chertkow, H., Bub, D., and Seidenberg, M. (1989). Priming and semantic memory loss in Alzheimer's disease *Brain and Language*, **36**, 420–6.

Cohen, R. L. (1981). On the generality of some memory laws. *Scandinavian Journal of Psychology*, **22**, 267–82.

Craik, F. I. M., Byrd, M., and Swanson, J. M. 1987). Patterns of memory loss in three elderly samples. *Psychology and Aging*, **2**, 79–86.

Davis, P. E. and Mumford, S. J. (1984). Cued recall and the nature of the memory disorder in dementia. *British Journal of Psychiatry*, **144**, 383–6.

Dick, M. B., Kean, M. L., and Sands, S. (1989*a*). Memory for internally generated words in Alzheimer-type dementia: Breakdown in encoding and semantic memory. *Brain and Cognition*, **9**, 88–108.

Dick, M. B., Kean, M.-L., and Sands, S. (1989*b*). Memory for action events in Alzheimer-type dementia: Further evidence of an encoding failure. *Brain and Cognition*, **9**, 71–87.

Diesfeldt, H. F. A. (1984). The importance of encoding instructions and retrieval cues in the assessment of memory in senile dementia. *Archives of Gerontology and Geriatrics*, **3**, 51–7.

Fuld, P. A., Masur, D. M., Blau, A. D., Crystal, H., and Aronson, M. K. (1990). Object-memory evaluation for prospective detection of dementia in normal functioning elderly: Predictive and normative data. *Journal of Clinical and Experimental Neuropsychology*, **12**, 520–8.

Gollin, E. S. and Sharps, M. J. (1988). Facilitation of free recall by categorical blocking depends on stimulus type. *Memory and Cognition*, **16**, 539–44.

Granholm, E. L. and Butters, N. (1988). Associative encoding and retrieval in Alzheimer's disease. *Brain and Cognition*, **7**, 335–47.

Hanley-Dunn, P. and McIntosh, J. L. (1984). Meaningfulness and recall of names by young and old adults. *Journal of Gerontology*, **39**, 583–5.

Hart, R. P., Kwentus, J. A., Hamer, R. M., and Taylor, J. R. (1987). Selective reminding procedure in depression and dementia. *Psychology and Aging*, **2**, 111–15.

Hartman, M. (1991). The use of semantic knowledge in Alzheimer's disease: Evidence for impairments of attention. *Neuropsychologia*, **29**, 213–28.

Herlitz, A. and Viitanen, M. (1991). Semantic organization and verbal episodic memory in patients with mild and moderate Alzheimer's disease. *Journal of Clinical and Experimental Neuropsychology*, **13**, 559–74.

Herlitz, A., Adolfsson, R., Bäckman, L., and Nilsson, L.-G. (1991). Cue utilization following different forms of encoding in mildly, moderately, and severely demented patients with Alzheimer's disease. *Brain and Cognition*, **15**, 119–30.

Herlitz, A., Lipinska, B., and Bäckman, L. (1992). Utilization of cognitive support for episodic remembering in Alzheimer's disease. In *Memory functioning in dementia* (ed. L. Bäckman), pp. 73–96. North-Holland, Amsterdam.

Herlitz, A., Hill, R. D., Fratiglioni, L., and Bäckman, L. (1995). Episodic memory and visuospatial ability in detecting and staging dementia in a community-based sample of very old adults. *Journal of Gerontology: Medical Sciences*, **50**, 107–13

Hill, R. D., Wahlin, Å., Winblad, B., and Bäckman, L. (1995). The role of demographic and lifestyle variables in utilizing cognitive support for episodic remembering among very old adults. *Journal of Gerontology: Psychological Sciences*, **50**, 219–27.

Hodges, J. R., Salmon, D. P., and Butters, N. (1991). The nature of the naming deficit in Alzheimer's and Huntington's disease. *Brain*, **114**, 1547–58.

Hodges, J. R., Salmon, D. P., and Butters, N. (1992). Semantic memory impairment in Alzheimer's disease: Failure of access or degraded knowledge. *Neuropsychologia*, **30**, 301–14.

Hultsch, D. F. and Dixon, R. A. (1983). The role of pre-experimental knowledge in text processing in adulthood. *Experimental Aging Research*, **9**, 17–22.

Huppert, F. A. (1994). Memory function in dementia and normal aging—dimension or dichotomy? In *Dementia and normal aging* (ed. F. A. Huppert, C. Brayne, and D. O'Connor), pp. 291–330. Cambridge University Press, Cambridge.

Karlsson, T:, Bäckman, L., Herlitz, A., Nilsson, L.-G., Winblad, B., and Österlind, P.-O. (1989). Memory improvement at different stages of Alzheimer's disease. *Neuropsychologia*, **27**, 737–42.

Kopelman, M. D. (1989). Remote and autobiographical memory, temporal context memory, and frontal atrophy in Korsakoff and Alzheimer patients. *Neuropsychologia*, **27**, 437–60.

Kopelman, M. D. (1992). Storage, forgetting, and retrieval in the anterograde and retrograde amnesia of Alzheimer dementia. In *Memory functioning in dementia* (ed. L. Bäckman), pp. 45–72. North-Holland, Amsterdam.

Lawson, J. S. and Barker, M. G. (1968). The assessment of nominal dysphasia in dementia: The use of reaction-time measures. *British Journal of Medical Psychology*, **41**, 411–14.

Lipinska, B., Bäckman, L., and Herlitz, A. (1992). When Greta Garbo is easier to remember than Stefan Edberg: Influences of prior knowledge on recognition memory in Alzheimer's disease. *Psychology and Aging*, **7**, 214–20.

Lipinska, B., Bäckman, L., Mäntylä, T., and Viitanen, M. (1994). Effectiveness of self-generated cues in early Alzheimer's disease. *Journal of Clinical and Experimental Neuropsychology*, **16**, 809–19.

Mäntylä, T. (1986). Optimizing cue effectiveness: Recall of 500 and 600 incidentally learned words. *Journal of Experimental Psychology: Learning, Memory, and Cognition*, **12**, 66–71.

Mäntylä, T. and Nilsson, L.-G. (1983). Are my cues better than yours? Uniqueness and reconstruction as prerequisites for optimal recall of verbal material. *Scandinavian Journal of Psychology*, **24**, 303–12.

Martin, A. (1987). Representation of semantic and spatial knowledge in Alzheimer's patients: Implications for models of preserved learning in amnesia. *Journal of Clinical and Experimental Neuropsychology*, **9**, 191–224.

Martin, A. and Fedio, P. (1983). Word production and comprehension in Alzheimer's disease: The breakdown of semantic knowledge. *Brain and Language*, **19**, 124–41.

Martin, A., Brouwers, P., Cox, C., and Fedio, P. (1985). On the nature of the verbal memory deficit in Alzheimer's disease. *Brain and Language*, **25**, 323–41.

Masur, D. M., Fuld, P. A., Blau, A. D., Crystal, H., and Aronson, M. K. (1990). Predicting development of dementia in the elderly with the selective reminding test. *Journal of Clinical and Experimental Neuropsychology*, **12**, 529–38.

Mitchell, D. B., Hunt, R. R., and Schmitt, F. A. (1986). The generation effect and reality monitoring: Evidence from dementia and normal aging. *Journal of Gerontology*, **41**, 79–84.

Morris, R. G. and Kopelman, M. D. (1986). The memory-deficits in Alzheimer-type dementia: A review. *Quarterly Journal of Experimental Psychology*, **38**, 575–602.

Nebes, R. D. (1989). Semantic memory in Alzheimer's disease. *Psychological Bulletin*, **106**, 377–94.

Nebes, R. D. (1992). Cognitive dysfunctions in Alzheimer's disease. In *Handbook of aging and cognition* (ed. F. I. M. Craik and T. A. Salthouse), pp. 373–446. Erlbaum, Hillsdale, NJ.

Nelson, T. O., Metzler, J., and Reed, D. A. (1974). Role of details in the long-term recognition of pictures and verbal descriptions. *Journal of Experimental Psychology*, **102**, 184–6.

Paivio, A. and Csapo, K. (1973). Picture superiority in free recall: Imagery or dual coding? *Cognitive Psychology*, **5**, 175–200.

Randolph, C. (1991). Implicit, explicit, and semantic memory functions in Alzheimer's disease and Huntington's disease. *Journal of Clinical and Experimental Neuropsychology*, **13**, 25–42.

Rissenberg, M. and Granzer, M. (1986). Picture superiority in free recall: The effects of normal aging and primary degenerative dementia. *Journal of Gerontology*, **41**, 64–71.

Sagar, H. J., Cohen, N. J., Sullivan, E. V., Corkin, S., and Growdon, J. H. (1988). Remote memory function in Alzheimer's disease and Parkinson's disease. *Brain*, **111**, 185–206.

Shimamura, A. P., Salmon, D. P., Squire, L. R., and Butters, N. (1987). Memory dysfunction and word priming in dementia and amnesia. *Behavioral Neuroscience*, **101**, 347–51.

Slamecka, N. J. and Graf, P. (1978). The generation effect: Delineation of a phenomenon. *Journal of Experimental Psychology: Human Learning and Memory*, **4**, 592–604.

Spoehr, K. T. and Lehmkuhle, S. W. (1982). *Visual information processing*. Freeman, San Francisco.

Storandt, M. and Hill, R. D. (1989). Very mild senile dementia of the Alzheimer-type: II. Psychometric test performance. *Archieves of Neurology*, **46**, 383–6.

Strauss, M. W., Weingartner, H., and Thompson, K. (1985). Remembering words and how often they occurred in memory-impaired patients. *Memory and Cognition*, **13**, 507–10.

Tulving, E. and Thomson, D. M. (1973). Encoding specificity and retrieval processes in episodic memory. *Psychological Review*, **80**, 352–73.

Wahlin, Å., Bäckman, L., Mäntylä, T., Herlitz, A., Viitanen, M., and Winblad, B. (1993). Prior knowledge and face recognition in a community-based sample of healthy, very old adults. *Journal of Gerontology: Psychological Sciences*, **48**, 54–61.

Watts, F. N., Dalgleish, T., Bourke, P., and Healy, D. (1990). Memory deficit in clinical depression: Processing resources and the structure of materials. *Psychological Medicine*, **20**, 345–9.

Weingartner, H. and Silberman, E. (1982). Models of cognitive impairment: Cognitive changes in depression. *Psychopharmacology Bulletin*, **18**, 27–42.

Weingartner, H., Kaye, W., Smallberg, S., Ebert, M. H., Gillin, J. C., and Sitaram, N. (1981). Memory failures in progressive idiopathic dementia. *Journal of Abnormal Psychology*, **90**, 187–96.

Welsh, K. A., Butters, N., Hughes, J. P., Mohs, R. C., and Heyman, A. (1992). Detection and staging of dementia in Alzheimer's disease: Use of the neuropsychological measures developed for the consortium to establish a registry for Alzheimer's disease. *Archives of Neurology*, **49**, 448–52.

Worden, P. E. and Sherman-Brown, S. S. (1983). A word-frequency cohort effect in young versus elderly adults' memory for words. *Developmental Psychology*, **19**, 521–30.

SEVEN

Implicit memory

David P. Salmon and Christine Fennema-Notestine

Episodic and semantic memory impairment is an early and ubiquitous feature of dementia of the Alzheimer type (AD; see Chapters 5, 6, and 8). Numerous studies of episodic memory (memory for events and episodes that remains tightly linked to the context in which it was originally acquired) have shown that patients with AD have a deficit in learning new information (Buschke and Fuld 1974; Masur *et al.* 1989; Moss *et al.* 1986; Wilson *et al.* 1983) and in retaining over time what little information they do acquire (Butters *et al.* 1988; Moss *et al.*, 1986; Troster *et al.* 1993; Welsh *et al.* 1991). Similarly, studies of semantic memory (general knowledge, rules, and procedures that are highly overlearned and essentially context free) suggest that patients with AD suffer a loss of semantic knowledge (Chertkow and Bub 1990; Hodges *et al.* 1992), or a disruption of semantic organization (Chan *et al.* 1993*a*, *b*, 1995; Salmon and Chan 1994), early in the course of the disease.

Most of the studies examining episodic and semantic memory in patients with AD have relied on tasks which require a conscious and explicit attempt to learn and retain new information (episodic memory) or to recall information from a long-standing pre-existing store (semantic memory). Recently, however, some interest has turned to the performance of these patients on memory tasks which do not require conscious recollection, but rather allow knowledge to be expressed implicity through the facilitation of performance on some task due simply to prior exposure to stimulus materials (priming) or through improvement in performance on a particular motor or cognitive task with repeated practice (skill learning) (Graf and Schacter 1985, 1987; Salmon and Butters 1995; Schacter 1987; Squire 1987).

The growing interest in priming and skill learning in patients with AD stems from neuropsychological and neurobiological evidence that explicit (or declarative) and implicit (or non-declarative or procedural) memory may be mediated by distinct neural systems. Numerous studies have shown, for example, that these two forms of memory are differentially affected in patients with circumscribed amnesia arising from damage to medial temporal lobe (hippocampus, entorhinal cortex) or midline diencephalic brain structures (for review, see Squire 1987). Although patients with amnesia exhibit severe deficits in explicit memory on episodic memory tasks, these same patients retain the ability to benefit from the prior presentation of information on priming tasks (Cermak *et al.* 1985; Gardner *et al.* 1973; Graf *et al.* 1984; Shimamura 1986; Shimamura and Squire 1984; Warrington and Weiskrantz 1968, 1970) and can learn and retain new visuomotor and cognitive-based skills normally (Brooks and Baddeley 1976; Cermak *et al.* 1973; Cohen and Squire 1980; Corkin 1968).

The preserved implicit memory abilities of patients with circumscribed amnesia suggests that this form of memory does not rely on the same medial temporal and diencephalic brain structures that are thought to mediate explicit memory. Unfortunately, however, the study of amnesic patients can tell us little more about the psychobiological bases of implicit memory. Only through the careful investigation of patients with damage to brain regions other than those involved in circumscribed amnesia will a fuller understanding of the neurology of implicit memory be possible. Thus, studies of implicit memory in patients with Alzheimer's disease and other dementing illnesses have been carried out to determine if unique patterns of preserved and impaired implicit memory abilities are associated with the particular brain pathology that occurs in each disease.

The present chapter will describe some of the recent research concerning implicit memory in patients with Alzheimer's disease or related dementing disorders and will discuss the implications of this research for our understanding of the neuropsychological bases of this form of memory. Priming and its relationship to semantic memory will be the focus of the first part of the chapter, while motor and cognitive skill learning will be covered in the second part. Finally, the dissociation of priming and skill learning in patients with different forms of dementing illnesses, and different sites of neural damage, will be discussed.

PRIMING

Studies of priming in AD patients have employed two general methodologies: repetition and associative priming. Repetition priming refers to a procedure in which a stimulus is presented and after some interval (ranging from fractions of a second to minutes or hours), the original stimulus, or some degraded form of the original stimulus, is presented again. The initial presentation of the stimulus is assumed to produce some activation that facilitates its subsequent processing. This facilitation is reflected by faster processing of the stimulus on its second presentation or by an enhanced ability to identify the stimulus in its degraded form.

Some investigators have further divided repetition priming into perceptual (or data-driven) and conceptual (or concept-driven) types (Blaxton 1989; Roediger and Blaxton 1987). Perceptual priming involves processes that operate at the level of the visual or auditory form of a target stimulus. This type of priming is not affected by the particular meaning or content of the stimulus, but can be influenced by manipulations of its surface features (such as changes in modality or typeface). Conceptual priming, in contrast, does involve processes that operate at the level of the meaning or content of a target stimulus, and is influenced by manipulations of the depth of conceptual analysis of the stimulus.

Associative priming refers to a procedure in which a stimulus is presented and after some interval a lexically or semantically related stimulus is presented. In this procedure, the presentation of the first stimulus is assumed to activate the second stimulus through their lexical or semantic association (that is to say through spreading activation within the semantic network). Activation of the second stimulus facilitates its processing in some task, such as deciding whether it is a word or non-word. Because associative priming relies on activation of a stimulus through its associations rather than through its direct presentation (as in repetition priming), it is conceptual in nature.

The various tasks that have been used to assess priming in patients with AD often do not exclusively engage either conceptual or perceptual processes. Rather, both types of processing may contribute to normal priming performance, with the relative contribution of each depending on the specific features of the task. Priming effects in normal individuals and amnesic patients on the widely used, word-stem completion task (see below), for example, have been shown to be greater following elaborative processing of a semantic, rather than a physical, feature of the stimuli during study (indicating a conceptual processing component), but also greater when the stimuli are presented in the same modality, rather than in different modalities, at study and test (indicating a perceptual processing component) (Carlesimo 1994).

Keeping in mind the caveat that both conceptual and perceptual processes may contribute to priming effects in many tasks, we will first discuss repetition and associative priming in AD patients on tasks that are heavily weighted toward conceptual processes. We will then turn the discussion to repetition priming in AD patients on primarily perceptually based tasks.

Conceptual priming

Two of the first studies to examine priming in patients with AD (Shimamura *et al.* 1987; Salmon *et al.* 1988) compared their performance to those of Huntington's disease (HD) patients, alcoholic

Korsakoff's (AK) syndrome patients with circumscribed amnesia, and normal control subjects on a word-stem completion task previously used by Graf and colleagues (Graf *et al.* 1984). In this task, subjects were first exposed to a list of ten target words (for example motel, abstain) and asked to rate each word in terms of its 'likeability'. Following two presentations and ratings of the entire list, the subjects were shown three-letter stems of words (for example mot, abs) that were not on the presentation list and asked to complete the stems with the 'first word that comes to mind'. Half of the stems could be completed with previously presented words, while the other half were used to assess baseline guessing rates. Other lists of words were used to assess the subjects' ability at free recall and recognition.

Although all three patient groups were severely and equally impaired on free recall and recognition of presented words, the AK and HD patients exhibited intact stem-completion priming. In comparison, the AD patients showed little or no tendency to complete the word stems with previously presented words. That is, for the AD patients the presentation-rating procedure failed to generate the transient memory traces needed for this form of implicit memory. Similar deficits in the stem-completion priming performance of AD patients have been reported by many investigators (Bondi *et al.* 1993; Heindel *et al.* 1989; Keane *et al.* 1991; Perani *et al.* 1993; Randolph 1991; but see Deweer *et al.* 1994; Huberman *et al.* 1994).

Salmon and colleagues (Salmon *et al.* 1988) also compared the priming performance of AD, HD, and control subjects on a semantic priming test which employed a paired-associate procedure. In this task, subjects were first asked to judge categorically or functionally related word pairs (for instance bird—robin, needle—thread) and later to 'free-associate' to the first words of the previously presented pairs and to words that were not presented as part of the paired associates. The results with this priming task showed that AD patients were significantly less likely to produce the second word of the semantically related pair than were the other two subject groups. In fact, the priming score for the AD patients did not differ from baseline guessing rates.

A similar free-association procedure was used by Brandt *et al.* (1988) to assess verbal priming in AD patients. These investigators first read a list of ten stimulus words to AD and NC subjects. After a short delay, an unrelated free-association task was administered in which the subject was asked say a word in response to a probe word read by the experimenter. For half of the probe words, a previously presented stimulus word was the third most common associate according to normative data. The other half of the probe words were not associated with any of the ten stimulus words. Priming of the stimulus words was demonstrated in the NC subjects by their increased tendency to produce the previously presented stimulus words as the primary associate in the free-association task. Patients with AD also showed a slightly increased tendency to produce the previously presented words, but this priming was impaired relative to that of the NC subjects.

The studies of priming in AD patients described above were among the first to demonstrate significant deficiencies in long-term priming in any neurologically impaired patient group, and suggest that priming may be mediated by neural substrates that are selectively disrupted in Alzheimer's disease. Since AD patients, and not HD or amnesic patients, evidence marked pathology in temporal, parietal, and frontal association cortices (Brun 1983; Terry and Katzman 1983) (see Chapter 13), impaired priming may be the result of damage to those neocortical association areas which are presumed to store the representations of semantic memory. This cortical damage in AD patients may result in a breakdown in the organization of semantic knowledge that is necessary to support priming. That is, the hierarchical associative network underlying semantic knowledge may have deteriorated sufficiently in the AD patients to limit greatly the capacity of available cues to activate traces of previously presented stimuli. For example the cue 'bird' may not evoke an unconscious activation of the categorical associate 'robin' on the semantic priming task because the association between the two words has been greatly weakened. Similarly, the association in semantic memory between the word stem 'mot' and the word 'motel' on the lexical priming task may have been sufficiently disrupted to negate the facilitating effect of the word's presentation.

Further support for the notion that abnormal priming in AD patients is related to their semantic memory deficit is provided by several recent investigations that examined priming through the use of semantically based, Event Related Potentials (ERP). A number of studies have shown that the amplitude of the N400 component of the ERP that is elicited as an individual reads or listens to meaningful material is sensitive to semantic and associative relationships among lexical items (Kutas and Hillyard 1980, 1983, 1984). Specifically, N400 amplitude is typically larger when a subject hears or sees a word that is incongruous with the semantic context that preceded it (provided by a word or sentence; for instance, 'The bird ate the *nail*') than when the word matches its context (for example 'The hammer hit the *nail*'). This suggests that the N400 component might serve as a reliable index of semantic priming.

Using an ERP semantic priming paradigm, Iragui and colleagues (Iragui *et al.*, in press) compared the N400 component of young normal control subjects, elderly normal control subjects, and patients with AD. In this study, a sentence was read to the subject and the final word of the sentence, which could be congruous or incongruous with the context provided by the sentence, was presented visually. Subjects were asked to read the final word aloud as quickly as possible. The results showed that the N400 component of the ERP produced by AD patients occurred later and was broader and of lower amplitude than those of either control group.

In a related study, Schwartz *et al.* (in press) found similar abnormalities in the N400 component of AD patients who were performing a task in which they first heard a category name and then were shown a related or an unrelated target item and required to press a key to indicate whether or not the target item was a member of the category. The AD patients also performed abnormally in terms of the behavioural reaction time data; however, these data indicated greater than normal priming (hyperpriming) in the AD patients. The results of this study, in conjunction with those from the study by Iragui *et al.*, are consistent with the notion that AD patients suffer a decline in their ability to analyse and integrate semantic information, and that this deficit is related to abnormal semantic or conceptual priming.

Although the above interpretation of the priming deficit of AD patients is consistent with their known semantic memory impairment (for review, see Salmon and Chan 1994), several studies have cast some doubt upon this interpretation by demonstrating that, under certain conditions, AD patients can exhibit normal performance on semantic or conceptual priming tasks. One such study, recently reported by Fennema-Notestine *et al.* (1994), examined verbal priming in AD patients using a homophone spelling bias task. In the initial phase of this study, it was determined that across two test sessions normal control (NC) subjects, AD patients, and amnesic patients all spontaneously shifted their preferred spelling on approximately 30% of homophonic words. With this baseline rate of shifting in mind, subjects were asked to spell a series of homophonic words (to establish the initial spelling preference) and then to spell these words again a few minutes later after they had been biased against their preference by presenting the homophone within a semantic context. For example if a subject's preferred spelling had initially been *son*, he or she was asked in the second phase to spell this word immediately after having heard *moon* and *stars*. Conversely, if their preferred spelling had been *sun*, they were biased with *father* and *daughter* in the second phase. After the biasing trails, all subject groups tended to shift to their non-preferred spelling on approximately 60% of the homophonic words. This doubling of the shift to non-preferred spelling by the biasing presentation suggests that the semantic relationship between the biasing and target words was intact enough in the AD patients to activate the non-preferred spelling to a normal level.

Additional evidence of intact semantic or conceptual priming in patients with AD was provided by Gross *et al.* (1990). These investigators reasoned that the semantic structure necessary to support priming may be intact in patients with AD, but, unlike normal individuals, they fail to process fully the target words at a semantic level during the initial orienting phase of the long-term priming task. To examine this possibility, Grosse *et al.* (1990) administered a stem-completion priming task to AD patients in which the encoding demands were increased at the time of initial word presentation. These investigators employed a task for stimulus presentation in which subjects were required to complete sentence frames (for instance 'He hit the nail with a . . .?') with the single best fit word (for example 'hammer'). In the test phase, three letter words stems of the best fit words and distractor words were presented in a stem-completion task. The authors proposed that this sentence completion task more effectively ensured that target stimuli were fully and elaboratively processed at a semantic level than in the 'likeability-judgement' or naming tasks used in previous studies.

On the stem-completion task, AD patients correctly completed 36% of targets that they had accessed during the stimulus presentation task, while correctly completing only 18% of the distractor items (baseline performance). Similarly, the NC subjects correctly completed 34% of targets during the stem-completion task, and 20% of the distractor items. Thus, there was no significant difference between the groups in stem-completion priming.

Partridge *et al.* (1990) obtained similar results by changing the nature of the orienting task in the stem-completion paradigm to a task which would increase the likelihood of semantic processing of the target words. Rather than judging the likeability of the target words during the presentation phase of the task (as in the studies by Salmon *et al.* 1988 and Shimamura *et al.* 1987), AD patients were required to supply the meaning of each word, thus ensuring that the semantic properties of the words had been analysed. With this procedure, Partridge *et al.* observed normal levels of stem-completion priming in AD patients.

The results of the studies by Grosse *et al.* (1990) and by Partridge *et al.* (1990) indicate that when patients with AD are required to attend to the semantic aspects of the target stimulus they exhibit normal stem-completion priming. However, the interpretation of the results of these studies is complicated by several methodological issues. For example, AD subjects who were unable to perform the semantic encoding task were eliminated from the Partridge *et al.* (1990) study, and these may have been the very subjects with semantic–memory deterioration who would have exhibited impaired priming on the stem-completion task. In addition, the sentence frame task used by Grosse *et al.* (1990) resulted in considerably less priming in control subjects than usually observed in other studies that have used the stem-completion procedure. In Grosse *et al.*'s study the NC and AD subjects' priming was only 14% and 18% above baseline completion levels, respectively. While the level of priming exhibited by the AD patients is comparable to the 16% increase above baseline noted by Heindel *et al.* (1989), and similar to the increases reported by Shimamura *et al.* (1987) and Salmon *et al.* (1988), the 14% increase for NC subjects is far below the 40–50% increase for NC subjects reported in other studies of stem-completion priming (Graf *et al.* 1984; Heindel *et al.* 1989; Shimamura *et al.* 1987; Salmon *et al.* 1988). Finally, neither of these studies directly compared the 'likeability-judgement' and 'semantic-processing' orienting tasks, so alternative explanations for the differences in Grosse *et al.*'s and Partridge *et al.*'s results and those of Shimamura *et al.* (1987) and Salmon *et al.* (1988) (for instance subject differences) cannot be ruled out.

It should also be noted that the results of the studies by Grosse *et al.* (1990), Partridge *et al.* (1990), and Fennema-Notestine *et al.* (1994) do not necessarily indicate that semantic memory is completely intact in patients with AD. As suggested by Grosse *et al.* (1990), AD patients may have a defective semantic network that requires the target stimulus to be presented in a richer semantic context to achieve the level of activation necessary for normal priming. In addition, Fennema-Notestine *et al.* (1994) point out that different tasks place different demands on semantic memory, and that there are likely to be degrees of semantic degradation in patients with AD. Thus, if a given AD patient has only partial deterioration of semantic memory, the semantic processing demands of the task will determine whether or not normal priming will be observed.

Other studies that demonstrate normal semantic or conceptual priming in patients with AD (for review, see Nebes 1989) suggest that previous findings of impaired priming may be related to a deficiency in controlled, effortful retrieval processes, rather than to semantic deterioration. According to this view, semantic knowledge is intact in patients with AD, but can only be accessed in a normal fashion through automatic retrieval processes.

A number of investigators have examined priming in AD patients using tasks that involve 'automatic' cognitive processing such as naming or prounciation, or that measure priming over extremely short time intervals (less than 400 msec) that preclude the use of controlled processes such as expectancy or semantic matching. In a study by Nebes *et al.* (1984), for example, a given word was preceded (by approximately 500 msec) either by a semantically related word (primed trials) or by an unrelated word (unprimed trials), and priming was measured by the difference in naming latencies between primed and unprimed trials. The results of this study showed that both the AD patients and control subjects had a slight and equivalent facilitation in naming (or pronunciation) latency when a word was preceded by a semantic associate (that is, semantic priming). Based on these data, Nebes *et al.* concluded that priming and semantic memory are normal in AD patients when they are assessed with techniques which rely solely upon automatic information processing.

A number of subsequent studies have examined priming and semantic memory in patients with AD using naming (reading or pronunciation) and lexical decision tasks that are thought to involve automatic processes. Ober *et al.* (1991), for example, examined priming in AD patients with a naming procedure similar to the one used by Nebes *et al.* (1984) and with a lexical decision procedure (both with 250 msec interstimulus intervals). In the lexical decision task, a series of letter strings is presented visually, and the subject is asked to indicate, as quickly as possible, whether or not each string represents a real word. Pairs of prime and target words (for instance spinach, lettuce) are embedded in the series, and priming is reflected by the facilitation of the subject's reaction time in making the word/non-word decision when a target item is preceded by a related prime relative to when it is preceded by an unrelated prime. Ober *et al.* observed no significant differences in the magnitude of priming exhibited by the AD patients and elderly normal control subjects on either type of task. These results are difficult to interpret, however, because in a number of the many semantic conditions that were employed in this study, either the AD patients or normal control subjects failed to show any significant priming. Because this appeared to occur randomly within both groups, the tasks may have lacked the sensitivity to measure semantic priming effects consistently.

In another study, Albert and Milberg (1989), like Ober *et al.* (1991), found no significant difference in the magnitude of priming exhibited by AD patients and elderly normal control subjects in a lexical decision task (with a 500 msec interstimulus interval) when priming was defined as the absolute difference in reaction times when the target word was primed or not primed. However, because the AD patients were slower and had significantly longer reaction times than the control subjects in all conditions, Albert and Milberg re-examined priming in their study after taking the AD patients' general slowing into account by using proportional priming scores. These scores were calculated by dividing the difference score (unprimed minus primed reaction times) by a baseline measure of reaction time (reaction time to the unprimed item). When proportional priming scores were analysed, it became evident that AD patients exhibited significantly less priming than the control subjects, suggesting that they had difficulty with the semantic processing required by this task.

Several additional studies that employed lexical decision or naming (reading) tasks have revealed abnormal priming in AD patients, even though these tasks are thought to minimize the use of controlled, effortful access of semantic memory. Ober and Shenaut (1988), for example, observed no significant priming in AD patients on a lexical decision task (with a 1000 msec interstimulus interval) in which target words were primed by semantically related words. Similarly, Glosser and Friedman (1991), using a threshold oral reading task, found that AD patients were impaired on a short-term priming task when the prime and target words were semantically related (for example sheep—goat), but not when they were only lexically related (for instance cottage—cheese). In a number of other studies using a lexical decision or naming procedure, abnormal priming in AD patients was reflected by significantly *greater* than normal semantic priming (hyperpriming) (Balota and Duchek 1991; Chenery *et al.* 1994; Chertkow *et al.* 1989, 1994; Hartman 1991; Nebes *et al.* 1989).

Although this latter abnormality is difficult to interpret, Martin (1992) has suggested that these hyperpriming effects in AD patients may be the direct result of underspecified, overgeneralized semantic representations created by the loss of item-specific attributes. In this view, AD patients are not able to distinguish between items that are closely related in semantic memory (such as robin and finch) because their knowledge of detailed attributes (such as respective size and colourings of the birds) no longer exists. Thus, activating one representation in the semantic memory of an AD patient serves to activate to the same degree all other representations with which it has become generalized. For example the activation of 'robin' may activate 'finch' to the same extent since the overgeneralized representation essentially imposes the same meaning on both items. Once this overgeneralization has occurred, semantic priming (for example robin—finch) virtually becomes repetition priming (for instance robin—robin) for the AD patient. Because repetition priming effects are almost always larger than semantic priming effects, AD patients exhibit greater than normal priming (hyperpriming) in the semantic priming task.

Although far from uniform, the results of the studies reviewed above suggest that, under at least some conditions, abnormal conceptually based priming effects can be observed in patients with AD. This abnormality can take the form of deficient priming, as on stem-completion and free-association priming tasks, or may be manifested as hyperpriming, as on short-term priming tasks that use naming or lexical decision procedures. Although the mechanisms that underlie the conceptual priming deficit of AD patients remain unknown, some evidence suggests that it may be related to a deterioration of semantic memory. Other factors, however, such as deficient effortful retrieval processes or a general decline in the ability to activate representations (see Salmon and Heindel 1992), may be involved.

Perceptual priming

Studies consistently demonstrate normal repetition priming in patients with AD when procedures are used that allow priming to occur at a perceptual level. Several studies, for example, have demonstrated normal repetition priming effects on the speed with which AD patients are able to read geometrically transformed script (Deweer *et al.* 1993; Grober *et al.* 1992; Moscovitch *et al.* 1986). Similarly, normal repetition priming has been observed in patients with AD on a task in which subjects were required to identify briefly presented words, half of which had been presented previously in an unrelated reading task (Keane *et al.* 1991). Priming was reflected in this study by a shorter exposure time necessary to identify previously presented words relative to words not previously seen. The AD patients' normal perceptual repetition priming ability occurred despite their impairment on a stem-completion task that was similar to that employed by Shimamura *et al.* (1987).

Normal perceptually based repetition priming was also observed in AD patients in several studies of semantic priming that included a repetition priming component as a secondary feature of the experimental design. Balota and Duchek (1991), for example, used a semantic priming paradigm in which the latency to read semantically related triads (for instance kidney—organ—heart) was assessed on two consecutive blocks of trials. Repetition priming could be assessed by comparing subjects' reading speeds for the same triads across the two presentations. The results of such an analysis revealed no significant difference between AD patients and elderly normal control subjects in the magnitude of the decrease in reaction time to name target items in the second block relative to the first block. In a similar study, Ober and Shenaut (1988) assessed repetition priming in a relatively indirect manner within a semantic lexical-decision priming paradigm. In this study, the repetition of items occurred as an inevitable consequence of within-subject counterbalancing of items. That is, all target items were repeated within each block of trials so that each target word could serve as its own baseline in the semantic priming task. When repetition priming was assessed by comparing the first and second presentations of the target word, AD patients and normal control subjects exhibited equivalent facilitation of their lexical decisions.

Finally, normal perceptually based repetition priming effects were observed in AD patients in several studies that examined real-time cognitive processing with event-related brain potentials (ERP) (Friedman *et al.* 1992; Rugg *et al.* 1994). In both studies a continuous list of words was presented and the subject was required to respond with a keypress to any animal names that appeared in the list. Repetition priming was examined in non-target (namely non-animal) words that were repeated after lags of either 1 or 6 intervening items (Rugg *et al.* 1994) or that averaged 14 intervening items (Friedman *et al.* 1992). Repetition priming was revealed by a greater positivity within a set of complex ERP components for repeated items than for unrepeated items. There were no significant differences in repetition priming between the AD patients and normal elderly control subjects in either study.

The preservation of perceptually based repetition priming in patients with AD suggests that this form of priming occurs independently of the brain regions that are damaged by Alzheimer's disease. Consistent with this suggestion, Gabrieli, Fleischman, and colleagues (Fleischman *et al.* 1995; Gabrieli *et al.* in press) have recently presented evidence that perceptually based priming may be mediated by a putative visual memory mechanism (similar to the presemantic Perceptual Representation System proposed by Tulving and Schacter 1990) in the right occipital cortex, a brain area not prominently affected by Alzheimer's disease. These investigators examined explicit memory and perceptual identification priming in a patient (M.S.) with a left homonymous hemianopia due to a right hemisphere temporal lobectomy performed as treatment for pharmacologically intractable epilepsy. Despite normal performance on a visually based explicit recognition memory test, patient M.S. was impaired on a perceptual identification priming test similar to that used by Keane *et al.* (1991).

Preserved perceptually based repetition priming in AD patients may also have important implications for the variability in their performance across studies of verbal priming. As mentioned previously, several investigators (e.g. Carlesimo 1994; Keane *et al.* 1991; Tulving and Schacter 1990) have suggested that most verbal priming tasks involve both a semantic (namely conceptual) and a presemantic perceptual processing component, but that the relative contribution of each component varies across tasks. As the demands of priming tasks become more heavily weighted towards perceptual processing, the performance of patients with AD may approach normal. Thus, AD patients may exhibit normal priming on a perceptual identification task that can be performed solely on the basis of perceptual processes, some residual (albeit, less than normal) priming on a stem-completion priming task that invokes both conceptual and perceptual processes, and almost no priming on a paired-associate priming task that precludes the use of perceptual processes and is solely dependent on conceptual processes.

SKILL LEARNING

In contrast to the variability in the performance of AD patients on various priming tasks, studies consistently demonstrate that the ability to acquire and retain motor-based skills (that is to say procedural learning) is preserved in these patients. In an initial study, for example, Eslinger and Damasio (1986) compared the ability of AD patients and aged-matched normal control subjects to learn the motor skills underlying a pursuit rotor task. In this task, subjects were required to maintain contact between a hand-held stylus and a rotating metallic disc. The amount of time the stylus was kept in contact with the disc on each 20-second trial was measured across five trials. The results of this study showed that the AD patients' performance on the pursuit rotor task improved significantly across trials, and at the same rate as that of the control subjects.

In addition to this and several other demonstrations of AD patients' preserved ability to learn the skilled motor behaviour underlying performance on the pursuit rotor task (Bondi *et al.* 1993; Heindel *et al.* 1988, 1989); Gabrieli *et al.* (1993) recently showed that these patients were able to acquire and retain normally the visuomotor skills necessary to trace a pattern seen in mirror-reversed view. Similarly, a number of investigators have reported that AD patients acquire the visuoperceptual skills necessary to read mirror-reversed text in a normal fashion (Deweer *et al.* 1993; 1994, Huberman *et al.* 1994; Perani *et al.* 1993).

In order to understand better the neurological correlates of skill learning, Heindel *et al.* (1988) compared the ability of AD, HD, and circumscribed amnesia patients to learn the pursuit rotor task. To ensure that any observed group differences in skill acquisition would not be attributable to ceiling or floor effects, the initial levels of performance among the groups was equated by manipulating the difficulty (namely the speed of rotation of the disc) of the task. Consistent with Eslinger and Damasio's (1986) findings, with practise AD patients exhibited rapid and extensive motor learning that was equivalent to that of amnesic patients and normal control subjects. The HD patients, in contrast, were impaired in learning this motor skill, which suggests that this form of implicit memory may be mediated by a corticostriatal system that is severely compromised in HD (Bruyn *et al.* 1979)

As suggested by Heindel *et al.* (1988), the neostriatal damage suffered by HD patients may lead to a deficiency in developing the motor programmes that are necessary to perform the pursuit rotor task. In learning a motor skill, appropriate movements comprising the target skill must be combined in a correct temporal sequence (a motor programme). In the early stages of learning a motor skill, an elementary closed-loop negative feedback system is employed in which new motor commands are generated in direct response to visually perceived errors. As motor programmes are acquired and modified through practise, a sequence of movements can be organized in advance of their performance (rather than simply responding to errors) and smooth, coordinated motor performance ensues. If, as suspected, the neostriatal damage in the HD patients precludes their developing motor programmes, these patients may demonstrate some improvement in the early stages of motor skill acquisition by relying upon their error-correction mode of performance. However, their inability to generate new motor programmes would prevent them from adopting the more effective predictive mode of performance utilized by AD patients, amnesics, and normal control subjects.

Although Heindel *et al.* (1988) found no significant relationship between the severity of HD patients' primary motor dysfunction and their ability to learn the pursuit rotor task, some concern about this potential confound remained. To address this concern, Heindel *et al.* (1991) examined the performance of demented patients on another form of procedural learning that is thought to rely on the development of motor programmes, but that is much less reliant than the pursuit rotor task on overt movement. This form of procedural learning, classical adaptation-level effects observed in a weight judgement task (Benzig and Squire 1989), involves a task in which AD and HD subjects are first exposed either to a relatively heavy (heavy bias) or a relatively light (light bias) set of weights, and are later asked to rate the heaviness of a standard set of 10 weights using a 9-point scale. In this study, patients with AD and normal control subjects both perceived the standard set of weights as heavier following the light bias trials and lighter following the heavy bias trials, despite the AD patients' poor explicit memory for the initial biasing session. In contrast, the weight judgements of the HD group were not significantly influenced by prior exposure to relatively heavy or light weights.

The results with the weight biasing task are of particular interest since the perceptual biasing may involve the modification of programmed movement parameters. A number of studies (see review by Jones 1986) have demonstrated that the perception of weight is normally mediated by centrally generated motor commands rather than by peripheral sensory information. The sensation of heaviness is then influenced by discrepancies between the intended, or programmed, force and the actual force needed to lift an object. Prior exposure to relatively heavy or light weights (the biasing trials) may result in an increase or decrease in the amount of force programmed for lifting weights, which would then lead to an illusory decrease or increase in the perceived heaviness of the standard set of weights. Thus, the impaired weight biasing performance of the HD patients, like their skill learning deficits shown with the pursuit rotor task, may be due to a motor programming deficit resulting from neostriatal dysfunction.

In a related study, Paulsen *et al.* (1993) recently compared the performance of AD patients, HD patients, and normal elderly control subjects on a perceptual adaptation task involving laterally displaced vision. In this task, subjects were required to point to a target while wearing distorting prisms that shifted the perceived location of objects 20 degrees to the right or left. Quantitative indices of pointing accuracy were obtained under several conditions. First, baseline performance was assessed without prisms or visual feedback regarding accuracy. Second, pre-adaptation performance was assessed with prisms and without visual feedback. Third, a series of 30 adaptation trials were carried out with prisms and visual feedback. Fourth, post-adaptation performance was assessed with prisms and without visual feedback. Finally, after-effects were assessed without prisms or visual feedback. It is generally believed that adaptation to such lateral spatial distortion is mediated by modification of central motor programmes (involved in directed movements) following visual feedback regarding accuracy of intended movements. The results of this study demonstrated that AD patients exhibited normal adaptation to the prisms after visual feedback, and normal negative after-effects when the prisms were removed. In contrast, HD patients failed to exhibit normal adaptation or negative after-effects on this task. It should be noted that the HD patients' prism adaptation performance was not associated with extra-pyramidal motor impairment, but was significantly correlated with the severity of their dementia. Thus, their motor skill learning deficit appears to be a feature of their cognitive loss and not a consequence of their basic motor disability.

Visuomotor skill learning in demented patients has been further examined with a serial reaction time task developed by Nissen and Bullemer (1987). The serial reaction time task is a four-choice procedure in which a subject must respond as quickly as possible to the illumination of one of four lights, each located immediately above a corresponding response key. During the first four blocks of trials, the stimuli are presented in a particular 10-item sequence that is repeated ten times in each block. The stimuli are presented in a new random sequence during the fifth block of trials. Procedural learning is reflected in a reduction in response latency over the first four blocks of trials as the subject benefits from the sequence repetition. An increase in response time is anticipated on the fifth block of trials (the new random sequence) if the initial response time decline is due to learning of the stimulus sequence rather than to learning non-specific aspects of the task. Amnesic patients demonstrate a normal decline in response latency over the first four blocks of this task and a normal increase in response latency during the random sequence trial (Nissen and Bullemer 1987). The decline in response latency on the repeated sequence suggests that these amnesic patients learn and retain the sequence despite an inability to recall it explicitly.

Several recent studies have examined the performance of AD and HD patients on this serial reaction time task. In two studies (Grafman *et al.* 1990; Knopman and Nissen 1987), patients with AD were found to respond generally slower than NC subjects on this task, but demonstrated the same rate of decline in response latency over the blocks of trials with a repeating sequence, and a normal increase in response latency when a random sequence was presented (but see Ferraro *et al.* 1993). In contrast to the AD patients' normal procedural learning on this task, Knopman and Nissen (1991) found that HD patients were impaired. The HD patients demonstrated significantly less decline in response latency than age-matched controls over the repeating sequence trials, and showed less increase in response latency than controls during the block of trials in which a new random stimulus sequence was presented.

The results of these studies of procedural learning and memory in AD, HD, and amnesic patients suggest that the ability to acquire motor and cognitive-based skills is not dependent upon the medial temporal, diencephalic, or cortical association areas affected in AD or circumscribed amnesia. Rather, these abilities appear to be critically dependent upon the neostriatal structures damaged in Huntington's disease and perhaps other subcortically based dementing disorders (such as Parkinson's disease).

DISSOCIATIONS WITHIN IMPLICIT MEMORY

When considered together, the studies of priming and skill learning reviewed in this chapter indicate that a dissociation exists between AD and HD patients in their patterns of impaired and preserved implicit memory abilities. Patients with AD are impaired on some tests of long-term priming that are performed normally by HD patients. In contrast, HD patients are impaired on many skill learning tasks that are easily mastered by AD patients.

To examine this apparent dissociation directly within a single investigation, Heindel *et al.* (1989) compared the performance of patients with circumscribed amnesia, AD, HD, and Parkinson's disease (PD) on skill learning and verbal priming tasks. Motor skill learning was assessed with the pursuit rotor task, and long-term verbal priming was evaluated in the same patients with the stem-completion procedure used by Salmon *et al.* (1988). Although amnesics performed normally on both tasks, a double dissociation was observed between AD and HD patients on the two implicit memory tasks. The AD patients were severely impaired on verbal priming but showed normal acquisition of the pursuit rotor skill; the HD patients showed the opposite relationship. The performance of the PD patients was dependent upon whether they were demented or not. Demented PD patients were impaired on both implicit memory tasks, whereas the non-demented PD patients were intact on both tests. For both the HD and PD patients, their impairments on the motor skill learning task correlated with their degree of dementia, not with the severity of their motor deficits (chorea, bradykinesia, rigidity, tremor).

This double dissociation between HD and AD patients on the verbal priming and pursuit rotor tasks provides strong evidence that various forms of implicit memory depend upon different neuroanatomical substrates. While the HD patients' impairment on the pursuit rotor task is certainly consistent with the proposed association between the acquisition of motor skills and the neostriatum, the AD patients' deficiencies on verbal priming (and semantic memory in general) may be attributable to the neocortical damage associated with this disorder.

CONCLUSIONS

As our knowledge of implicit memory in demented patients has grown over the past ten years, it has become increasingly clear that this form of memory is not subserved by a single brain system. As described above, various types of implicit learning and memory are differentially affected in dementing disorders that differ in their sites of neural damage. Furthermore, the relationship between the particular region of neural damage and the type of implicit memory affected in demented patients is consistent with the notion that implicit memory is mediated by those brain structures that are directly engaged in processing information during learning of a given task (Squire 1987). Thus, patients with HD who have damage to the basal ganglia structures that are involved in processing motor information have difficulty in implicitly learning and retaining new motor skills. Similarly, patients with AD who have damage in neocortical regions that are thought to process semantic information are impaired on some verbal priming tasks. Further delineation of the neurological bases of implicit memory should be possible with continued study of this form of memory in patients with Alzheimer's disease and other dementing disorders.

ACKNOWLEDGEMENTS

The preparation of this manuscript was supported in part by NIA grants AG-05131 and AG-12963, and NIMH grant MH-48819, to the University of California at San Diego.

REFERENCES

Albert, M. and Milberg, W. (1989). Semantic processing in patients with Alzheimer's disease. *Brain and Language*, **37**, 163–71.

Balota, D. A. and Duchek, J. M. (1991). Semantic priming effects, lexical repetition effects, and contextual disambiguation effects in healthy aged individuals and individuals with senile dementia of the Alzheimer's type. *Brain and Language*, **40**, 181–201.

Benzig, W. C. and Squire, L. R. (1989). Preserved learning and memory in amnesia: Intact adaptation-level effects and learning of stereoscopic depth. *Behavioral Neuroscience*, **103**, 538–47.

Blaxton, T. A. (1989). Investigating dissociations among memory measures: Support for a transfer-appropriate processing framework. *Journal of Experimental Psychology: Learning, Memory, and Cognition*, **15**, 657–68.

Bondi, M. W., Kaszniak, A. W., Rapsak, S. Z., and Butters, M. A. (1993). Implicit and explicit memory following anterior communicating artery aneurysm rupture. *Brain and Cognition*, **22**, 213–29.

Brandt, J., Spencer, M., McSorley, P., and Folstein, M. F. (1988). Semantic activation and implicit memory in Alzheimer disease. *Alzheimer Disease and Associated Disorders*, **2**, 112–19.

Brooks, D. N. and Baddeley, A. D. (1976). What can amnesic patients learn? *Neuropsychologia*, **14**, 111–22.

Brun, A. (1983). An overview of light and electron microscopic changes. In *Alzheimer's disease*, (ed. B. Reisberg), pp. 37–47. The Free Press, New York.

Bruyn, G. W., Bots, G., and Dom, R. (1979). Huntington's chorea: Current neuropathological status. In *Advances in neurology*, Vol. 23: *Huntington's disease*, (ed. T. Chase, N. Wexler, and A. Barbeau), pp. 83–94. Raven Press, New York.

Buschke, H. and Fuld, P. A. (1974). Evaluating storage, retention, and retrieval in disordered memory and learning. *Neurology*, **24**, 1019–25.

Butters, N., Salmon, D. P., Cullum, C. M., Cairns, P., Troster, A. I., Jacobs, D. *et al.* (1988). Differentiation of amnesic and demented patients with the Wechsler Memory Scale – Revised. *The Clinical Neuropsychologist*, **2**, 133–44.

Carlesimo, G. A. (1994). Perceptual and conceptual priming in amnesic and alcoholic patients. *Neuropsychologia*, **32**, 903–21.

Cermak, L. S., Lewis, R., Butters, N., and Goodglass, H. (1973). Role of verbal mediation in performance of motor tasks by Korsakoff patients. *Perceptual and Motor Skills*, **37**, 259–62.

Cermak, L. S., Talbot, N., Chandler, K., and Wolbarst, L. R. (1985). The perceptual priming phenomenon in amnesia. *Neuropsychologia*, **23**, 615–22.

Chan, A. S., Butters, N., Paulsen, J. S., Salmon, D. P., Swenson, M. R., and Maloney, L. T. (1993*a*). An assessment of the semantic network in patients with Alzheimer's disease. *Journal of Cognitive Neuroscience*, **5**, 254–61.

Chan, A. S., Butters, N., Salmon, D. P., and McGuire, K. A. (1993*b*). Dimensionality and clustering in the network of patients with Alzheimer's disease. *Psychology and Aging*, **8**, 411–19.

Chan, A. S., Butters, N., Salmon, D. P., Johnson, S. A., Paulsen, J. S., and Swenson, M. R. (1995). Comparison of the semantic networks in patients with dementia and amnesia. *Neuropsychology*, **9**, 177–86.

Chenery, H. J., Ingram, J. C. L., and Murdoch, B. E. (1994). The effect of repeated prime-target presentation in manipulating attention-induced priming in persons with dementia of the Alzheimer's type. *Brain and Cognition*, **25**, 108–27.

Chertkow, H. and Bub, D. (1990). Semantic memory loss in dementia of Alzheimer's type. *Brain*, **113**, 397–417.

Chertkow, H., Bub, D., and Seidenberg, M. (1989). Priming and semantic memory loss in Alzheimer's disease. *Brain and Language*, **36**, 420–46.

Chertkow, H., Bub, D., Bergman, H., Bruemmer, A., Merling, A., and Rothfleisch, J. (1994). Increased semantic priming in patients with dementia of the Alzheimer's type. *Journal of Clinical and Experimental Neuropsychology*, **16**, 608–22.

Cohen, N. and Squire, L.R. (1980). Preserved learning and retention of pattern analyzing skills in amnesia: Dissociation of knowing how and knowing that. *Science*, **210**, 207–10.

Corkin, S. (1968). Acquisition of motor skill after bilateral medial temporal lobe excision. *Neuropsychologia*, **6**, 255–65.

Deweer, B., Pillon, B., Michon, A., and Dubois, B. (1993). Mirror reading in Alzheimer's disease: Normal skill learning and acquisition of item-specific information. *Journal of Clinical and Experimental Neuropsychology*, **15**, 789–804.

Deweer, B., Ergis, A. M., Fossati, P., Pillon, B., Boller, F., Agid, Y. *et al.* (1994). Explicit memory, procedural learning and lexical priming in Alzheimer's disease. *Cortex*, **30**, 113–26.

Eslinger, P.J. and Damasio, A.R. (1986). Preserved motor learning in Alzheimer's disease: Implications for anatomy and behavior. *Journal of Neuroscience*, **6**, 3006–9.

Fennema-Notestine, C., Butters, N., Heindel, W.C., and Salmon, D.P. (1994). Semantic homophone priming in patients with dementia of the Alzheimer type. *Neuropsychology*, **8**, 579–87.

Ferraro, F. R., Balota, D. A., and Connor, L. T. (1993). Implicit memory and the formation of new associations in nondemented Parkinson's disease individuals and individuals with senile dementia of the Alzheimer type: A serial reaction time (SRT) investigation. *Brain and Cognition*, **21**, 163–80.

Fleischman, D.A., Gabrieli, J.D.E., Reminger, S., Rinaldi, J., Morrell, F., and Wilson, R. (1995). Conceptual priming in perceptual identification for patients with Alzheimer's disease and a patients with right occipital lobectomy. *Neuropsychology*, **9**, 187–97.

Friedman, D., Hamberger, M., Stern, Y., and Marder, K. (1992). Event-related potentials (ERPs) during repetition priming in Alzheimer's patients and young and older controls. *Journal of Clinical and Experimental Neuropsychology*, **14**, 448–62.

Gabrieli, J. D. E., Corkin, S., Mickel, S. F., and Growdon, J. H. (1993). Intact acquisition and long-term retention of mirror-tracing skill in Alzheimer's disease and global amnesia. *Behavioral Neuroscience*, **107**, 899–910.

Gabrieli, J. D. E., Fleischman, D. A., Keane, M. M., Reminger, S. L., and Morrell, F. Double dissociation between memory systems underlying explicit and implicit memory in the human brain. *Psychological Science* (In press).

Gardner, H., Boller, F., Moreines, J., and Butters, N. (1973). Retrieving information from Korsakoff patients: Effects of categorical cues and reference to the task. *Cortex*, **9**, 165–75.

Glosser, G. and Friedman, R.B. (1991). Lexical but not semantic priming in Alzheimer's disease. *Psychology and Aging*, **6**, 522–7.

Graf, P. and Schacter, D. (1985). Implicit and explicit memory for new associations in normal and amnesic subjects. *Journal of Experimental Psychology: Learning, Memory and Cognition*, **11**, 501–18.

Graf, P. and Schacter, D. (1987). Selective effects of interference on implicit and explicit memory for new associations. *Journal of Experimental Psychology: Learning, Memory and Cognition*, **13**, 45–53.

Graf, P., Squire, L., and Mandler, G. (1984). The information that amnesic patients do not forget. *Journal of Experimental Psychology: Human Learning and Memory*, **10**, 164–78.

Grafman, J., Weingartner, H., Newhouse, P. A., Thompson, K., Lalonde, F., Litvan, I. *et al.* (1990). Implicit learning in patients with Alzheimer's disease. *Pharmacopsychiatry*, **23**, 94–101.

Grober, E., Ausubel, R., Sliwinski, M., and Gordon, B. (1992). Skill learning and repetition priming in Alzheimer's disease. *Neuropsychologia*, **30**, 849–58.

Grosse, D. A., Wilson, R. S., and Fox, J. H. (1990). Preserved word-stem-completion priming of semantically encoded information in Alzheimer's disease. *Psychology and Aging*, **5**, 304–6.

Hartman, M. (1991). The use of semantic knowledge in Alzheimer's disease: evidence for impairments of attention. *Neuropsychologia*, **29**, 213–28.

Heindel, W., Butters, N., and Salmon, D. (1988). Impaired learning of a motor skill in patients with Huntington's disease. *Behavioral Neuroscience*, **102**, 141–7.

Heindel, W., Salmon, D., Shults, C., Walicke, P., and Butters, N. (1989). Neuropsychological evidence for multiple implicit memory systems: A comparison of Alzheimer's, Huntington's and Parkinson's disease patients. *Journal of Neuroscience*, **9**, 582–7.

Heindel, W., Salmon, D., and Butters, N. (1991). The biasing of weight judgments in Alzheimer's and Huntington's disease: A priming or programming phenomenon? *Journal of Clinical and Experimental Neuropsychology*, **13**, 189–203.

Hodges, J. R., Salmon, D. P., and Butters, N. (1992). Semantic memory impairment in Alzheimer's disease: Failure of access or degraded knowledge? *Neuropsychologia*, **30**, 301–14.,

Huberman, M., Moscovitch, M., and Freedman, M. (1994). Comparison of patients with Alzheimer's and Parkinson's disease on different explicit and implicit tests of memory. *Neuropsychiatry, Neuropsychology, and Behavioral Neurology*, **7**, 185–93.

Iragui, V., Kutas, M., and D. P. Salmon. Event-related brain potentials during semantic categorization in normal aging and senile dementia of the Alzheimer's type. *Electroencophalography and Clinical Neurophysiology* (in press).

Jones, L. A. (1986). Perception of force and weight: Theory and research. *Psychological Bulletin*, **100**, 29–42.

Keane, M. M., Gabrieli, J. D. E., Fennema, A. C., Growdon, J. H., and Corkin, S. (1991). Evidence for a dissociation between perceptual and conceptual priming in Alzheimer's disease. *Behavioral Neuroscience*, **105**, 326–42.

Knopman, D. S. and Nissen, M. J. (1987). Implicit learning in patients with probable Alzheimer's disease. *Neurology*, **37**, 784–8.

Knopman, D. S. and Nissen, M. J. (1991). Procedural learning is impaired in Huntington's disease: Evidence from the serial reaction time test. *Neuropsychologia*, **29**, 245–54.

Kutas, M. and Hillyard, S. A. (1980). Reading senseless sentences: Brain potentials reflect semantic incongruity. *Science*, **207**, 203–5.

Kutas, M. and Hillyard, S. A. (1983). Event related brain potentials to grammatical errors and semantic anomalies. *Memory and Cognition*, **11**, 539–50.

Kutas, M. and Hillyard, S. A. (1984). Brain potentials during reading reflect work expectancy and semantic association. *Nature*, **307**, 161–3.

Martin, A. (1992). Degraded knowledge representations in patients with Alzheimer's disease: Implications for models of semantic and repetition priming. In *Neuropsychology of memory* (2nd edn), (ed. L. Squire and N. Butters), pp. 220–32. The Guilford Press, New York.

Masur, D. M., Fuld, P. A., Blau, A. D., Thal, L. J., Levin, H. S., and Aronson, M. K. (1989). Distinguishing normal and demented elderly with the selective reminding test. *Journal of Clinical and Experimental Neuropsychology*, **11**, 615–30.

Moscovitch, M., Winocur, G., and McLachlan, D. (1986). Memory as assessed by recognition and reading time in normal and memory-impaired people with Alzheimer's disease and other neurological disorders. *Journal of Experimental Psychology: General*, **115**, 331–47.

Moss, M. B., Albert, M. S., Butters, N., and Payne, M. (1986). Differential patterns of memory loss among patients with Alzheimer's disease, Huntington's disease and alcoholic Korsakoff's syndrome. *Archives of Neurology*, **43**, 239–46.

Nebes, R. D. (1992). Cognitive dysfunction in Alzheimer's disease. In *The handbook of aging and cognition* (ed. F. I. M. Craik and T. Salthouse), pp. 373–446. Lawrence Erlbaum Associates, Hillsdale, NJ.

Nebes, R., Martin, D., and Horn, L. (1984). Sparing of semantic memory in Alzheimer's disease. *Journal of Abnormal Psychology*, **93**, 321–30.

Nebes, R. D., Brady, C. B., and Huff, F. J. (1989). Automatic and attentional mechanisms of semantic priming in Alzheimer's disease. *Journal of Clinical and Experimental Neuropsychology*, **11**, 219–30.

Nissen, M. J. and Bullemer, P. (1987). Attentional requirements of learning: Evidence from performance measures. *Cognitive Psychology*, **19**, 1–32.

Ober, B. A. and Shenaut, G. K. (1988). Lexical decision and priming in Alzheimer's disease. *Neuropsychologia*, **26**, 273–86.

Ober, B. A., Shenaut, G. K., Jagust, W. J., and Stillman, R. C. (1991). Automatic semantic priming with various category relations in Alzheimer's disease and normal aging. *Psychology and Aging*, **6**, 647–60.

Partridge, F., Knight, R., and Feehan, M. (1990). Direct and indirect memory performance in patients with senile dementia. *Psychological Medicine*, **20**, 111–18.

Paulsen, J. S., Butters, N., Salmon, D. P., Heindel, W. C., and Swenson, M. R. (1993). Prism adaptation in Alzheimer's and Huntington's disease. *Neuropsychology*, **7**, 73–81.

Perani, D., Bressi, S., Cappa, S. F., Vallar, G., Alberoni, M., Grassi, F. *et al.* (1993). Evidence of multiple memory systems in the human brain. *Brain*, **116**, 903–19.

Randolph, C. (1991). Implicit, explicit and semantic memory functions in Alzheimer's disease and Huntington's disease. *Journal of Clinical and Experimental Neuropsychology*, **13**, 479–94.

Roediger, H. L. and Blaxton, T. A. (1987). Effects of varying modality, surface features, and retention interval on priming in word fragment completion. *Memory and Cognition*, **15**, 379–88.

Rugg, M. D., Pearl, S., Walker, P., Roberts, R. C., and Holdstock, J. S. (1994). Word repetition effects in event-related potentials in healthy young and old subjects, and in patients with Alzheimer-type dementia. *Neuropsychologia*, **32**, 381–98.

Salmon, D. P. and Butters, N. (1995). Neurobiology of skill and habit learning. *Current Opinion in Neurobiology*, **5**, 184–90.

Salmon, D. P. and Chan, A. S. (1994). Semantic memory deficits associated with Alzheimer's disease. In *Neuropsychological explorations of memory and cognition: Essays in honor of Nelson Butters* (ed. L. S. Cermak), pp. 61–76. Plenum Press, New York.

Salmon, D. P. and Heindel, W. C. (1992). Impaired priming in Alzheimer's disease: Neuropsychological implications. In *Neuropsychology of memory* (2nd edn), (ed. L. R. Squire and N. Butters), pp. 179–87. Guilford Press, New York.

Salmon, D., Shimamura, A., Butters, N., and Smith, S. (1988). Lexical and semantic priming deficits in patients with Alzheimer's disease. *Journal of Clinical and Experimental Neuropsychology*, **10**, 477–94.

Schacter, D. (1987). Implicit memory: History and current status. *Journal of Experimental Psychology: Learning, Memory and Cognition*, **13**, 501–17.

Schwartz, T. J., Kutas, M., Butters, N., Paulsen, J. S., and Salmon, D. P. Electrophysiological insights into the nature of the semantic deficit in Alzheimer's disease. *Neuropsychologia* (in press).

Shimamura, A. P. (1986). Priming effects in amnesia: Evidence for a dissociable memory function. *Quarterly Journal of Experimental Psychology [A]*, **38**, 619–44.

Shimamura, A. and Squire, L. (1984). Paired-associate learning and priming effects in amnesia: A neuropsychological study. *Journal of Experimental Psychology: General*, **113**, 556–70.

Shimamura, A., Salmon, D., Squire, L., and Butters, N. (1987). Memory dysfunction and word priming in dementia and amnesia. *Behavioral Neurosciences*, **101**, 347–51.

Squire, L. (1987). *Memory and brain.* Oxford University Press, New York.

Terry, R. D. and Katzman, R. (1983). Senile dementia of the Alzheimer type. *Annals of Neurology*, **14**, 497–506.

Troster, A. I., Butters, N., Salmon, D. P., Cullum, C. M., Jacobs, D., Brandt, J. *et al.* (1993). The diagnostic utility of savings scores: Differentiating Alzheimer's and Huntington's diseases with the logical memory and visual reproduction tests. *Journal of Clinical and Experimental Neuropsychology*, **15**, 773–88.

Tulving, E. and Schacter, D. (1990). Priming and human memory systems. *Science*, **247**, 301–6.

Warrington, E. K. and Weiskrantz, L. (1968). New method of testing long-term retention with special reference to amnesic patients. *Nature*, **217**, 972–4.

Warrington, E. K. and Weiskrantz, L. (1970). Amnesic syndrome: Consolidation or retrieval? *Nature*, **228**, 628–30.

Welsh, K., Butters, N., Hughes, J., Mohs, R., and Heyman, A. (1991). Detection of abnormal memory decline in mild cases of Alzheimer's disease using CERAD neuropsychological measures. *Archives of Neurology*, **48**, 278–81.

Wilson, R. S. Bacon, L. D., Fox, J. H., and Kaszniak, A. W. (1983). Primary and secondary memory in dementia of the Alzheimer type. *Journal of Clinical Neuropsychology*, **5**, 337–44.

EIGHT

Semantic processing

John D. W. Greene and John R. Hodges

INTRODUCTION

Memory is almost always the first aspect of cognition to become impaired in Alzheimer-type dementia (AD); anterograde episodic impairment occurs initially, and in many ways the pattern of memory loss resembles that seen in the classic amnesic syndrome. One of the most apparent differences between the amnesic syndrome and AD is, however, the impairment of semantic memory seen in the latter. It was previously claimed that semantic memory became impaired only in more advanced AD, but recent research suggests that semantic memory is impaired very early in the disease, at least in the majority of cases (Hodges and Patterson 1995). In this review we begin with an introduction to the concept of semantic memory and its organization, before turning to the central issue of semantic memory impairment in AD. We conclude with a short section on semantic dementia: there is growing awareness of this syndrome in which patients show a progressive, yet relatively pure, loss of semantic memory, although it is likely that most patients with semantic dementia have non-Alzheimer pathology (Hodges *et al.* 1992*a*, 1994, 1995; Snowden *et al.* 1989, 1994).

WHAT IS SEMANTIC MEMORY?

The term semantic memory refers to the component of long-term memory which represents our knowledge of objects, facts, and concepts, as well as words and their meaning (Tulving 1972, 1983). In contrast to episodic memory, semantic memory is culturally shared, not temporally specific and to a large extent acquired early in life. In short, semantic memory is the database which gives meaning to our sensory experience. Tasks dependent on intact semantic memory include object naming, generation of definitions for spoken words, word–picture matching, the generation of exemplars on category fluency tests (animals, vegetables, etc.), and answering general knowledge based questions (for instance 'What is the boiling point of water?', 'Does an elephant eat meat?' etc.).

In an attempt to overcome the linguistic confounds inherent in these tasks, picture–picture matching tests have also been developed such as the Pyramids and Palm Trees Test in which subjects are required to match conceptually related pictures (Howard and Patterson 1992); for instance, the target picture of an Egyptian pyramid is presented above a drawing depicting a palm tree and one depicting a fir tree, and the subject is asked to judge which one goes with the pyramid. A similar matching test has also been used by McCarthy and Warrington (1990*a*).

All of these tasks employ explicit means of testing semantic memory, that is the subject is asked to retrieve some aspect of knowledge and to 'declare' the knowledge explicitly. In addition, a number of implicit tests of semantic 'knowledge' have been employed which use various priming paradigms (for example word-stem completion, speeded naming, lexical decision, etc.). Such tasks may reveal evidence of supposedly intact semantic representations even when patients show gross impairment on explicit tasks (see Moss *et al.* 1995). The issue of whether patients with AD show defective, normal, or even enhanced (hyper-) priming remains highly controversial and is reviewed elsewhere in this book (see Chapter 7). The remainder of our chapter deals with performance of AD patients on tests of explicit semantic knowledge only.

THE ORGANIZATION OF SEMANTIC MEMORY

There has been considerable controversy regarding the internal architecture of semantic memory, that is whether there is separate representation of knowledge relating to different sensory modalities, or to different conceptual categories, or both (Allport 1985; Caramazza *et al.* 1990; McCarthy and Warrington 1988; Patterson and Hodges 1995; Saffran and Schwartz 1994; Warrington and McCarthy 1987; Warrington and Shallice 1984).

Models of semantic memory can be divided into those that assume that there is a unitary amodal store of semantic knowledge which is accessed by all modalities of input (such as the Organised Unitary Content Hypothesis (OUCH) of Caramazza *et al.* 1990 and those which hypothesize separate modality-specific stores of semantic knowledge (McCarthy and Warrington 1990*b*; Shallice 1988; Warrington 1975; Warrington and Shallice 1984). According to the OUCH model, modality-specific effects arise either because of selective disorders within the appropriate input systems (the separate structural form systems for objects and words), or because objects and words differ in the extent to which their physical forms yield information about their nature and function (for example the perceptual features of an object like a fork are informative about its function, whereas the sound of the word 'fork' is not).

By contrast, in modality-specific semantic models, knowledge about objects—acquired primarily through the visual domain—and knowledge about words—acquired verbally—is largely represented in separate systems; thus modality-specific disorders in these models can be attributable to central semantic impairments. Warrington and McCarthy (1987, 1988) have argued that knowledge can be fractionated both by modality and category, with some patients having semantic disorders restricted, for instance, to visual knowledge of living things. Finally, a sort of hybrid model proposed by Chertkow and colleagues (1990, 1992) also argues for two central semantic systems, but differentiated by type of information rather than a strict visual/verbal modality split. The 'identification semantics' system represents knowledge necessary, and sufficient, for identifying familiar objects and activating their names. In the case of natural kinds (animals, fruits, etc.), such information is largely physical (shape, size, colour, etc.), but for man-made objects, identification semantics may include functional attributes. Other semantic knowledge, such as encyclopaedic facts and associative information (such as where an animal lives, what it eats, etc.) is represented independently in an amodal system which can be accessed by both words and pictures/objects. Chertkow *et al.* have claimed that the typical pattern of semantic impairment in AD is selective loss of associative information with relative preservation of identification semantics. Clearly much remains to be resolved in this controversial area.

EVIDENCE FOR SEMANTIC MEMORY IMPAIRMENT IN AD

We shall now consider the evidence that there is semantic memory impairment in AD, as well as the question of how early in the course of AD it occurs, and whether it is due to an access or storage deficit. Performance on tests of category fluency and naming has been studied most extensively and will be discussed prior to the use of more comprehensive semantic memory test batteries.

Category fluency

AD patients show impairment on tests of sustained verbal fluency early in the course of the disease. Verbal fluency is, however, a complex task dependent upon several cognitive processes including attention and retrieval strategies, working memory, intact semantic stores, and phonological processes. In the case of initial letter fluency (in which subjects are asked to generate as many words as possible within one minute beginning with a certain letter, typically F, A, and S), the phonologically based word store is clearly critical, whereas category fluency (the generation of words from defined semantic categories such as animals, fruit, vehicles, etc.) depends on the intactness of semantic memory (Butters *et al.* 1987; Hodges *et al.* 1992*b*; Martin and Fedio 1983).

There has been some controversy concerning the relative impact of AD on letter and category fluency. Controls tend to perform less well on letter fluency than on category fluency (Hodges *et al.* 1990; Monsch *et al.* 1992, 1994; Rosser and Hodges 1994). Whereas some workers have found equal impairment on both types of fluency test in AD (Ober *et al.* 1985; Rosen 1980), the majority have found disproportionate impairment on category fluency tests (Hodges *et al.* 1990; Martin and Fedio 1983; Monsch *et al.* 1992; Rosser and Hodges 1994; Weingartner *et al.* 1993). This suggests a breakdown in the semantic component of the task. Comparison of patient groups, matched for overall level of dementia, has shown that AD selectively impairs category fluency, whereas in Huntington's disease and progressive supranuclear palsy (Steele–Richardson–Olszewski syndrome), the normal pattern of relatively worse performance on letter fluency is maintained (Rosser and Hodges 1994). Chan *et al.* (1993), using a multidimensional scaling technique, have recently shown that the impairment in category fluency performance reflects a fundamental change in the structure of the semantic representations.

Naming

Conclusions regarding the locus of pathology in anomic patients may be reached by analysis of the pattern of naming errors. It is agreed that normal naming proceeds in a series of basic stages (Coslett and Saffran 1989; Gainotti *et al.* 1981; Kohn and Goodglass 1985; Ratcliffe and Newcombe 1982; Riddoch *et al.* 1988). The first stage is perceptual in which analysis of the structural features of the target picture or object occurs. There follows a semantic stage in which the visual percept accesses identifying semantic knowledge. Next is the lexical stage in which the correct phonological form of the target word that corresponds to the semantic concept is retrieved. Finally, there is an articulatory stage.

Naming errors of different types result from breakdown at these stages (Kohn and Goodglass 1985). Perceptual errors indicate a defect at the visual analysis stage (for example 'football' for 'orange'). Superordinate naming errors imply severe loss of semantic information such that only broad category knowledge is accessible (for instance 'fruit' for 'orange'), whereas semantic-associative errors suggest that although some more specific knowledge is available, this is inadequate to generate an accurate descriptive response (such as 'juicy' for 'orange'). Semantic within-category errors are more difficult to interpret (for example 'banana' for 'orange'); when this label is reserved for responses which are clearly distinct from the target visually then it can be assumed that the defect is at a late stage of the semantic process. If accurate circumlocutory responses occur (such as 'It's tasty, has lots of pips and comes from abroad' for 'orange') then it can be assumed that appropriate activation of the semantic knowledge network has occurred, but that the correct target word cannot be accessed. Phonological paraphasias imply impaired assembly of phonological information.

Although there have been consistent demonstrations of impaired object naming in AD, a number of claims have been made regarding the nature of the naming deficit; while early studies suggested a primary perceptual deficit as the major cause of the naming disorder (Kirshner *et al.* 1984), more recent investigators have favoured a central semantic defect (Bayles and Tolmoeda 1983; Bowles *et al.* 1987; Hodges *et al.* 1991; Huff *et al.* 1986; Martin and Fedio 1983; Smith *et al.* 1989). The evidence supporting the latter hypothesis derives, to a large extent, from the analysis of the types of error produced. Hodges *et al.* (1991) found that both spontaneous and cued naming were significantly impaired. AD patients tended to make semantic-superordinate and semantic-associative errors. They also found that the pattern of naming errors evolved over time; as the patients' overall performance fell, the proportion of both semantic and visually based errors increased. These finding suggest that in the early stages of AD the anomia reflects breakdown in semantic memory, but as the disease progresses, perceptual problems also contribute.

Henderson *et al.* (1990) also addressed the issue of whether the lexico-semantic deficits causing anomia in AD are due to lexical access or loss of information. From the consistency of responses over time, they concluded that anomia in AD is due to a loss of semantic information.

Word–picture matching, probed knowledge, and other tests of semantic memory

The evidence from error analyses points to a defect within the semantic system, but is rather indirect. More convincing evidence would be if there were consistent impairment of knowledge for the same items across tests which access knowledge via different modalities (for example picture naming, picture–name matching, generating verbal descriptions in response to the item's name, etc.). The technique of testing knowledge of items across a range of semantic categories, both within and across modalities, has been applied in detail to individual cases with semantic memory loss, mostly resulting from herpes simplex encephalitis (Sartori and Job 1988; Warrington and Shallice 1984), and in semantic dementia (Hodges *et al.* 1995). In the context of AD, Huff *et al.* (1986) showed a significant correlation between anomia and word comprehension for the same exemplars in a selected group of patients. Chertkow and co-workers (1990, 1992) extended these findings and confirmed a significant item-by-item correspondence between comprehension (picture–word matching) and name production. Their patients also showed a significantly greater ability to answer detailed probe questions concerning items whose pictures they named correctly. Further evidence of impaired semantic memory in AD includes defective ranking of object attributes (Grober *et al.* 1985).

The semantic battery approach

The nature of the semantic deficit can be addressed more extensively by the use of integrated semantic batteries, testing knowledge of items common to the various tests (Fig. 8.1). This approach has been adopted in our studies (Hodges and Patterson 1995; Hodges *et al.* 1992*a*, *b*). The battery of tests, all employing one consistent set of stimulus items, was designed to assess input to and output from central representational knowledge about the same group of items via different sensory modalities. It contains 48 items from three categories of animals (land animals, sea creatures, and birds) and three categories of man-made items (household items, vehicles, and musical instruments) matched for category prototypicality and word frequency. They were chosen from the corpus of line drawings by Snodgrass and Vanderwart (1980). In brief, the original five sub-tests consisted of;

1. Category fluency for each of the six main categories plus two lower order categories (breeds of dog and types of boat).
2. Naming of all 48 line drawings with cueing.
3. Picture sorting at superordinate (living vs. man-made), category (land animal vs. bird vs. water creature; household item vs. vehicle vs. musical instrument), and subordinate (e.g. fierce vs. non-fierce animal; native vs. foreign; kitchen vs. non-kitchen item; electrical vs. non-electrical, etc.) levels.
4. Picture pointing to spoken word using within-category arrays (the original battery used arrays of six items all from the same category, such as land animals, but in the subsequent version we now use

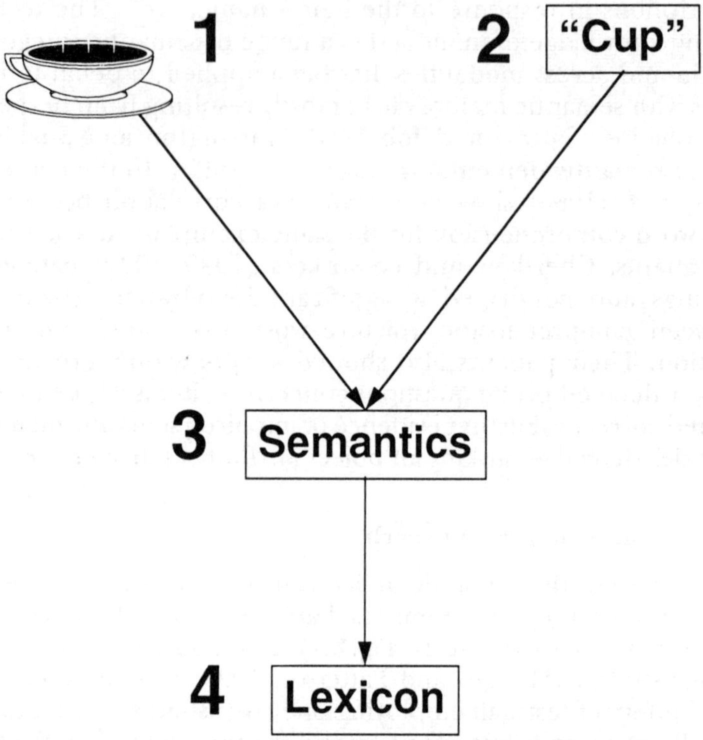

Components employed by individual tests	
Category fluency	3,4
Picture naming	1,3,4
Word-picture matching	2,3,1
Generation of definitions	2,3, 4
Naming to description	3,4
Picture sorting	3

FIG. 8.1 Use of the semantic battery to assess input to and output from the semantic system using a consistent set of stimuli across different tests.

arrays of eight which contain two foils not otherwise included in the test battery).

5. Generation of verbal definitions in response to the spoken name of the item (e.g. 'Tell me everything you can about a rhinoceros'; 'penguin'; 'guitar' etc.). The following two sub-tests have been added since the battery was developed:
6. Naming in response to the verbal description (e.g. 'What do you call the large African animal with a curved horn on its head?').

7. Semantic feature questions—for each item we designed eight questions such that four questions explore knowledge of physical features (size, shape, colour, etc.) and four probe associative non-perceptual knowledge (habitat, diet, uses, etc.).

In our 1992 study, we found that there was significant semantic memory impairment in AD on all the sub-tests of the semantic battery (Hodges *et al.* 1992*b*). The pattern of the results suggested a loss of semantic knowledge rather than a disorder of semantic access. This conclusion was based upon three lines of evidence. First, the finding of preserved superordinate knowledge on the picture sorting and definitions tests, together with the suggestion of a disproportionate reduction in the generation of exemplars from the lower order categories on the fluency test (that is relatively greater impairment for the category 'dogs' than for the category 'animals'). Second, the finding of a marked frequency effect, in that AD patients were more impaired at naming less familiar items. Third, and perhaps most persuasively, the demonstration of item-by-item correspondence across a number of sub-tests. In other words, the AD patients showed a significant correspondence between the individual items that they were unable to name and those that produced errors on the picture matching-to-spoken word test. Similarly there was item-specificity between naming and sorting, and between naming and the ability to generate adequate definitions in response to spoken names. Analysis of the exemplars produced on the category fluency tests and performance on the naming test showed that unnamed items were very rarely produced in the free recall condition. These results combined offered strong evidence in favour of semantic memory loss in AD.

A similar approach has been taken by Bayles *et al.* who have devised a battery of tests, using the same thirteen exemplars across a range of tasks including naming, auditory comprehension, category recognition, and pantomime expression (Bayles *et al.* 1990, 1991). They have emphasized the difficulty in interpreting performance across tests with very different demands, some of which have high chance levels due to their multiple-choice format. Clearly further longitudinal studies based on a larger corpus of items are required.

REMOTE MEMORY: THE CONTRIBUTION OF SEMANTIC IMPAIRMENT TO TESTS OF FACE AND NAME IDENTIFICATION

Famous face and famous name tests have been used to study the remote memory impairment seen in AD (Beatty *et al.* 1988; Greene and Hodges 1996; Hodges *et al.* 1993; Wilson *et al.* 1981). Prior to discussing their results, a brief description of the model of face and name processing which has been widely applied to the analysis of patients with prosopagnosia will be given (Bruce and Young 1986; Valentine *et al.* 1991).

In this model, the correct naming of a famous face depends upon four basic stages of processing. First, a stage of visual processing (or structural encoding) in which a complex percept of the face is built up, presumably in visual association areas. Next, the structural description is recognized as familiar by matching it to the store of unknown familiar faces—breakdown at this level of the 'face recognition unit' is the deficit postulated to occur in classic prosopagnosia in which patients fail to recognize people from their faces but usually identify

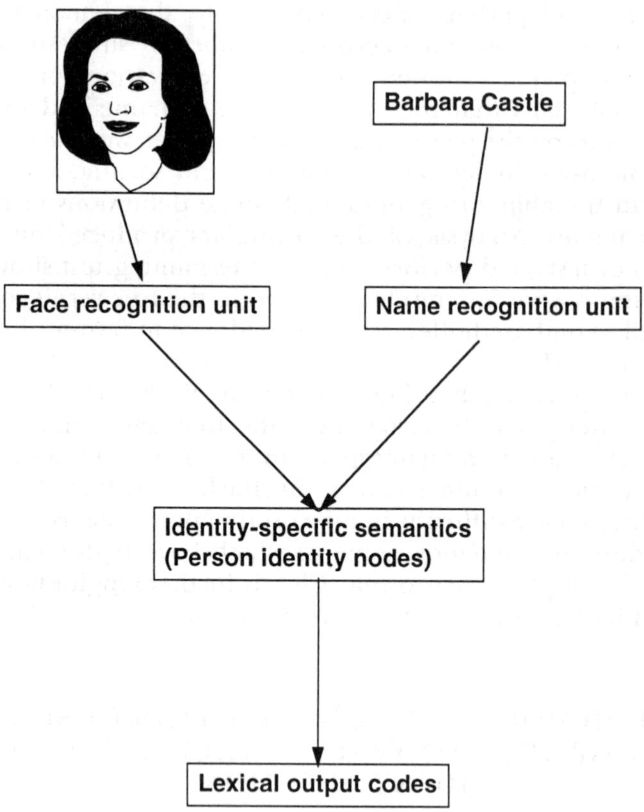

FIG. 8.2 The functional model of face and name reognition (from Valentine *et al.* 1991).

the same individuals from their voice, clothing, or gait. In the third stage, person-specific semantic information associated with the face is activated. Lastly, there is the stage of name retrieval followed by phonological and articulatory processing. This sequential processing model is almost identical to that proposed for naming of objects except that each face is unique and cannot be identified unless there is an exact match between the structural description and recognition unit. Impairment of the face recognition unit, semantic store, or lexicon can lead to impaired recognition, identification, and naming, respectively.

This model has more recently been updated to incorporate the identification of people from their names (Burton and Bruce 1992, 1993; Valentine *et al.* 1991). Recognizing a name as familiar involves unique name recognition units, analogous to face recognition units. These subsequently activate semantic knowledge regarding why the person is famous.

In an attempt to explore the nature of the cognitive deficit underlying AD patients' failure to identify famous faces, Hodges *et al.* (1993) tested recognition (in arrays consisting of famous and non-famous faces), naming, identification (the ability to provide person-specific details about unnamed faces), and cued naming using semantic and first-name cues. The AD patients were impaired in all test conditions. Performance in all five conditions declined with disease severity, but this effect did not reach significance in the recognition and naming with phonological (first-name) cues. A number of lines of converging evidence suggested that the primary deficit was not in name access, but instead represented a loss of stored semantic knowledge about the person represented. First, the patients named and identified a significantly smaller proportion of faces that they recognized as famous than did controls; second, at no stage was identification superior to spontaneous naming; and third, semantic cueing did not aid performance.

We have recently (Greene and Hodges 1996) extended these studies to include famous names as well as famous faces. At a cognitive level, the deficit in face and name processing involved primarily identification and naming, although recognition was also involved to a lesser extent. This suggested that so-called 'face and name recognition units' are mildly affected, but that the deficit primarily involves semantic knowledge of famous persons and post-semantic processing. We also found a strong concordance between performance on the face and name identification tasks, implying that these tasks tap a common pool of person-specific semantic knowledge. However, famous face and name identification correlated poorly with general semantic tasks. It appears, therefore, that person-based knowledge and general semantic knowledge are represented separately. Further support for this assertion comes from the findings in a patient with focal right temporal lobe atrophy presenting with a progressive loss of person-based semantics but sparing general semantic knowledge (Evans *et al.* 1995).

HOW EARLY IN AD DOES SEMANTIC IMPAIRMENT OCCUR?

It is not clear how early in the course of the disease, and how consistently, the defect in semantic memory occurs. Most studies of semantic memory in AD have concerned patients with well-established disease (e.g. Hodges *et al.* 1992*b*; Martin and Fedio 1983; or have deliberately selected patients with evidence of semantic memory impairment for investigation (e.g. Chertkow and Bub 1990). Moreover, virtually all studies (with the exception of Bayles *et al.* 1991 and Chertkow and Bub 1990) have considered group data only, rather than adopting a multiple single-case strategy. We have recently (Hodges and Patterson 1995) addressed these issues. Semantic memory is mildly, though significantly, impaired at the very earliest stages of AD, designated minimal (MMSE > 24) in our studies, but becomes a major feature of AD in later stages of the disease. The semantic impairment in early disease is largely due to a consistent impairment across the range of tests in a subgroup of individuals.

WHICH TESTS OF SEMANTIC MEMORY ARE IMPAIRED FIRST IN AD?

It is particularly interesting to study cases of AD with very mild semantic impairment as they give greater insight into the structure of semantic memory than those with more pervasive impairment. In a recent study (Hodges and Patterson 1995), we have shown that the most mildly demented group (designated minimal AD) were impaired on category fluency, picture naming, naming to description, answering semantic features questions, and the Pyramids and Palm Trees Test. There was no significant impairment on word–picture matching and picture sorting tests. All of the tests in the battery share, in common, the fact that the central semantic representation of that item must be activated in order to achieve the correct response. Hence, the ability to name pictures, to match a spoken word to the correct picture from an array of semantically related items (for example 'Point to the tiger' when shown eight foreign-land animals), and to answer similar types of questions ('Does a rhinoceros have a horn?', 'Does it eat meat?', etc.)

all require access to semantic memory. In addition, each individual task depends upon additional and different subsidiary processes. In the case of picture naming and word–picture matching, for instance, there is a succession of essential pre-semantic perceptual processing stages. Naming pictures and naming to description depend upon additional post-semantic (phonological and articulatory) stages.

Of the tests from the semantic battery on which the minimal AD subgroup showed significant impairment, three of the four have, in common, that they require a spoken output. This might lead one to the conclusion either that verbally based semantic knowledge is selectively impaired early in AD, or alternatively that such patients show a post-semantic language output disorder. There are three reasons for doubting that either of the latter explanations is likely to be correct, and for concluding instead that the impairment reflects an actual breakdown in semantic memory. The first is that it is likely that the pattern observed in the minimal AD patients reflects, at least in part, the order of task difficulty. Another is that minimal AD patients were impaired on the Pyramids and Palm Trees Test (Howard and Patterson 1992), the three-picture version of which can be considered a test of non-verbal semantic knowledge, suggesting that there is a central semantic deficit in AD. The third line of evidence is the close item-by-item correspondence in individual patients' performance across semantically based tests, which can reasonably be explained only on the basis of a breakdown in semantic memory itself rather than a failure of access (for a fuller discussion of this topic see Chertkow *et al.* 1992 and Hodges *et al.* 1992*b*).

We suggest, therefore, that useful tests for the detection of subtle semantic deficits in clinical practice are category fluency, naming of pictures and from verbal descriptions, and the Pyramids and Palm Trees Test.

IS THE SEMANTIC IMPAIRMENT IN AD A STORAGE OR ACCESS PROBLEM?

There has been considerable controversy regarding whether impaired performance by AD patients on semantic memory tests is due to degradation of the representations within semantic memory or a failure of procedures yielding access to that representation. Some researchers have claimed that the deficits found on tests of semantic memory may primarily reflect impaired access to semantic memory (for review see Bayles *et al.* 1991; Nebes 1989) but the majority of investigators support the explanation which hypothesizes a breakdown in the structure of semantic memory (Chan *et al.* 1993; Chertkow and Bub 1990; Hodges *et al.* 1992*b*; Martin and Fedio 1983). For instance, in both the studies by Chertkow and colleagues (1990, 1992) and that by Hodges *et al.* (1992*b*) there was a highly significant item-by-item correspondence between AD subjects; performance on picture naming and on other tests designed specifically to probe for semantic knowledge about the same items.

A number of criteria have been suggested to adjudicate between these disorders of access and of stored knowledge, including item-specific consistency of errors, susceptibility to priming, a marked word frequency effect, and hierarchically modulated loss from more detailed to more general knowledge (Shallice 1988; Warrington and Shallice 1984).

More modern parallel distributed processing-based models of semantic organization bring into question the validity of these distinctions (Farah and McClelland 1991; Patterson and Hodges 1995). Since it is no longer held that semantic knowledge is organized hierarchically, but rather represented in the form of distributed features, there is no a priori reason to believe that a loss of features, rather than disruption of access, would cause differential effects. Moreover, there is some evidence that a disorder of access to phonological forms from semantics may cause item-specific consistency (Funnell and Hodges 1991), which obviously casts some doubt upon this criterion for deciding between loss of representation and impaired access to such representations.

In conclusion, the current evidence from performance on explicit tasks points to a loss of knowledge, although we suspect that this distinction may not hold up to further scrutiny, a point which has been made by Rapp and Caramazza (1993).

CATEGORY-SPECIFICITY IN AD

It is now well established that some patients with semantic memory impairment, usually in the context of herpes simplex viral encephalitis, may have a disproportionate loss of knowledge about living, as opposed to man-made, things (Laurent *et al.* 1990; Pietrini *et al.* 1988; Sartori and Job 1988; Sartori *et al.* 1993; Silveri and Gainotti 1988; Warrington and Shallice 1984). Patients with the reverse dissociation have also been reported (Hillis and Caramazza 1991; Sacchett and Humphreys 1992; Warrington and McCarthy 1983, 1987). The interpretation of these findings is, however, more controversial, but most authorities now agree that these patterns reflect the differential weighting of perceptual and function attributes in the representation of natural vs. artefactual objects (Farah and McClelland 1991; McCarthy and Warrington 1988; Patterson and Hodges 1995). The issue of the most appropriate matching of items in tests of semantic memory, as most man-made objects are rated as more familiar than the majority of animals, has also added to the difficulty in interpreting the reported dissociations (Funnell 1995; Funnell and Sheridan 1992; Stewart *et al.* 1992). If we assume that the representation of items from the natural world is in some way distinct, both cognitively and neurologically, then it is possible that AD could systematically impair knowledge of natural (or artefactual) things. Silveri *et al.* (1991) reported that AD patients were worse at naming, and on a verbal associates recognition task, for living things. We have been unable to replicate this finding using a more comprehensive battery of tests in a larger group of patients (Hodges *et al.* 1992*b*; Hodges and Patterson 1995).

SEMANTIC DEMENTIA

Although we consider this condition to be cognitively and pathologically separate from Alzheimer's disease, we mention it here briefly on account of the insight it provides into the organization of semantic memory and the independence of semantic memory from other cognitive modules. This condition affects semantic memory while leaving all other cognitive abilities relatively intact (Hodges *et al.* 1992*a*, 1994; Saffran and Schwartz 1994; Snowden *et al.* 1989, 1994). The term semantic dementia was chosen to convey the concept of profound and pervasive semantic deterioration which disrupts factual memory and knowledge, language and object recognition.

Patients usually present complaining that they have 'forgotten' the names of things or people. Relatives notice their declining vocabulary and word-finding difficulties. This clinical syndrome is characterized by fluent dysphasia with severe anomia, reduced vocabulary and prominent impairment of single-word comprehension. Category fluency is impaired early in the course of the disease, but letter-based fluency is characteristically well preserved. Semantic memory tests, such as those in our semantic memory test battery, reveal a radically impoverished knowledge about a range of living and man-made items. In contrast, the sound-based (phonological) and grammatical aspects of spoken language are largely preserved, as is comprehension of syntactically complex commands. Reading shows a pattern of surface dyslexia (namely a selective impairment in the ability to read words with irregular spelling to sound correspondence, such as pint, island, with the production of regularization errors).

Perhaps the most striking contrast to AD is the relative preservation of autobiographical and episodic memory, certainly in the early stages of the disorder. The distinction between affected semantic memory and preserved episodic memory is most clearly seen in the area of remote memory. Personal semantic memory is lost, with preservation of personal episodic memory. However, the laying down of new episodic memories is likely to be seriously impaired with progression of the semantic deficit as semantic memory must ultimately subserve other memory processes.

Non-verbal memory, perceptual, and visuospatial abilities are also consistently preserved. In some cases, behavioural and personality changes may supervene, with features of the Kluver–Bucy syndrome such as hyperphagia and sexual disinhibition.

Radiological investigation have shown marked focal temporal neocortical atrophy particularly involving the inferior and middle temporal gyri, with relative sparing of the hippocampus. Functional imaging by SPECT appears more sensitive in early cases showing hypoperfusion of the dominant temporal lobe (Hodges *et al.* 1992*a*; Sinnatamby *et al.* in press; Snowden *et al.* 1989). The pathological data is, as yet, limited but two of the earliest reported patients (then termed selective impairment of semantic memory) studied by Warrington (1975) were later shown to have Pick's disease (Cummings and Duchen 1981). A similar patient with Pick's pathology was reported by Graff-Radford *et al.* (1990) and one of our patients (JL) recently died and was shown to have atypical Pick's pathology (Hodges *et al.* 1995).

Although it remains possible that semantic dementia represents an atypical focal form of Alzheimer's disease, the current evidence suggests that this is unlikely and that most patients have Pick's disease.

THE NEURAL BASIS OF SEMANTIC MEMORY

Unlike episodic memory (Squire 1982), the neural substrate of semantic memory has been poorly defined. Semantic memory probably relies on neural networks, distributed over broad areas of cerebral cortex bilaterally. However, the region of most importance appears to be the inferolateral areas of temporal neocortex, more so on the left (Damasio *et al.* 1990; Patterson and Hodges 1995).

Cases of semantic dementia have shown consistent imaging (Hodges *et al.* 1992*a*; Patterson *et al.* 1994; Snowden *et al.* 1992; Tanabe *et al.* 1993; Tyrrell *et al.* 1990) and pathological abnormalities (Graff-Radford *et al.* 1990; Neary *et al.* 1993) in the temporal lobes. The areas most involved appear to be the temporal neocortex, with an emphasis on the inferior and middle temporal gyri and the polar region. More medial temporal structures (the hippocampus, parahippocampal gyrus, and subiculum) are relatively spared.

Cases of semantic memory loss due to herpes simplex viral encephalitis have also implicated the temporal neocortex (Bakchine *et al.* 1986; Damasio *et al.* 1985; De Renzi *et al.* 1987; McCarthy and Warrington 1992; Pietrini *et al.* 1988; Sartori and Job 1988; Sartori *et al.* 1993; Warrington and Shallice 1984) and similar conclusions regarding localization of semantic memory have been reached in studies of head-injured subjects (Behrmann and Bub 1992; Bub *et al.* 1985, 1988).

Thus, there is converging evidence that the temporal lobe plays a critical role in semantic memory. It is unclear, however, exactly which temporal lobe structures are consistently involved in semantic dementia, and whether there is regional or lateralized specialization of function. Some cases have had bilateral temporal lobe atrophy, while in others the atrophy has been confined to the left (Hodges *et al.* 1992*a*).

Given what is already known about the localization of verbal vs. non-verbal cognitive abilities, one hypothesis is that patients with left-sided pathology will have impairment in verbal semantic knowledge with relative preservation of non-verbally based knowledge, while for those with right-sided disease, the opposite pattern would be found. The current evidence is conflicting (Patterson and Hodges 1995) some patients with left-sided pathology (on MRI and PET) have shown both verbal and non-verbal impairments, while one recently studied case with selective right temporal lobe atrophy (Evans *et al.* 1995) presented with progressive prosopagnosia which evolved into a loss of person-specific knowledge.

There is overwhelming evidence that semantic memory is impaired in AD; this appears to be due a deficit of storage rather than of access. Although semantic memory relies on a distributed neuro-anatomical system, the temporal neocortex, particularly of the dominant hemisphere, is important. The development of semantic impairment in AD, and the stage of the illness at which this occurs, is likely to reflect spread of AD pathology to these areas.

REFERENCES

Allport, A. (1985). Distributed memory, modular subsystems and dysphasia. In *Current perspectives in dysphasia* (ed. S. K. Newman and R. Epstein), pp. 32–60. Churchill Livingstone, Edinburgh.

Bakchine, S., Chain, F., and Lhermitte, F. (1986). Syndrome de Kluver—Bucy humain complet apres une encephalite a herpes simplex type 2. *Revue Neurologique*, **142**, 126–32.

Bayles, K. A. and Tolmoeda, D. K. (1983). Confrontational naming impairment in dementia. *Brain and Language*, **19**, 98–114.

Bayles, K. A., Tomoeda, C. K., and Trosset, M. W. (1990). Naming and categorical knowledge in Alzheimer's disease: the process of semantic memory deterioration. *Brain and Language*. **39**, 498–510.

Bayles, K. A., Tomoeda, C. K., Kasniak, A. W., and Trosset, M. W. (1991). Alzheimer's disease effects on semantic memory: loss of structure or impaired processing. *Journal of Cognitive Neuroscience*, **3**, 166–82.

Beatty, W. W., Salmon, D. P., Butters, N., Heindel, W. C., and Granholm, E. L. (1988). Retrograde amnesia in patients with Alzheimer's disease or Huntington's disease. *Neurobiology of Ageing*, **9**, 181–6.

Behrmann, M. and Bub, D. (1992). Surface dyslexia and dysgraphia: dual routes, single lexicon. *Cognitive Neuropsychology*, **9**, 209–51.

Bowles, N. L., Obler, L. K., and Albert, M. L. (1987). Naming errors in healthy aging and dementia of the Alzheimer type. *Cortex*, **23**, 519–24.

Bruce, V. and Young, A. W. (1986). Understanding face recognition. *British Journal of Psychology*, **77**, 305–27.

Bub, D., Cancelliere, A., and Kertesz, A. (1985). Whole-word and analytic translation of spelling to sound in a nonsemantic reader. In *Surface dyslexia* (ed. K. Patterson, J. C. Marshall, and N. Coltheart), pp.15–34. Erlbaum, London.

Bub, D., Black, S., Hampson, E., and Kertesz, A. (1988). Semantic encoding of pictures and words: some neuropsychological observations. *Cognitive Neuropsychology* **5**, 27–66.

Burton, A. M. and Bruce, V. (1992). I recognise your face but I can't remember your name: a simple explanation? *British Journal of Psychology* 45–61.

Burton, A. M. and Bruce, V. (1993). Naming faces and naming names: exploring an interactive activation model of person recognition. *Memory*, **1**, 457–80.

Butters, N., Granholm, E., Salmon, D. P., Grant, I., and Wolfe, J. (1987). Episodic and semantic memory: a comparison of amnesic and demented patients. *Journal of clinical and Experimental Neuropsychology*. **9**, 479–97.

Caramazza, A., Hillis, A. E., Rapp, B. C., and Romani, C. (1990). The multiple semantics hypothesis: multiple confusions. *Cognitive Neuropsychology*, **7**, 161–89.

Chan, A. S., Butters, N., Paulson, J. S., Salmon, D. P., Swenson, M., and Maloney, L. (1993). An assessment of the semantic network in patients with Alzheimer's disease. *Journal of Cognitive Neuroscience*, **5**, 254–61.

Chertkow, H. and Bub, D. (1990). Semantic memory loss in dementia of Alzheimer's type. *Brain*, **113**, 397–417.

Chertkow, H., Bub, D., and Caplan, D. (1992). Constraining theories of semantic memory processing: evidence from dementia. *Cognitive Neuropsychology*, **9**, 327–65.

Coslett, H. B. and Saffran, E. M. (1989). Preserved object recognition and reading comprehension in optic aphasia. *Brain*, **112**, 1091–110.

Cummings, J. L. and Duchen, L. W. (1981). Kluver—Bucy syndrome in Pick's disease: clinical and pathological correlations. *Neurology*, **31**, 1415–22.

Damasio, A. R., Eslinger, P. J., Damasio, H., Van Hoesen, G. W., and Cornell, S. (1985). Multimodal amnesic syndrome following bilateral temporal and basal forebrain damage. *Archives of Neurology*, **42**, 252–9.

Damasio, A.R., Damasio, H., Tranel, D., and Brandt, J.P. (1990). Neural regionalisation of knowledge access: preliminary evidence. In *Symposia on Quantitative Biology*, Vol. 55, pp. 1039–47. Laboratory Press, Cold Spring Harbor.

De Renzi, E., Liotti, M., and Nichelli, P. (1987). Semantic amnesia with preservation of autobiographic memory: a case report. *Cortex*, **23**, 575–97.

Evans, J. J., Heggs, A. J., Antoun, N., and Hodges, J. R. (1995). Progressive prosopagnosia associated with selective right temporal lobe atrophy: a new syndrome? *Brain*, **118**, 1–13.

Farah, M. J. and McClelland, J. L. (1991). A computational model of semantic memory impairment: Modality specificity and emergent category specificity. *Journal of Experimental Psychology: General*, **120**, 339–57.

Funnell, E. (1995). From objects to properties: Evidence for spreading semantic activation in a case of semantic dementia. *Memory*, **3**, 497–519.

Funnell, E. and Hodges, J. R. (1991). Progressive loss of access to spoken word forms in a case of Alzheimer's disease. *Proceedings of the Royal Society London B*, **243**, 173–9.

Funnell, E. and Sheridan, J. (1992). Categories of knowledge: unfamiliar aspects of living and non-living things. *Cognitive Neuropsychology*, **9**, 135–54.

Gainotti, G., Miceli, G., Caltagirone, C., Silveri, M. C., and Masullo, C. (1981). The relationship between type of naming error and semantic-lexical discrimination in aphasic patients. *Cortex*, **17**, 401–9.

Graff-Radford, N. R., Damasio, A. R., Hyman, B. T., Hart, M. N., Tranel, D., Damasio, H., *et al.*, (1990). Progressive aphasia in a patient with Pick's disease: a neuropsychological, radiologic, and anatomic study. *Neurology*, **40**, 620–6.

Greene, J. D. W. and Hodges, J. R. (1996). Identification of famous faces and names in early Alzheimer's disease, *Brain*, **119**, 111–28.

Grober, E., Buschke, H., Kawas, C., and Fuld, P. (1985). Impaired ranking of semantic attributes in dementia. *Brain and Language*, **26**, 276–86.

Henderson, V. W., Mack, W., Freed, D. M., Kempler, D., and Andersen, E. S. (1990). Naming consistency in Alzheimer's disease. *Brain and Language*, **39**, 530–8.

Hills, A. E. and Caramazza, A. (1991). Category-specific naming and comprehension impairment—a double dissociation. *Brain*, **114**, 2081–94.

Hodges, J. R. and Patterson, K. (1995). Is semantic memory consistently impaired early in the course of Alzheimer's disease? Neuroanatomical and diagnostic implications. *Neuropsychologia*, **33**, 441–59.

Hodges, J. R., Salmon, D. P., and Butters, N. (1990). Differential impairment of semantic and episodic memory in Alzheimer's and Huntington's diseases: a controlled prospective study. *Journal of Neurology, Neurosurgery and Psychiatry*, **53**, 1089–95.

Hodges, J. R., Salmon, D. P., and Butters, N. (1991). The nature of the naming deficit in Alzheimer's and Huntington's disease. *Brain*, **114**, 1547–58.

Hodges, J. R., Patterson, K., Oxbury, S., and Funnell, E. (1992*a*). Semantic dementia: progressive fluent aphasia with temporal lobe atrophy. *Brain*, **115**, 1783–806.

Hodges, J. R., Salmon, D. P., and Butters, N. (1992*b*). Semantic memory impairment in Alzheimer's disease: failure of access or degraded knowledge? *Neuropsychologia*, **30**, 310–11.

Hodges, J. R., Salmon, D. P., and Butters, N. (1993). Recognition and naming of famous faces in Alzheimer's disease: a cognitive analysis. *Neuropsychologia*, **31**, 775–88.

Hodges, J. R., Patterson, K., and Tyler, L. K. (1994). Loss of semantic memory: implications for the modularity of mind. *Cognitive Neuropsychology*, **11**, 505–42.

Hodges, J. R., Graham, N., and Patterson, K. (1995). Charting the progression in semantic dementia: implications for the organisation of semantic memory. *Memory*, **3**, 463–95.

Howard, D. and Patterson, K. (1992). *Pyramids and Palm Trees: a test of semantic access from pictures and words.* Thames Valley Publishing Company, Bury St Edmunds, Suffolk.

Huff, F. J., Corkin, S., and Growdon, J. H. (1986). Semantic impairment and anomia in Alzheimer's disease. *Brain and Language*, **28**, 235–49.

Kirshner, H. S., Webb, W. G., and Kelly, M. P. (1984). The naming disorder of dementia. *Neuropsychologia*, **22**, 23–30.

Kohn, S. E. and Goodglass, H. (1985). Picture-naming in aphasia. *Brain and Language*, **24**, 266–83.

Laurent, B., Allegri, R. F., Michel, D., Trillet, M., Naegele-Faure, B., Foyatier, N. *et al.* (1990). Post-herpetic encephalitis with lateralised lesions: long-term neuropsychological study of 9 cases. *Revue Neurologique (Paris).* **146** (11), 671–81.

McCarthy, R. A. and Warrington, E. K. (1988). Evidence for modality-specific meaning systems in the brain. *Nature*, **334**, 428–30.

McCarthy, R. A. and Warrington, E. K. (1990*a*). *Cognitive neuropsychology: a clinical introduction.* Academic Press, San Diego.

McCarthy, R. A. and Warrington, E. K. (1990*b*). Evidence for modality-specific meaning systems in the brain. *Nature*, **334**, 428–30.

McCarthy, R. A. and Warrington, E. K. (1992). Actors but not scripts: the dissociation of people and events in retrograde amnesia. *Neuropsychologia*, **30** (7), 633–44.

Martin, A. and Fedio, P. (1983). Word production and comprehension in Alzheimer's disease: the breakdown of semantic knowledge. *Brain and Language*, **19**, 124–41.

Monsch, A. U., Bondi, M. W., Butters, N., Salmon, D. P., Katzman, R., and Thal, L. J. (1992). Comparisons of verbal fluency tasks in the detection of dementia of the Alzheimer type. *Archives of Neurology*, **49**, 1253–8.

Monsch, A. U., Bondi, M. W., Butters, N., Pauslen, J. S., Salmon, D. P., Brugger, P. *et al.* (1994). A comparison of category and letter fluency in Alzheimer's disease and Huntington's disease. *Neuropsychologia*, **8**, 25–30.

Moss, H. E., Tyler, L. K., Hodges, J. R., and Patterson, K. E. (1995). Exploring the loss of semantic memory in semantic dementia: evidence from a primed monitoring study. *Neuropsychology*, **9**, 16–26.

Neary, D., Snowden, J. S., and Mann, D. M. A. (1993). The clinical pathological correlates of lobar atrophy. *Dementia*, **4**, 154–9.

Nebes, R. B. (1989). Semantic memory in Alzheimer's disease. *Psychological Bulletin*, **106**, 377–94.

Ober, B. A., Koss, E., Friedland, R. P., and Delis, D. C. (1985). Processes of verbal memory failure in Alzheimer-type dementia. *Brain and Cognition*, **4**, 90–103.

Patterson, K. E., Graham, N., and Hodges, J. R. (1994). The impact of semantic memory loss on phonological representations. **6** (1), 57–69.

Patterson, K. E. and Hodges, J. R. (1995). Disorders of semantic memory. In *Handbook of memory disorders* (ed. A. Baddeley, B. A. Wilson, and F. Watts), pp. 167–86. John Wiley & Sons, Chichester.

Pietrini, V., Nertempi, P., Vaglia, A., Revello, M. G., Pinna, V., and Ferro-Milone, F. (1988). Recovery from herpes simplex encephalitis: selective impairment of specific semantic categories with neuroradiological correlation. *Journal of Neurology, Neurosurgery and Psychiatry*, **51**, 1284–93.

Rapp, B. and Caramazza, A. (1993). On the distinction between deficits of access and deficits of storage: a question of theory. *Cognitive Neuropsychology*, **10**, 113–41.

Ratcliffe, G. and Newcombe, F. (1982). Object recognition: some deductions from the clinical evidence. In *Normality and pathology in cognitive functions* (ed. A. W. Ellis), pp. 147–71. Academic Press, London.

Riddoch, M. J., Humphreys, G. W., Coltheart, M., and Funnell, E. (1988). Semantic systems or system? Neuropsychological evidence re-examined. *Cognitive Neuropsychology*, **5**, 3–25.

Rosen, W. (1980). Verbal fluency in ageing and dementia. *Journal of Clinical Neuropsychology*, **2**, 135–46.

Rosser, A. and Hodges, J. R. (1994). Initial letter and semantic category fluency in Alzheimer's disease, Huntington's disease and progressive supranuclear palsy. *Journal of Neurology, Neurosurgery and Psychiatry*, **57**, 1389–94.

Sacchett, C. and Humphreys, G. W. (1992). Calling a squirrel a squirrel but a canoe a wig-wam: a category-specific deficit for artefactual objects and body parts. *Cognitive Neuropsychology*, **9**, 73–86.

Saffran, E.M. and Schwartz, M.F. (1994). Of cabbages and things: semantic memory from a neuropsychological perspective – a tutorial review. In *Attention and performance XV*, (ed. C. Umilta and M. Moscovitch). Lawrence Erlbaum, Hove.

Sartori, G. and Job, R. (1988). The oyster with four legs: a neuropsychological study on the interaction of visual and semantic information. *Cognitive Neuropsychology*, **5**, 105–32.

Sartori, G., Job, R., Miozzo, M., Zago, S., and Marchiori, G. (1993). Category-specific form-knowledge deficit in a patient with Herpes Simple virus encephalitis. *Journal of Clinical and Experimental Neuropsychology*, **15**, 280–99.

Shallice, T. (1988). *From neuropsychology to mental structure*. Cambridge University Press, Cambridge.

Silveri, M. C. and Gainotti, G. (1988). Interaction between vision and language in category-specific semantic impairment. *Cognitive Neuropsychology*, **3**, 677–709.

Silveri, M. C., Daniele, A., Giustolisi, L., and Gainotti, G. (1991). Dissociation between knowledge of living and nonliving things in dementia of the Alzheimer type. *Neurology*, **41**, 545–6.

Sinnatamby, R., Antoun, N. A., Freer, C. E. L., Miles, K. A., and Hodges, J. R. The neuroradiological findings in primary progressive aphasia: a comparison of CT, MRI and cerebral perfusion SPECT. *Neuroradiology*, (In press).

Smith, S. R., Murdoch, B. E., and Chenery, H. J. (1989). Semantic abilities in dementia of the Alzheimer type: 1. Lexical semantics. *Brain and Language*, **36**, 314–24.

Snodgrass, J. G. and Vanderwart, M. (1980). A standardised set of 260 pictures: normal for name agreement, familiarity and visual complexity. *Journal of Experimental Psychology: General*, **6**, 174–215.

Snowden, J. S., Goulding, P. J., and Neary, D. (1989). Semantic dementia: a form of circumscribed cerebral atrophy. *Behavioural Neurology*, **2**, 167–82.

Snowden, J. S., Neary, D., Mann, D. M. A., Goulding, P. J., and Testa, H. J. (1992). Progressive language disorder due to lobar atrophy. *Annals of Neurology*, **31**, 174–83.

Snowden, J., Griffiths, H., and Neary, D. (1994). Semantic dementia: Autobiographical contribution to preservation of meaning. *Cognitive Neuropsychology*, **11**, 265–88.

Squire, L. R. (1982). The neuropsychology of human memory. *Annual Review of Neuroscience*, **5**, 241–73.

Stewart, F., Parkin, A. J., and Hunkin, N. M. (1992). Naming impairments following recovery from Herpes simplex encephalitis: category-specific? *Quarterly Journal of Experimental Psychology*, **44A**, 261–84.

Tanabe, H., Nakagawa, Y., Ikeda, M., Kazui, H., Yamamoto, H., Ikejiri, Y. *et al.* (1993). The neural substrate of the semantic memory for words. *Journal of Clinical and Experimental Neuropsychology*, **15**, 395.

Tulving, E. (1972). Episodic and semantic memory. In *Organisation of memory* (ed. E. Tulving and W. Donaldson), pp. 381–403. Academic Press, New York.

Tulving, E. (1983). *Elements of episodic memory*. Clarendon Press, Oxford.

Tyrrell, P. J., Warrington, E. K., Frackowiak, R. S. J., and Rossor, M. N. (1990). Heterogeneity in progressive aphasia due to focal cortical atrophy. A clinical and PET study. *Brain*, **113**, 1321–36.

Valentine, T., Bredart, S., Lawson, R., and Ward, G. (1991). What's in a name? Access to information from people's names. *European Journal of Cognitive Psychology*, **3**, 147–76.

Warrington, E. K. (1975). Selective impairment of semantic memory. *Quarterly Journal of Experimental Psychology*, **27**, 635–57.

Warrington, E. K. and McCarthy, R. A. (1983). Category-specific access dysphasia. *Brain*, **106**, 859–78.

Warrington, E. K. and McCarthy, R. A. (1987). Categories of knowledge: Further fractionation and an attempted integration. *Brain*, **110**, 1273–96.

Warrington, E. K. and McCarthy, R. A. (1988). The fractionation of retrograde amnesia. *Brain and Cognition*, **7**, 184–200.

Warrington, E. K. and Shallice, T. (1984). Category specific semantic impairments. *Brain*, **107**, 829–54.

Weingartner, H. J., Kawas, C., Rawlings, R., and Shapiro, M. (1993). Changes in semantic memory in early stage Alzheimer's disease patients. *The Gerontologist*, **33**, 637–43.

Wilson, R. S., Kaszniak, A. W., and Fox, J. H. (1981). Remote memory in senile dementia. *Cortex*, **17**, 41–8.

NINE

Reading disorder in Alzheimer-type dementia

Jane L. Mathias

INTRODUCTION

An association between the impairment of language and dementia was first reported in Prichard's (1837) description of a group of dementing patients who experienced a progressive loss of memory, reasoning, and language comprehension (see Breitner and Folstein, 1984). Language impairments which specifically affect the reading abilities of dementing patients were later noted by Alzheimer (1907) in what was to become the first documented case of Alzheimer's Disease. Notably, Alzheimer observed comprehension problems which affected the patient's understanding of language and, when referring to reading, stated that the patient '... went from one line into another, reading the letters or reading with a senseless emphasis' (p. 110). More recently, difficulties in the comprehension of written material have been shown to be one of the first symptoms to be noticed both by patients with Alzheimer-type dementia (AD) (Cogan 1987; Sadun *et al.* 1987) and their caregivers (Bayles and Tomoeda 1991).

Despite the subjective accounts of patients and their caregivers, and early references to the existence of language comprehension and reading problems, there is a surprising lack of research examining the reading deficits associated with AD. Even fewer studies have systematically assessed these deficits using a cognitive neuropsychological approach. The following review will commence by examining a widely adopted model of language and the routes by which reading can theoretically occur. Research evidence from a variety of studies, only some of which adopt a strictly cognitive neuropsychological framework, will then be presented. General studies which establish the presence of reading difficulties will be reviewed first, followed by studies dealing specifically with the ability of AD patients to read words, irregular words (with and without contextual cues) and non-words. Sentence reading and comprehension will not be examined here because of the paucity of research in these areas. The implications of this research literature for a theoretical explanation of reading deficits in AD will then be examined. Finally, methodological problems and directions for future research will be discussed.

It is important to note that the ability to read is dependent upon a number of sensory, perceptual, and cognitive processes. In particular, semantic memory is closely linked to the lexical storage of words, understanding of meaning, knowledge of syntax, and our ability to store complex verbal information long enough for it to be processed from written input to spoken output. Moreover, sensory and perceptual problems have been found to account for the reading disturbances experienced by some patients with AD (Levine *et al.* 1993; Sadun *et al.* 1987). Thus, while this chapter focuses on the language processes that are specific to reading, it is important to remain mindful of the complex interplay between these different systems.

MODELS OF READING

A number of models of language and reading have attempted to identify the mental processes which underlie the recognition and production of spoken and written words (for example, Coltheart 1987; Ellis 1982; Ellis and Young 1988; Kay *et al.* 1992). Although there are subtle differences between the specific details of these models, there is a large degree of consensus concerning the alternative routes by which reading can theoretically occur. For the purposes of this review, the Ellis and Young (1988) model shown in Fig. 9.1 will be used as the basis for examining the reading deficits of AD patients. Essentially, the Ellis and Young model, and others of this type, claim that reading commences in the *visual analysis system* which is designed to identify the letters of a word and to note the position of each letter within that word (Ellis and Young 1988). The processing that occurs in this system involves feature analysis which produces an abstract output, with a single identifier for all fonts and cases of a particular letter (Coltheart 1987; Friedman *et al.* 1993). The visual analysis system can operate on both words and non-words (Coltheart 1987).

The abstract identities from the visual analysis system are then transmitted to the *visual (or orthographic) input lexicon*, which contains representations for each word, together with their non-semantic properties (such as word frequency) (Coltheart 1987); enabling a word to be recognized and identified. Non-words or words not previously encountered do not have an entry in this lexicon. Output from the visual input lexicon can activate word meanings which are stored in the *semantic system*, allowing a reader to comprehend a familiar written word (Ellis and Young 1988). The semantic system is thought to be used for understanding both written and spoken words.

The *speech (or phonological) output lexicon* makes the spoken form of a word available to a person in response to activation from the semantic system or directly from the speech input lexicon (Ellis and Young

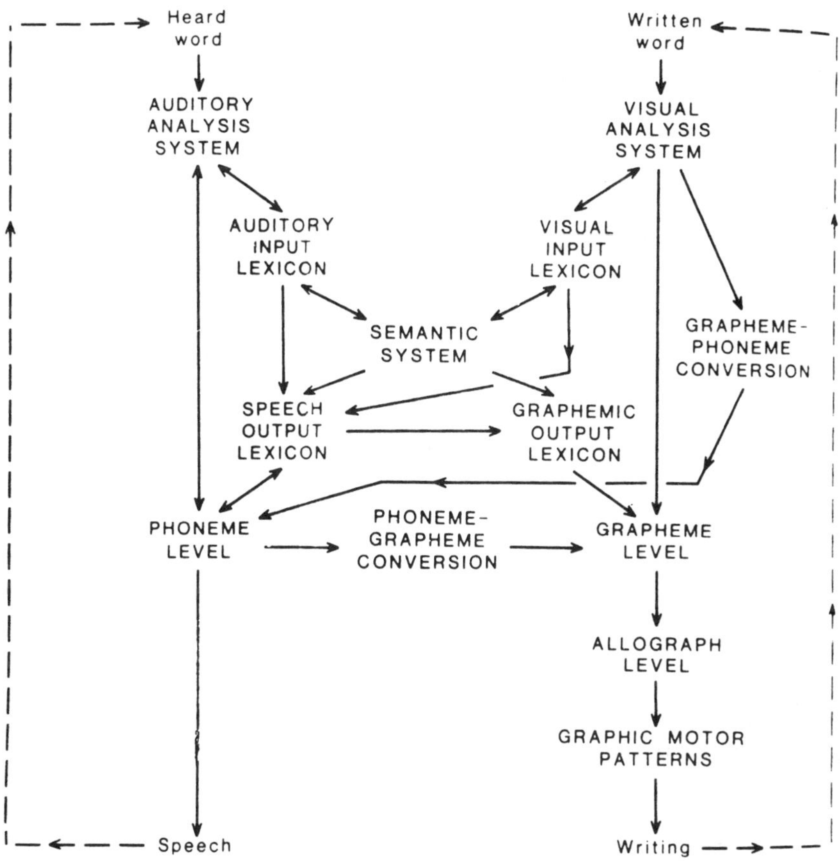

FIG. 9.1 Model of language provided by Ellis and Young (1988).

1988). The *phoneme level* is the final stage and is responsible for guiding speech production. In the process of reading, this module receives input from either the speech output lexicon or from the *grapheme-to-phoneme conversion* mechanism. The latter is a sub-lexical route that allows unfamiliar words or non-words to be read aloud by dividing a word into the constituent letters or letter groups (grapheme) and translating them into their corresponding sounds (phonemes). This route will allow a person to read unfamiliar words and non-words but results in the reader using regular pronunciations for irregular words and non-words.

Thus, according to most models, reading is thought to occur in one of three ways. First, there is the *semantic route* whereby information passes from the visual analysis system to the visual input lexicon, semantic system, and speech output lexicon. This is thought to be the normal route for skilled reading and is one which allows the reader to understand the meaning of the text. A second *lexical route* involves a direct connection between the visual input lexicon (which allows the recognition of familiar words) and the speech output lexicon (which provides their pronunciation). Using this route, words are effectively 'sight-read' and are correctly identified and pronounced without activating their meanings. Finally, a *sub-lexical route* uses grapheme-to-phoneme conversion rules, enabling a person to read unfamiliar words and non-words by 'sounding them out'. It is thought that this route is predominantly used when a person is learning to read.

READING AND LANGUAGE DEFICITS IN AD

General overviews of language dysfunction in AD can be found in reviews by Hart (1988), Miller (1989), and Thompson (1987) (see also Emery, Chapter 10, this volume). This section briefly reviews a number of correlational studies which have specifically examined the relationship between reading and other language impairments in patients with AD.

Murdoch *et al.* (1987) have attempted to document the range of language deficits shown by AD patients using tests of verbal expression, repetition, auditory comprehension, reading, writing, and articulation. With the exception of articulation, all language categories showed significant positive correlations with one another. Overall, AD patients showed preserved repetition, fluent but empty speech, diminished comprehension, impaired reading and writing abilities, and were likened to patients with transcortical sensory aphasia. They concluded that all AD patients showed some degree of language impairment and that all aspects of language showed some decline. Moreover, the pattern of deficits suggested that semantic abilities were more severely affected than phonemic and syntactic skills.

Sevush *et al.* (1993) have recently factor analysed the scores of a large group of AD patients on a range of cognitive tests, including measures of short- and long-term memory, orientation, language (spontaneous speech, comprehension, repetition, oral reading, writing, and naming), praxis, calculation, word fluency, left–right discrimination, and abstract thinking. Two orthogonal factors were extracted, collectively accounting for 63 per cent of the variance. Factor 1 was largely defined by language skills (except naming) together with left-right discrimination and digit span, while Factor 2 was defined by long-term memory, orientation, naming, and abstract thinking. Age of disease onset and

Factor 1 scores were positively correlated, indicating that patients who developed AD earlier performed more poorly on these language tasks. The reverse was true of Factor 2. Sevush *et al.* have therefore demonstrated that reading problems form part of a more general language impairment and have also suggested that these language deficits may manifest themselves differently in early- and late-onset patients.[1] Like the previous study, Roudier *et al.* (1991) performed a principal components analysis on a range of cognitive tasks which were administered to AD patients. The six-factor orthogonal solution was interpreted as including the following factors: abstract mental operation, orientation and memory, production, visuoperceptual ability, reading and writing, and constructional praxis. More specifically, the reading and writing factor did not include loadings from the semantic measures which was taken to suggest that AD patients read using the lexical or sub-lexical routes.

Emery and Breslau (1988) assessed mild, moderate, and severe AD patients on a variety of oral language, reading, and non-verbal tests. The reading tasks included tests of sentence comprehension in addition to oral reading and the matching of spoken words to written words. Alzheimer's disease subjects performed more poorly than their matched controls on all tests of oral language, reading, and non-verbal skills (that is, calculation, apraxia). The reading comprehension task was performed most poorly, suggesting that the semantic system may be impaired. Other tasks which could be completed using the lexical route which by-passes the semantic system, such as spoken word–written word matching and reading commands, were less impaired; again supporting the notion that the lexical system may be less affected than the semantic system or that it is affected later in the course of AD. However, differences in the complexity of tasks which assessed sentence comprehension and reading commands may mean that this result reflects differences in task difficulty rather than differences in the reading processes required to complete these tasks (that is, lexical versus semantic processing).

To summarize, there is evidence to suggest that reading is one of a number of language skills to be impaired early in AD and that semantically mediated reading tasks may be more severely affected than those relying only on the lexical system. As will be seen, the specific nature of these reading deficits has largely been investigated by examining the word and non-word reading abilities of AD patients.

[1] It is not the purpose of this paper to debate the mixed evidence relating to differences between the impairments of early- and late-onset patients. Readers are referred to Sevush *et al.* (1993) for a more detailed discussion of this issue (see also Gray and Della Sala, Chapter 3, this volume).

WORD READING ABILITY

Although the ability to read individual letters is an important part of word (and non-word) reading ability, few studies appear to have formally established the integrity of the visual analysis system by assessing the letter reading ability of AD patients. One exception to this, is the study by Cummings (1986) who demonstrated that letter reading was '. . . remarkably resistant to disruption by the dementia' (p. 317). Therefore, it appears that any disruption to the reading abilities of AD patients cannot merely be attributed to problems of a perceptual nature and that any such reading deficits are more likely to have a cognitive basis.

Word reading has been used in a variety of contexts to examine the reading ability of AD patients. Bayles *et al.* (1991), for example, used a series of 11 different language tasks which use the same stimuli (single concepts, such as pencil, comb) in order to determine whether there is a concept specific loss of information from the semantic memory of AD patients. Tasks were designed to vary in terms of difficulty and their reliance on semantic memory, and were repeatedly administered over a number of years. Differences in difficulty level were confirmed by the performance profile of normal control subjects. Reading tasks included oral word reading, the provision of definitions to written words, and the selection of pictures to match printed words. Various analyses of the language tasks suggested that the deterioration in semantic memory was task-specific rather than concept-specific and, therefore, that a concept may be retained in semantic memory but appear to be lost because a task is too demanding. They concluded that it was only possible to determine whether a concept was lost from semantic memory when all possible tasks in which that concept is a stimulus have been failed by a patient. In addition, more difficult tasks were found to deteriorate first.

With respect to reading, Bayles *et al.* (1991) found that AD patients performed most poorly on the word definition task, followed by reading comprehension (assessed by matching pictures to printed words), with the oral reading of single words being least impaired. While both the word definition and reading comprehension tasks required access to the semantic system to be completed successfully, the oral reading task could also be completed via the lexical route. Moreover, the word definition task required the *recall* of material from semantic memory, whereas the comprehension task required only *recognition* memory. Thus, it appears that semantic memory deteriorates before lexical access, and that the task-specific deterioration in semantic memory (that is, poorer word definition than comprehension performance) is consistent with the view that recall is more difficult than recognition

(Hasher and Zacks 1979). However, the situation is further complicated by the fact that the reading comprehension task also required an intact visual object recognition system which, while not shown in Ellis and Young's model, is included in some other models of language processing (for example, Kay *et al.* 1991). This system is used for the recognition of pictures and seen objects, and is directly linked to the semantic system. The finding by Bayles *et al.* that AD patients performed more poorly on a picture/object naming task than the reading comprehension task, both of which use pictorial stimuli, may indiciate that the visual object recognition system is also impaired; thereby contaminating patients' reading comprehension performance. Alternatively, the picture/object naming task, like the word definition task, required subjects to *recall* information from semantic memory. The poorer performance of AD patients on the picture/object naming task may therefore be a consequence of differential task demands (that is, recall versus recognition memory).

Further evidence of the nature of the word reading deficit associated with AD has been provided by Glosser and Friedman (1991) who examined the lexical and semantic basis of word priming effects in oral reading. Subjects were provided with different types of primes, including words that were highly associated with one another but were semantically unrelated (such as queen and bee) and words that were sementically related but were not associated with one another (such as mouse and horse). Patients with AD were found to show word priming effects for the first of these types of word pairs but not for the second, supporting the view that knowledge of lexical associations is preserved despite damage to a person's knowledge of superordinate categories (that is, the semantic system). However, some caution must be exercised when interpreting this finding because it could be argued that the only exemplar provided of a highly associated item is in fact also semantically related (that is, queen is a subordinate category of bee).

Word reading has also been used by Schwartz *et al.* (1980) to determine the intact reading routes of a patient with progressive dementia, known as WLP. Specifically, WLP was found to be able to read regular and irregular words but was largely unable to match words to pictures. In addition, her success at sorting printed words into categories was greater when the stimuli were high-frequency words. Thus, her oral reading did not appear to be achieved via the semantic route. In order to establish that WLP was using the lexical reading route rather than grapheme-to-phoneme conversion rules, Schwartz *et al.* required her to read word pairs which were matched in spelling but differed in pronunciation (such as cost–post). Repeated testings over a one-year period showed that she was largely successful at this task, indicating that her lexical reading route was intact. Finally, WLP's ability to read non-words provided evidence that grapheme-to-phoneme conversion could be achieved and, therefore, that the sub-lexical route was also operative (Schwartz *et al.* 1979).

In a related area, Schwartz and Chawluk (1990) have provided a detailed examination of the deteriorating language skills of a dementing patient, Susan G., who was diagnosed at autopsy as having Pick's disease; a disease causing diffuse brain damage which is often clinically indistinguishable from AD (Kolb and Wishaw 1990). Susan G. could correctly pronounce 50 per cent of written words on first testing but this declined to 28 per cent six months later. High frequency words were significantly more likely to be read correctly but the accuracy of regular word pronunciations did not differ from irregular words. When first tested, her errors tended to be phonologically related words or non-word approximations to the target word. However, the errors were not typically those that would occur as a result of the application of grapheme-to-phoneme conversion rules. By the second testing, her errors were less closely related to the phonology of the target word, with two-syllable words tending to be read as two high frequency words (for example, ballet as ball game). To test her understanding of words, Susan G. was required to match written and spoken words, which were either strong or weak examples of different categories of objects, to their superordinate categories. She was unable to reliably perform this task using either the auditory or visual modality and her performance was affected by semantic variables (for example, strength of the exemplar and object category), suggesting that her semantic system was impaired. The integrity of the visual analysis system was established by showing that Susan G. could accurately discriminate between words, and non-words which orthographically resembled words. Overall, the combined language deficits of this patient were thought to result from problems located at the speech output lexicon together with a semantic deficit which limited access to this lexicon via the semantic route.

Finally, Sasanuma *et al.* (1992) examined the word reading and reading comprehension of Japanese kanji using three patients who were diagnosed as having probable dementia of the Alzheimer type. Kanji is a script in which the same character can have a number of alternative pronunciations depending on its context. Thus, the translation from orthography to phonology is word-specific. Moreover, kanji characters are not composed of phonemes and so they cannot be phonologically decomposed. Sasanuma *et al.* reported that these patients showed preserved word reading abilities despite poor reading comprehension and suggested that reading occurred via the lexical route. Furthermore, word comprehension declined over time more than pronunciation, implying that the semantic system is more vulnerable to the effects of AD than the lexical system.

READING OF IRREGULAR WORDS

In recent years, there has been a growing trend toward using the National Adult Reading Test (NART; Nelson 1982), or one of the derivatives (for example, NAART; Spreen and Strauss 1991; or NART-R; Crawford 1990), to estimate the premorbid intellectual functioning of patients with brain damage (Crawford 1989, 1992). Measures of this type require subjects to correcly read aloud a list of printed low-frequency irregular words, also known as exception words, which do not follow regular grapheme-to-phoneme conversion rules. These measures assume that the reading ability and intelligence are highly correlated in the normal population, and that this type of reading ability is relatively insensitive to brain damage (Sharpe and O'Carroll 1991). Successful completion of the task requires the reader to use either the semantic or lexical reading route, with the sub-lexical route leading to regularization errors. Studies which have attempted to establish the suitability of the NART for use with AD patients therefore provide a test of the integrity of the lexical and semantic reading routes.

A number of such studies have reported that NART performance is unrelated to dementia severity (Hart *et al.* 1986; O'Carroll and Gilleard 1986; Sharpe and O'Carroll 1991). Moreover, while some decline in reading performance is evident (Hart *et al.* 1986), NART performance appears to be less affected by dementia than is performance of the Vocabulary subscale of the WAIS and WAIS-R (Crawford *et al.* 1988; Sharpe and O'Carroll 1991). It has also been found that NART performance does not show a significant decline over a one-year period, further supporting the NART's relative resistance to dementia (O'Carroll *et al.* 1987).

In contrast, Fromm *et al.* (1991) have shown that NART performance is inferior in AD patients, declining significantly over time. They attribute the discrepancy between these results and those of the preceding studies largely to variations in patient sampling characteristics (for example, different levels of dementia severity and some dementia groups being of unspecified origin) but may also result from the use of a modified version of the NART (Paque and Warrington 1995). Fromm *et al.* (1991) interpret the decline in AD performance as reflecting a deterioration in the semantic system. In terms of Ellis and Young's (1988) model, however, the result is equally consistent with damage to the visual input lexicon which would affect both the semantic and lexical reading routes.

More recently, Paque and Warrington (1995) have reported a gradual decline in the NART scores of AD patients who were re-assessed after a minimum period of 10 months, while also noting that this decline in NART reading scores was less than on other formal tests of intelligence, particularly the WAIS-R Verbal IQ. In addition, they found that patients who had Verbal IQ scores that were lower than their Performance IQ scores had poorer NART scores from the outset and that these patients were more prone to deterioration in their reading performance over time. They conclude that the NART can be used to assess the premorbid intelligence of patients with AD where such patients have a Verbal IQ that is higher than their Performance IQ.

Patterson *et al.* (1994) have used both the NART and a list of monosyllabic monomorphemic exception words when examining the reading skills of patients with minimal, mild, and moderate AD. They found that AD patients showed significant impairments in their ability to read low frequency monosyllabic and monomorphemic exception words, when compared to regular words matched for length, frequency, and initial phoneme. Further more, they observed a decline in NART performance as a function of the severity of dementia. The most frequent type of reading errors that were noted for both the NART and simpler list of exception words were referred to as surface errors. These typically involved regularization errors which would occur as a consequence of attempting to apply grapheme-to-phoneme conversion rules to arrive at a pronunciation instead of using the semantic or lexical reading routes.

Although reading tasks which use exception words are able to determine whether the lexical reading routes are intact, they are not designed to formally test the integrity of the semantic system to determine whether reading is semantically mediated. Schwartz *et al.* (1980) have addressed this aspect by requiring their patient, WLP, to read irregular words (objects, colours, and body parts), and to sort them into their appropriate categories. WLP could not reliably categorize many object names that could be pronounced, indicating that the semantic system was compromised and that successful reading was likely to be achieved by the lexical route which bypasses the semantic system. The fact that WLP's mispronunciations of irregular words generally conformed to pronunciations that would result from the application of grapheme-to-phoneme conversion rules additionally suggests that the sub-lexical reading route was operative. Similarly, the dominant type of errors described by Fromm *et al.* (1991) (referred to as phonetically possible errors) indicates that AD patients resort, at times, to the use of grapheme-to-phoneme conversion rules, therefore leading to regularization errors. In summary, these results suggest that the sub-lexical reading route is relatively preserved in AD.

While the NART has been used widely to evaluate the preservation of reading skills in AD patients, it has been argued, conversely, that a failure to recognize words and accurately pronounce them is not conclusive evidence that the visual input lexicon is damaged (Beardsall and Huppert 1994). Instead, it is possible that the sub-lexical route is occasionally used when a word is not recognized as familiar, despite it having an intact lexical entry. In order to examine this possibility, Beardsall and Huppert have placed the NART stimuli into sentences to form the Cambridge Contextual Reading Test (CCRT); thereby providing additional semantic and syntactic cues to facilitate word recognition and pronunciation. Demented subjects (and poor normal readers) were found to perform better on CCRT than the NART. One explanation for this finding was that the sentence context assisted demented readers in identifying words as being familiar which then served to improve the chance of accessing the lexical entry for that word. Lexical access may therefore be facilitated by judging a word as familiar, in which case the provision of a context may provide information which enhances processing at the visual input lexicon stage. Given that demented subjects are not only impaired on tests of recall but also recognition (Christensen *et al.* 1992), it is conceivable that problems with recognition memory impair judgement of familiarity and, consequently, lexical access in this way. Alternatively, Beardsall and Huppert (1994) argue that contextual cues may increase the likelihood that patients use the semantic route which, by an unspecified means, results in more correct pronunciations. Given these alternative explanations, it is not possible to determine whether the semantic or lexical reading routes have been used when completing the CCRT. Moreover, the effects of semantic and syntactic cues are confounded in this task. This issue is further complicated by the fact that syntactic and semantic knowledge appear to be differentially sensitive to the effects of AD, with some evidence that syntax is better preserved (Kemper *et al.* 1993). Additional research is therefore needed to examine the influence of syntactic and semantic variables and comprehension in these tasks.

READING OF NON-WORDS

Although non-words are not normally encountered in everyday reading situations, they provide a means to test the integrity of the sub-lexical reading route, since theoretically they are read using grapheme-to-phoneme conversion rules. In patients with limited education, low frequency NART words essentially function as non-words. Clinical experience with the NART suggests that most errors in the pronunciation of irregular words made with AD patients are regularization errors. This may suggest that the grapheme-to-phoneme conversion process is relatively well preserved. Very few studies, however, have formally examined the non-word (or pseudoword) reading abilities of AD patients. One exception, is Rapcsak *et al.* (1989) who found that three out of 11 AD patients showed impaired reading of non-words while being able to read both regular and irregular words. This was referred to as phonological dyslexia, which is assumed to result from damage to the mechanism responsible for grapheme-to-phoneme conversion (Friedman *et al.* 1993; Rayner and Pallatsek 1989). As a consequence, reading can only occur via the semantic or lexical routes and so phonological dyslexics are not able to read unfamiliar words (regular or exception) or non-words. It is important to note that although the majority of AD patients showed preserved word-reading ability, reading comprehension of sentences was impaired in all 11 cases, further suggesting that the semantic system was damaged and that the lexical reading route remained intact.

Prior to this, Schwartz *et al.* (1979) described the case of WLP who could read regular and exception words, and non-words. The ability to read non-words was taken to indicate that the grapheme-to-phoneme conversion rules were intact. However, this interpretation was questioned by Friedman *et al.* (1992) who argued that another means by which to pronounce non-words is to use the lexical route to derive pronunciations which are based on the stored pronunciations of real words that are 'orthographic neighbours' of the non-word. If this were so, AD patients who were able to read words, should be able to read non-words except where the non-word had no neighbours (that is, no orthographically similar words to draw upon), in which case the non-word could only be read by the use of grapheme-to-phoneme conversion rules. Friedman *et al.* tested this hypothesis by administering several tasks using a range of different pseudowords to a group of AD patients who were known to be able to read regular and irregular words. They concluded that, on the whole, AD patients' ability to read pseudowords was well preserved except for those non-words which could only be pronounced using grapheme-to-phoneme conversion rules. These findings suggest that many pseudowords are read by AD patients using the lexical reading route by drawing upon orthographically similar real words as a guide. For pseudowords where there were no analogues, they were forced to use the sub-lexical route. However, the markedly poorer performance on such stimuli suggests that this route is compromised. This contradicts the findings of Schwartz *et al.* (1980) and Fromm *et al.* (1991) who provide evidence for an intact sub-lexical route in AD patients.

Finally, Patterson *et al.* (1995) demonstrated a decline in non-word reading ability with increasingly severe dementia. In addition, they found that the majority of errors made during this task took the form of lexicalization errors in which a non-word was given the pronunciation of an orthographically similar word. Thus, consistent with the findings of Friedman *et al.* (1993), the results of Patterson *et al.* (1995) suggest that the sub-lexical reading route appears to be increasingly compromised as the severity of dementia increases, and that the lexical reading route may be utilized by AD patients when attempting to derive word pronunciations for non-words that have the appearance of pseudowords (that is, they use common spelling patterns).

SUMMARY OF READING DEFICITS IN AD

To summarize, there is evidence to suggest that impaired reading is one of a number of language deficits experienced by AD patients (Emery and Breslau 1988; Murdoch *et al.* 1987; Sevush *et al.* 1993). More specifically, research examining the word-reading ability of AD patients (Bayles *et al.* 1991; Glosser and Friedman 1991; Sasanuma *et al.* 1992; Schwartz and Chawluk 1990; Schwartz *et al.* 1980) shows that these reading impairments are largely attributable to problems in the semantic system, the lexical system showing less marked deterioration. Thus, AD patients in the early stages of their illness are quite often able to read both regular and irregular words but frequently fail to comprehend their meaning. Reading, therefore, appears to occur via the lexical rather than the semantic or sub-lexical routes. There is also some suggestion that, like other aphasic groups, high-frequency words may be better preserved than low-frequency words (Schwarz and Chawluk 1990). In addition, word comprehension that is dependent upon recognition memory may be less vulnerable to damage than comprehension which is dependent upon the recall of information from memory (Bayles *et al.* 1991). On the basis of the evidence presented, it is not possible to determine whether the problems at the semantic level involve the storage or retrieval of information from memory, nor is it possible to evaluate whether syntax is also compromised. However, there is reason to believe that memory deficits limit the reading of AD patients at the semantic level and, to a lesser extent, at the lexical level.

The evidence concerning the integrity of the sub-lexical system is mixed. Both Schwarz *et al.* (1980) and Fromm *et al.* (1991) provide evidence of regularization errors when AD patients mispronounced irregular words, thereby suggesting that this reading route is intact. Rapcsak *et al.* (1989), on the other hand, found that a small number of AD patients could not pronounce non-words, and this was thought to result from damage to the grapheme-to-phoneme conversion rules. Similarly, Friedman *et al.* (1992) found that AD patients could not pronounce those pseudowords which could only be read by use of grapheme-to-phoneme conversion rules. Interestingly, the evidence favouring a functional sub-lexical route comes from words with irregular spellings while the evidence to the contrary comes from non-words, raising the possibility of a methodological artefact.

METHODOLOGICAL ISSUES AND FUTURE RESEARCH

It is apparent that research into the reading deficits of AD patients raises a number of methodological issues. For example, few investigations have formally adopted a cognitive neuropsychological approach as a means by which to converge on the specific language processes which are defective. One consequence of this is that many reading tasks use mental processes which are not unique to reading (such as the use of pictures to assess reading comprehension) and, in so doing, introduce the possibility that other defective non-reading processes may account for the performance deficits. Another consequence, is that some tasks which specifically assess reading are not constructed in a way that allows researchers to distinguish between alternative reading routes. The NART is one such example, since successful completion of this task means that the lexical and/or semantic routes may be operative. An investigation of reading comprehension is needed in order to distinguish between these possibilities. In addition, there needs to be a systematic investigation of the effects of various semantic, syntactic, and lexical variables (such as word frequency, imageability, grammatical class, word length, number of syllables) on the reading ability of AD patients in order to accurately determine the exact nature of the reading deficits caused by AD. A cognitive neuropsychological approach to research on the reading deficits of AD patients therefore has a valuable contribution to make to our understanding of the theoretical constructs underlying these deficits.

Finally, more careful consideration needs to be given to variations in task difficulty. One reason for this is that task difficulty seems important in determining whether AD patients are able to complete it or not (for example, recall memory tasks seem to be more difficult than recognition tasks). While this is noteworthy in itself, it is important that researchers do not falsely conclude, for example, that concepts are lost from semantic memory, or that lexical reading is preserved but semantic reading lost, because their measurement techniques confound task difficulty and specific mental processes.

REFERENCES

Alzheimer, A. (1907). Über eine eigenartige Erkrankung der Hirnrinde. *Allgemeine Zeitschrift für Psychiatrie und psychisch-gerichtlich Medicin*, **64**, 146–8. Translated by R.H. Wilkins and I.A. Brody (1969). Alzheimer's Disease, *Archives of Neurology*, **21**, 109–110.

Bayles, K.A. (1991). Age at onset of Alzheimer's Disease. *Archives of Neurology*, **31**, 155–216.

Bayles, K.A., and Tomoeda, C.K. (1991). Caregiver report of prevalence and appearance order of linguistic symptoms in Alzheimer's patients. *Gerontologist* **31**, 210–16.

Bayles, K.A., Tomoeda, C.K., Kaszniak, A., and Trosset, M.W. (1991). Alzheimer's Disease effects on semantic memory: Loss of structure or impaired processing? *Journal of Cognitive Neuroscience*, **3**, 166–82.

Beardsall, L. and Huppert, F.A. (1994). Improvement in NART word reading in demented and normal older persons using the Cambridge Contextual Reading Test. *Journal of Clinical and Experimental Neuropsychology*, **16**, 232–42.

Breitner, J.C.S. and Folstein, M.F. (1984). Familial Alzheimer Dementia: A prevalent disorder with specific clinical features. *Psychological Medicine*, **14**, 63–80.

Christensen, H., Maltby, N., Jorm, A.F., Creasey, H., and Broe, G.A. (1992). Cholinergic 'blockade' as a model of the cognitive deficits in Alzheimer's Disease. *Brain*, **115**, 1681–99.

Cogan, D.G. ,(1987). Alzheimer syndromes. *American Journal of Ophthalmology*, **104**, 183–4.

Coltheart, M. (1987). Functional architecture of the language-processing system. In *The cognitive neuropsychology of language*, (ed. M. Coltheart, G. Sartori, and R. Job). Lawrence Erlbaum, London.

Crawford, J. (1989). Estimation of premorbid intelligence: A review of recent developments. In *Developments in clinical and experimental neuropsychology*, (ed. J. Crawford and D. Parker). Plenum Press, New York.

Crawford, J.R. (1990). The estimation of premorbid intelligence. Unpublished Ph.D. thesis, University of Aberdeen.

Crawford, J.R. (1992). Current and premorbid intelligence measures in neuropsychological assessment. In *A handbook of neuropsychological assessment*, (ed. J.R. Crawford, W. McKinlay, and D. M. Parker), pp. 21–49. Lawrence Erlbaum, London.

Crawford, J.R., Parker, D.M., and Besson, J.A.O. (1988). Estimation of premorbid intelligence in organic conditions. *British Journal of Psychiatry*, **153**, 178–81.

Cummings, J.L., Houlihan, J.P., and Hill, M.A. (1986). The pattern of reading deterioration in dementia of the Alzheimer type: Observations and implications. *Brain and Language*, **29**, 315–23.

Ellis, A.W. (1982). Spelling and writing (and reading and speaking). In *Normality and pathology in cognitive functions*, (ed. A.W. Ellis), pp. 113–46. Academic Press, London.

Ellis, A.W., and Young, A.W. (1988). *Human cognitive neuropsychology.* Lawrence Erlbaum, Hove.

Emery, O.B. and Breslau, L.D. (1988). The problem of naming in SDAT: A relative deficit. *Experimental Aging Research*, **14**, 181–93.

Friedman, R.B., Ferguson, S., Robinson, S., and Sunderland, T. (1992). Discussion of mechanisms of reading in Alzheimer's Disease. *Brain and Language*, **43**, 400–13.

Friedman, R.F., Ween, J.E., and Albert, M.L. (1993). Alexia. In *Clinical neuropsychology*, (ed. K.M. Heilman and E. Valenstein), pp. 37–62. Oxford, New York.

Fromm, D., Holland, A.L., Nebes, R.D., and Oakley, M.A. (1991). A longitudinal study of word-reading ability in Alzheimer's Disease: Evidence from the National Adult Reading Test. *Cortex*, **27**, 367–76.

Glosser, G. and Friedman, R.B. (1991). Lexical but not semantic priming in Alzheimer's Disease. *Psychology and Aging*, **6**, 522–7.

Hart, S. (1988). Language and dementia: A review. *Psychological Medicine*, **18**, 99–112.

Hart, S., Smith, C.M., and Swash, M. (1986). Assessing intellectual deterioration. *British Journal of Clinical Psychology*, **25**, 119–24.

Hasher, L. and Zacks, R.T. (1979). Automatic and effortful processes in memory. *Journal of Experimental Psychology: General*, **108**, 356–88.

Kay, J., Lesser, R., and Coltheart, M. (1992). *Psycholinguistic Assessments of Language Processing in Aphasia.* Lawrence Erlbaum, Hove.

Kemper, S., LaBarge, E., Ferraro, R., Cheung, H., Cheung, H., and Storandt, M. (1993). On the preservation of syntax in Alzheimer's Disease. *Archives of Neurology*, **50**, 81–6.

Kolb, B. and Wishaw, I.Q. (1990). *Fundamentals of human neuropsychology.* (3rd edn). Freeman, New York.

Levine, D.N., Lee, J.M., and Fisher, C.M. (1993). The visual variant of Alzheimer's Disease: A clinicopathologic case study, *Neurology*, **43**, 305–13.

Miller, E. (1989). Language in dementia of the Alzheimer type. In *Developments in clinical and experimental neuropsychology*, (ed. J.R. Crawford and D.M. Parker), pp. 75–85. Plenum Press, New York.

Mohs, R.C., Kim, Y., Johns, C.A., Dunn, D.D., and Davis, K.L. (1986). Assessing changes in Alzheimer's Disease: Memory and language. In *Clinical memory assessment of older adults*, (ed. L.W. Poon), pp. 149–55. American Psychological Association, Washington.

Murdoch, B.E., Chenery, H.J., Wilks, V., and Boyle, R.S. (1987). Language disorders in dementia of the Alzheimer type. *Brain and Language*, **31**, 122–37.

Nelson, H.E. (1982). *National Adult Reading Test: Test Manual.* NFER-Nelson, Windsor.

O'Carroll, R.E., Baikie, E.M., and Whittick, J.E. (1987). Does the National Adult Reading Test hold in dementia? *British Journal of Clinical Psychology*, **26**, 315–16.

O'Carroll, R.E. and Gilleard, C.J. (1986). Estimation of premorbid intelligence in dementia. *British Journal of Clinical Psychology*, **25**, 157–8.

Paque, L. and Warrington, E.K. (1995). A longitudinal study of reading ability in patients suffering from dementia. *Journal of the International Neuropsychological Society*, **1**, 517–24.

Patterson, K., Graham, N., and Hodges, J.R. (1994). Reading in dementia of the Alzheimer type: A preserved ability? *Neuropsychology*, **8**, 395–407.

Rapcsak, S.A., Arthur, S.A., Bliklen, D.A., and Rubens, A.B. (1989). Lexical agraphia in Alzheimer's Disease. *Archives of Neurology*, **46**, 65–8.

Rayner, K., and Pallatsek, A. (1989) *The psychology of reading*. Prentice Hall, Englewood Cliffs, New Jersey.

Roudier, M., Marcie, P., Podrabinek, N., Lamour, Y., Payan, C., Fermanian, J., and Boller, F. (1991). Cognitive functions in Alzheimer's Disease: Interaction of cognitive domains. *Developmental Neuropsychology*, **7**, 231–41.

Sadun, A.A., Borchert, M., De Vita, E., Hinton, D.R., and Bassi, C.J. (1987). Assessment of visual impairment in patients with Alzheimer's Disease. *American Journal of Ophthalmology*, **104**, 113–20.

Sasanuma, S., Sakuma, N., and Kitaro, K. (1992). Reading kanji without semantics: Evidence from a longitudinal study of dementia. *Cognitive Neuropsychology*, **9**, 465–86.

Schwartz, M.R.F. and Chawluk, J.B. (1990). Deterioration of language in progressive aphasia: A case study. In *Modular deficits in Alzheimer-type dementia*, (ed. M.F. Schwartz), pp. 245–96. MIT, Cambridge, Mass.

Schwartz, M.F., Marin, O.S.M., and Saffran, E.M. (1979). Dissociations of language function in dementia: A case study. *Brain and Language*, **7**, 277–306.

Schwartz, M.F., Saffran, E.M., and Marin, O.S.M. (1980) Fractionating the reading process in dementia: Evidence for word-specific print-to-sound associations. In *Deep dyslexia*, (ed. M. Coltheart, K. Patterson, and J.C. Marshall), pp. 259–69. Routledge & Kegan Paul, London.

Sevush, S., Leve, N., and Brickman, A. (1993). Age at disease onset and pattern of cognitive impairment in probable Alzheimer's Disease. *Journal of Neuropsychiatry and Clinical Neuroscience*, **5**, 66–72.

Sharpe, K., and O'Carroll, R. (1991). Estimating premorbid intellectual level in dementia using the National Adult Reading Test: A Canadian study. *British Journal of Clinical Psychology*, **30**, 381–4.

Spreen, O., and Strauss, E. (1991). *A compendium of neuropsychological tests*. Oxford University Press, New York.

Thompson, I.M. (1987). Language in dementia. Part 1: A review. *International Journal of Geriatric Psychiatry*, **2**, 145–61.

Wechsler, D. (1981). Manual for the Revised Wechsler Adult Intelligence Scale (WAIS-R). Psychological Corporation, New York.

TEN

Language functioning

V. Olga B. Emery

INTRODUCTION

The focus of this chapter is on language in Alzheimer-type dementia (AD). To create a context for the discussion of language structure and function in Alzheimer disorder, first there will be a brief description of some defining features of this dementing illness. AD is a progressive and diffuse encephalopathy resulting in the slow death of the brain (American Psychiatric Association 1994; Wisniewski *et al.* 1994). This progressive dementia is a syndrome, a final common symptomatic pathway, and not a homogeneous disease (Emery and Oxman 1994*a, b*). Put another way, AD is a phenotype (Emery 1988*a*) or final presentation, rather than a single disease entity.

Confirmation of diagnosis for this age-correlated dementia syndrome is, at present, contingent on neuropathologic findings: neuritic plaques, neurofibrillary tangles, granulovacuolar degeneration, amyloid angiopathy, loss of neurones, and atrophy of the brain (National Institute on Aging 1995; Selkoe *et al.* 1985). It appears that for some time prior to diagnosis, lesions accumulate below a threshold for producing clinical symptoms. Neuropathologic studies suggest that a pathologic process may begin with the abnormal processing of amyloid β-precursor protein and deposition of β-amyloid fibrils; pericytes-microglia appear to be cells engaged in the formation of amyloid fibrils, although the role of amyloid fibril-associated proteins is not clear (Selkoe *et al.* 1985; Wisniewski *et al.* 1992 1994). Accordingly, AD might be, at least in part, a function of β-protein amyloidosis. Beta-amyloid appears when amyloid precursor protein (APP) is broken down in an abnormal way, possibly because of a defect in the APP molecule or a reduction in the activity of enzymes that catalyse normative breakdown (Haass *et al.* 1991; National Institute on Aging 1995; Wegiel and Wisniewski 1990; Wisniewski *et al.* 1994). Amyloid precursor protein is produced by many body tissues and might function to maintain the growth of nerve cells or preserve connections between them. Factors leading to abnormal processing of amyloid β-precursor protein and the formation of β-amyloid fibrils also appear to result in abnormal phosphorylation of tau, with subsequent formation of neurofibrillary tangles in some neurones (Haass *et al.* 1991; Wisniewski *et al.* 1994).

The term Alzheimer's disease was used originally to describe a progressive dementia in patients with presenile or early onset of symptoms (before 65 years of age) (Alzheimer 1907). Since the late 1960s, primarily because of histopathologic observations that neuropathologic markers are also found in the brains of dementia patients with late-onset symptomatology, these early- and late-onset disorders came to be regarded as a single, homogeneous disease entity (Blennow *et al.* 1990, 1991, 1994). However, because neuropsychologic symptoms, neurochemical deficits, and neuropathologic changes may be more virulent or severe (Alexopoulos and Nambudiri 1994; Blennow *et al.* 1990, 1991, 1994; Filley *et al.* 1986; Mesulam 1982; Seltzer and Sherwin 1983) in early-onset compared with late-onset Alzheimer's syndrome (Emery 1985, 1988*b*; Emery and Breslau 1987*a*), some investigators question the validity of combining these disorders (Alexopoulos and Nambudiri 1994; Blennow *et al.* 1990, 1991, 1994; Emery 1985, 1988*b*; Emery and Breslau 1987*a*,*b*; Emery and Oxman 1994*b*; Gottfries *et al.* 1990; Sourander and Sjogren 1970). Careful analysis of studies concluding that no significant differences exist between early-onset and late-onset Alzheimer dementia often reveals a methodologic error, whereby symptom severity has been compared out of context with disease course (see also Agnew, Chapter 15). The existence of neurofibrillary tangles and neuritic plaques is not a sufficient basis for a conjoint nosologic construction, because tangles and plaques are also found in normal ageing (Jagust 1994; Jobst *et al.* 1994; Oxman and Baynes 1994; Roth *et al.* 1966). Because the quantitative parameter of the degree of tangles and plaques is used to separate normal ageing from Alzheimer's syndrome, reliable degree differences should also serve to keep nosologically distinct early-onset Alzheimer's disease from late-onset Alzheimer's disease. The quantitative variable of degree of neuropsychologic, neurochemical, and neuropathologic changes, when recast into the frame of temporality, becomes disease-course acceleration.

Blennow and colleagues (1991, 1994) have provided evidence for two distinct clinical subgroups of AD for which age of onset correlates significantly with degree of memory disturbance, dominance of temporoparietal symptoms (including language deficits), blood–brain barrier function, frequency of leukoaraiosis, frequency of vascular factors, and degree of confusional symptoms. Other possible parameters for the subtyping of AD include depression (Emery 1988*a*, 1992, 1994; Emery and Oxman 1994*a*, *b*; Kral 1983; Kral and Emery 1989; Mulsant and Zubenko 1994) and/or psychosis (Mulsant and Zubenko 1994), serotonergic deficits (Arora *et al.* 1991), myoclonic and extrapyramidal signs, and clinically obvious aphasia (Kirshner 1994; Kirshner *et al.* 1984a; Mesulam 1987; Tyrrell *et al.* 1990). Also, there appears to be a distinct subtype at the interface between AD and vascular dementia, which is currently neither validly defined nor subsumed under existing categories of AD or vascular dementia (Emery *et al.* 1993, 1994, 1995; see also Agnew, Chapter 15)

This spectrum approach to AD is quite relevant for this chapter because as the literature pertaining to language (as well as other neuropsychological variables) in AD is analysed, one finds some conflicting conclusions across studies that might be better comprehended and integrated were it understood that there are probably a number of subtypes of AD. These, as yet, undefined subtypes probably present somewhat variably despite having fundamental Alzheimer characteristics in common. Thus, with a spectrum framework in mind, we can move on to the next sections of this chapter in which language in AD is analysed; there will be an effort to bring into focus the fundamental features of language in AD that cut across possible subtype and stage-of-progression variations.

LANGUAGE CONSTRUCTS

Language is a system of codes, evolved for the purpose of communication. The use of language involves the processes of encoding and decoding symbols and signs. Also, language is a system of rules requiring the mental processing and integration of varying forms and sets of relationships. Language involves the induction of an underlying set of rules, which can generate an indefinite number of statements (Emery 1985, 1986). Accordingly, language is a cognitive activity which permits one to say new things, never before heard or rehearsed, which nevertheless conform to the rules, and which are comprehensible to others knowing those rules.

Before describing language processing in AD, I would like to define some major language terms that will be used. A review of research on language function in AD shows that the major language variables investigated—for example naming, syntax, and semantics—represent categories or levels of the semiotic system (deSaussure 1966; Newmeyer 1980; Yngve 1986). Nevertheless, these language variables are most often investigated piecemeal and outside the context of the semiotic hierarchy. This lack of embeddedness in the hierarchical components of semiotic theory has made it difficult to get a clear picture, both within and across studies, of the *relative* aspects of language deficits in AD. Thus one aim of this chapter is to pull together and organize research findings pertaining to language decrement in AD in the context of the semiotic hierarchy.

The hierarchy goes from simple to more complex linguistic units (corresponding roughly to sound, part of word/word, sentence, expressed meaning (Jakobson 1964). The semiotic categories are phonology, morphology, syntax, and semantics, with qualitative as well as quantitative differences at each hierarchical level (deSaussure 1966; Yngve 1986).

Phonology refers to phonetic and phonemic systems of language; both systems refer to the analysis of sound without reference to meaning (Darden 1974; deSaussure 1966). The main task of linguistics, as the scientific study of language, is the analysis of the relationship between sound and meaning (Yngve 1986). Phonology refers to the sound part of this relationship.

Morphology involves the analysis of morphemes (parts of words/ words), the smallest units of meaningful linguistic signalling; morphology never refers to phrases (Bloomfield 1933; Lederer 1980, 1984). The total stock of morphemes in a language is its lexicon. Two kinds of morphological analysis are (1) lexical or vocabulary competence (for example confrontation naming) and (2) word-internal morphological analysis (for example declension and conjugation involving word-internal changes) (Darden 1974, and personal communication; Lederer 1980).

Syntax is the analysis of the structure of phrases and sentences. Variables of syntax include differing sentence types, forms of substitution, linear word order, differing kinds of clauses, pronomial and prepositional usage, and forms of propositional relations (Huck and Ojeda 1987; Yngve 1986). Variation of syntactic elements can be ordered on dimensions of concreteness–abstraction, alogicality–logicality, as well as other parameters of simplicity–complexity (Brown 1973; Chomsky 1979; Dale 1976; Emery 1982, 1985, 1986, 1993; Luria 1973, 1980; Newmeyer 1980; Svedelius 1897). Svedelius was one of the first linguists to delineate basic models of syntactic structures (syntagmas) on the parameter of complexity. Svedelius (1897) distinguished between simple narrative syntactic structure termed 'communication of actions or events' and more complex syntactic structures involving expression of logical forms and termed 'communication of relationships'. The 'communication of relationships' represents grammatical structures which arose last of all in the history of language, and represents greater syntactic structural complexity (Brown 1973; Chomsky 1979; Dale 1976; Luria 1973, 1980; Slobin 1970; Svedelius 1897). This differentiation of syntactic models into the concrete, alogical, simple as opposed to abstract, logical, complex has served over time as the basis for the testing and discrimination of brain-damaged from normal populations in the seminal works of Goldstein (1942), Head (1926), Jackson (1884), Luria (1973, 1980), Monakow (1914), and others who found that organic brain deficits hinder mental processing of abstract, logical, complex syntactic forms.

Semantics, the final category of the semiotic hierarchy that will be discussed, refers to analysis and knowledge of meaning. Further, this semiotic rank includes the parameter of organization of meaning (Bayles and Kaszniak 1987). Semantics is the category of the semiotic hierarchy focused on the relationship between signs and that which they denote and connote, meaning that to which signs refer; hence, semantics has an intrinsic referential component (Jakobson 1964; Yngve 1986). Semantics is sometimes dichotomized into the two categories of 'semantics as meaning' and 'semantics as reference' (Akmajian *et al.* 1979; Bayles and Kaszniak 1987), however, careful consideration of this dichotomy reveals that, in fact, there is no meaning without knowledge of reference (that is, to what a word or larger grammatical unit refers to) and therefore, semantic reference needs to be subsumed, logically as well as by definition, under the overarching definition of semantics as meaning. Semantics as reference is a subset of semantics as meaning, and thus dichotomization is misleading and has led to confusion even in the literature on language function in AD, which will be described in the next sections. A second failure of class inclusion, which again leads to confusion in this field, stems from the fact that phonology, morphology, and syntax constitute a true hierarchy, whereas semantics cross-cuts both morphology and syntax; hence, semantics poses a problem for linguistic theory (Yngve, personal communication 1986), which has had a negative impact on research on morphologic, syntactic, and semantic processing in AD. Semantic processing can be analysed at both the level of the word or at the level of larger language units, thereby overlapping morphologic and syntactic ranks. Despite this overlap, semantics constitutes a separate rank of the semiotic hierarchy because of emergent properties of the rank (for instance organization of meaning), and in turn, morphology and syntax involve formal properties distinct from those of the semantic rank (deSaussure 1966; Huck and Ojeda 1987; Yngve 1986). Semantic processing at the level of larger units, such as the phrase or sentence, constitutes a more complex linguistic task than does semantic processing at the level of the word (Brown 1973). The issue of differing complexity demands of the different language tasks will be a recurrent issue in the description and analysis of language in the Alzheimer population.

Every level of the semiotic hierarchy involves a different relationship between the code and the context (Emery 1985). How do different diagnostic populations operate with code and context at the differing semiotic ranks? The semiotic categories provide a systematic and hierarchical context through which to analyse how patients with Alzheimer dementia operate with code and linguistic context.

LANGUAGE IN ALZHEIMER-TYPE DEMENTIA

The first reported case of Alzheimer's disease (Alzheimer 1907) involved a 51-year-old woman with significant language impairment. Despite the fact that Alzheimer himself included descriptions of language decrement in his hallmark case, reported almost 90 years ago, only relatively recently has a consistent interest in the diagnostic and prognostic functions of language in AD evolved (Kirshner *et al.* 1984*a*, *b*; Light and Burke 1993). Kertesz (1994) has pointed out that the first systematic studies of an Alzheimer population using standardized language tests were carried out by Bayles (1982) in a mildly impaired group of community-dwelling patients, by Emery (1982) in three severity groups of patients, and by Appell *et al.* (1982) in hospitalized in-patients.

Language deficit in AD is now recognized to occur in about 8–10% of patients as a major symptom early in the disease (Faber-Langendoen *et al.* 1988; Kertesz 1994; Kertesz *et al.* 1986), and it becomes the rule in advanced cases (Appell *et al.* 1982; Kertesz 1994). Kirshner and colleagues (1984*b*) describe language as an initial symptom, presaging the cortical degeneration of dementia of Alzheimer illness. Higher familial incidence might be associated with those cases where language disturbance is not just an early, but the presenting symptom (Folstein and Breitner 1982; Morris *et al.* 1984; Seltzer and Sherwin 1983). Several researchers have reported that prominent language symptoms are associated with the presenile form of AD (Blennow *et al.* 1990, 1991, 1994; Filley *et al.* 1986; Mesulam 1982; Seltzer and Sherwin 1983), but other investigators have not found onset to be a critical variable (Bayles 1991; Selnes *et al.* 1988). Disease course acceleration notwithstanding, a disturbance of language appears to be an intrinsic part of both Alzheimer's disease early- and late-onset and shows steady progression (Emery 1985, 1993). Ferm (1974) found that only 5% of over 100 AD patients, spanning both onset periods, had normative language capacity; language was impaired early in the disease and declined steadily. We will now examine these changes in more detail.

Phonologic decrement in Alzheimer-type dementia

As stated earlier, phonology refers to the phonetic and phonemic systems of a language. To define phonology further, 'phonetics' is the domain of sound without reference to meaning in which only sound producing processes are investigated. 'Phonemics' involves phonemes, which are not sounds *per se* (which is the domain of phonetics), but rather are features of sound, again without reference to meaning, which the speakers have been socialized to recognize and produce in actual speech sound (Darden 1974; Yngve 1986).

Phonologic knowledge has hardly been investigated in dementia populations, but is believed to remain relatively intact (Bayles and Boone 1982; Oxman and Baynes 1994; Whitaker 1976). The most noted aspect is 'phonemic paraphasia' (for example harmonita for harmonica) and is considered useful in the differential diagnosis of vascular dementia from AD (Moss and Albert 1988; Oxman and Baynes 1994). Overall, it appears that Alzheimer patients retain the ability to produce the sounds of their language and order them appropriately until they are in advanced stages of illness (Bayles and Kaszniak 1987; Emery 1982, 1985, 1993). Whitaker (1976) was the first to report the preservation of phonologic knowledge in an echolalic and severely demented woman who no longer was capable of producing meaningful language, but who nevertheless could correct errors spontaneously when asked to repeat phonologically anomalous sentences. Further, the neologisms of this patient conformed to the rules of English phonology (Whitaker 1976). Bayles and Kaszniak (1987) concluded that phonologic knowledge can be applied by AD patients who are incapable of meaningful communication. In an analysis of phonologic function in early-stage elderly AD patients, Patel and Satz (1994) reported, 'from bottom-up in the hierarchy of levels, it is clear that there are no deficits in phonetic articulation of word and sentence systems, that is, segmental sound combination and prosodic patterns' (p. 7 therein). Further, Patel and Satz conclude that there is preservation of phonology in AD, which applies also to orthographic structure, and that this 'cannot happen unless the phonologic and orthographic storage systems in lexical representation are intact and functional in SDAT' (1994, p. 7 therein).

Related to these findings is the ability of AD patients to continue to read orally (Cummings *et al.* 1986; Emery 1982, 1985). Because both the phonological and orthographic storage systems in lexical memory appear to remain active, preserved oral reading without comprehension in AD appears to involve both direct visual lexical access and graphophonological encoding.

Looking at phonologic processing in the context of working memory, Morris (1987) found that the processes underlying articulatory rehearsal in working memory remain spared in AD; the function of articulatory rehearsal in memory-span performance remains intact. The phonological store and the articulatory loop appear to be working, as evidenced by normal phonological-similarity and word-length effects on memory span.

In my own investigations (Emery 1982, 1985, 1988*a*, 1992, 1993, 1994; Emery and Breslau 1988, 1989), it was found that Alzheimer patients do best on language tasks requiring transmission, reception, or production of speech sounds without reference to meaning. This is consistent with the finding (Emery 1982, 1985) that the cognition decline due in AD involves the de-differentiation and desocialization, in which there occurs a separating of thought and meaning from sound. The sound components without reference to meaning appear to be the best preserved language function in AD.

Morphologic decrement in AD

Morphology is the semiotic level limited to parts of words and words, which are the smallest units of meaningful linguistic signalling. As previously mentioned, lexicon is a subset of morphology which refers to the totality of morphemes in a language. Morphologic language tasks include measures of lexical or vocabulary competence, for instance naming tasks. With few exceptions (e.g. Appell *et al.* 1982; Emery 1982, 1985, 1993; Emery and Breslau 1988, 1989; Kemper *et al.* 1993; Kempler 1984, 1991; Kempler *et al.* 1987), research on language in Alzheimer's syndrome has been focused primarily on naming impairment, formally termed nominal aphasia/dysphasia or anomia. Given the complexity of the language system and the many constraints on its investigation, it is interesting to see that there exists an overall consensus amongst the numerous investigators that naming impairment is prominent in Alzheimer patients (Appell *et al.* 1982; Bayles and Kaszniak 1987; Bayles and Tomoeda 1983; Butterworth *et al.* 1984; Critchley 1964; Emery 1985, 1988*a*, 1993; Emery and Breslau 1988; Huff 1993; Kertesz 1979, 1994; Kirshner 1994; Light and Burke 1993; Massman *et al.* 1994; Mathews *et al.* 1994; Patel and Satz 1994; Price *et al.* 1993; Stevens 1992). In one of the first extensive attempts at a systematic understanding of the language disturbance in Alzheimer disorder, Pearce and Miller (1973) state that a fundamental language deficit in Alzheimer patients is 'a poverty of speech due to the inaccessibility of the different vocabularies which are normally used in speech, writing, and reading' (p. 57 therein). In this same vein, Kertesz (1994) points out that the most commonly reported finding on language in Alzheimer's syndrome is 'an impoverishment of vocabulary and difficulty in finding words' (p. 125 therein). Irigaray (1967) found that parts of speech are impacted differentially; nouns are affected more than adjectives, and adjectives more than verbs. Several investigators have shown that words in common usage are more easily produced than are low-frequency words (e.g. Barker and Lawson 1968; Kertesz 1979; Miller and Hague 1975; Skelton-Robinson and Jones 1984). Non-linguistic factors have also been implicated in the naming impairment of Alzheimer patients. Naming proficiency increased when AD patients were permitted to handle stimulus objects (Hart 1988). In my own experience, AD patients have more difficulty correctly naming drawings of objects than they do the actual objects themselves, which points to some visual recognition component which is either additive or interactive in the naming problems of these patients (Emery, unpublished data). Indeed, studies that have systematically varied perceptual difficulties of objects in a naming task have shown a substantial effect on performance in AD patients (Kirschner *et al.* 1984*b*).

Looking at the earliest stage in the progression of Alzheimer disorder, Miller (1977) reported that 'the first changes to be noticed are usually a general poverty of vocabulary and range of expression; the speech becomes concrete, circumlocutory, and repetitive . . . dysphasic signs may also appear at some stage of illness' (p. 61 therein). Similarly, Kertesz (1994) concluded that the early stage of AD is marked by word-finding difficulties and circumlocutions with normally fluent articulated speech. This early naming impairment appears on the surface to be similar to anomic aphasia (Albert 1980; Hier *et al.* 1985; Kertesz 1979, 1994).

Turning now to longitudinal data, two longitudinal studies designed specifically for the investigation of changes in communicative function over time are the Chicago study (Kaszniak and Wilson 1985) and the Tucson study (Bayles 1985). In the Chicago study, 62 AD patients were evaluated annually for five years. This study found that mild to moderate naming impairment existed at initial evaluation, and performance on all naming tasks deteriorated during the course of the study. Most confrontation naming errors were perseverations of previously correct naming responses or terms semantically related to the target term (for example 'lock' for 'key'); phonemic substitutions were rare (Kaszniak and Wilson 1985). The Tucson study concluded that knowledge of vocabulary is significantly impaired early on and gradually deteriorates as dementia worsens; the Tucson study involved repeated measurements on 13 patients over 18 months (Bayles and Kaszniak 1987).

In summary, numerous studies have reliably shown that vocabulary becomes impoverished, speech concretized and circumlocutory, with confrontation naming progressively impaired in Alzheimer's syndrome. Consistent with this, it was found that good performance on morphologic tasks (as well as tasks from other semiotic levels) is related to low task demand, such as occurs when the correct answer is a high frequency term, cliche, stereotyped or overlearned expression (Emery 1985, 1988*a*, 1993).

A number of studies have found that the more complex morphologic task of generative naming/word fluency is significantly more impaired than confrontation naming, the impairment occurring earlier (see, for example, Bayles and Kaszniak 1987; Emery 1985, 1988*a*, 1993; Emery and Breslau 1988; Kertesz 1994; Pearce and Miller 1973). This finding, while robust, nevertheless has been a puzzle to researchers. Why does the AD patient experience greater processing demand when asked to name as many category constituents as possible (for instance animals, grocery items, clothing, and so forth), than when asked to name an object confronted with, or to fill in a missing term in a commonplace sentence? Addressing this issue, Emery and Breslau (1988) found that the answer lies in the greater inherent complexity of generative naming. Six variables are delineated which demonstrate that generative naming tasks, that is to say word fluency, are best regarded as 'meta-naming tasks' because generative naming:

(1) requires that many names/terms be generated as opposed to a single name or term;

(2) requires organization of names/terms into subsets, for instance wild animals, farm animals, for effective response;

(3) necessitates categorical attitude;

(4) necessitates maintenance of a cognitive set, namely must keep task requirement in mind over a longer period of time;

(5) hence, makes greater demand on memory;

(6) involves less constant stimulus and structural facilitation than do other kinds of naming tasks.

Thus, structural complexity of linguistic demand is an intervening variable between Alzheimer language function and linguistic tasks, making the task additionally one of executive function.

Finally, recently there have been a number of investigations attempting to uncover the nature of synthetic mechanisms underlying naming impairment (Butterworth *et al.* 1984; Huff 1993; Huff *et al.* 1986; Kertesz 1994; Kirshner 1994; Kirshner *et al.* 1984*a*, *b*; Massman *et al.* 1994; Mathews *et al.* 1994; Nicholas *et al.* 1985; Patel and Satz 1994; Price *et al.* 1993). This work has generated a number of hypotheses to explain the synthetic deficits underlying naming impairment in AD, the major hypotheses being semantic discrimination deficit, visual processing deficit, and lexical access, lexical recognition, lexical retrieval, and/or lexical selection deficits. Further, the interaction between cognitive deficits in both language and memory seems to configure the substrate underlying morphologic impairments in AD; the systemic interconnection of these cognitive processes becomes apparent in the context of organic brain syndromes (Emery 1994). Investigations designed to evaluate the relative contributions of these variables to the morphologic decrement in Alzheimer disorder are, as yet, inconclusive (Huff 1993; Kertesz 1994; Kirshner 1994; Light and Burke 1993; Massman *et al.* 1994; Patel and Satz 1994).

Syntactic decrement in AD

There are many investigations of naming impairment and other morphologic dimensions in AD showing these are prominent in the profile of language dysfunction. In contrast, only a few investigators have focused on the nomothetic study of syntax, and even among these there is disagreement as to whether syntactic function remains preserved in AD (Emery 1982, 1985, 1988*a*, 1993, 1994; Emery and Breslau 1988, 1989; Kemper *et al.* 1993; Kempler 1984, 1991; Kempler *et al.* 1987). Also, there exist several classical idiographic descriptions of language (including syntax) in dementia in general (for example Irigaray 1973; Schwartz *et al.* 1979; Whitaker 1976). A major problem encountered is that none of the standardized aphasia batteries measure syntax by isolating it as a specific test construct.

In what was probably the first nomothetic study of syntax in Alzheimer's syndrome, normal ageing, and pre-middle-age (Emery 1982, 1985) these populations were administered an adapted version of the Chomksy Test of Syntax (Chomsky 1979), the Test for Syntactic Complexity (Emery 1982, 1985, 1986), the Token Test (DeRenzi and Vignolo 1962; Spreen and Benton 1969), and the Boston Diagnostic Aphasia Examination (Goodglass and Kaplan 1972), along with measures from the Wechsler Memory Scale (Wechsler and Stone 1979), and measures of concrete operational thinking (Piaget 1952). The AD sample had a mean age of 80.3 years and the normal elderly a mean age of 83.4 years. All subjects were high school graduates; none had attended college. Variables of native birth, native language, native birth and language of parents, and occupation were controlled, as was literate socialization (Emery and Csikszentmihalyi 1981*a*). The Chomsky Test of Syntax (1979) was originally designed for children, but was adapted for this study of the elderly. It consists of four sub-tests, each of which is based on one of four syntactic conditions under which maximal complexity occurs, For example the true grammatical relationships that hold among words in a sentence are not expressed directly in the surface structure (for instance in Chomsky's 'Easy to See Test' the subject is presented with a blindfolded doll and asked, 'Is this doll easy to see or hard to see?'). The grammatical forms used in the Chomsky Test approach normative adult levels by age 10, but are absent in the grammar of 5-year-olds (Chomsky 1979). The Test for Syntactic Complexity was designed by Emery (1982, 1985, 1986) with the assistance of William Darden, PhD, Chair, Department of Linguistics, University of Chicago. The test consists of four sections which test comprehension of various syntactic relations that are complex and relatively late to develop (Brown 1973; Chomsky 1979; Dale 1976; Slobin 1970), namely:

1. Prepositions of time sequence, for example: 'Do you put on your stockings after your shoes?' 'What season comes before spring and after autumn?'
2. Passive subject-object discrimination, for example: 'The woman is seen by the man; who is seen and who did the seeing?' 'The dog was bitten by the cat; which animal bit the other and which was bitten?'
3. Possessive relationships of a reversible construction; for example: 'What is the relationship of your mother's sister to you?'; 'What is the relationship of your sister's mother to you?'; 'What is the relationship of your uncle's daughter to you?'; 'What is the relationship of your daughter's uncle to you?'.
4. Communication of narrative action events that are concrete and/or alogical, versus communication of abstract and/or logical relations of the same number of words per sentence, for example: 'John and Mary run to the hospital really fast' versus 'John runs faster than George but slower than Hamilton.'

The last syntactic section consisted of four pairs of communications of equal word-length per sentence, thus controlling for memory as an intervening variable (see Emery 1982, 1985). The linguistic data of this study were ordered within the hierarchical framework of the semiotic system (deSaussure 1966; Newmeyer 1980; Yngve, personal communication and 1986). In addition, data at the phonological, lexical-morphological, and semantic levels of linguistic operations were provided by the Token Test and Boston Diagnostic Aphasia Examination.

The results indicate that at no level of the semiotic hierarchy was the performance of the AD group comparable to the normal elderly or the pre-middle-aged. Nevertheless, the performance of the AD group varied markedly on different tasks; there was considerable gradation in performance corresponding to the semiotic ranks, with an inverse relationship between AD performance and task complexity and a direct relationship between good performance and early acquisition of a linguistic form in the developmental sequence of language.

In this section we are concerned with syntactic processing, and results from this study show unequivocally that elderly AD patients are very impaired in their processing of syntactic complexities. On all syntactic measures, the statistical differences between the AD sample and both normal elderly and pre-middle-aged were significant at the 0.0001 level. On the Test for Syntactic Complexity (TSC), mean scores for AD, normal elderly, and pre-middle-aged were, respectively, 5.4, 24.4, and 33.1 out of a maximal score of 36. Breaking down the AD mean score on the TSC into means by AD severity levels one finds that mild, moderate, and severe subgroup means were 11.3, 7.6, and 2.0, respectively. On the passive subject–object discrimination tasks of the TSC, the AD patients were unable to make correct passive subject–object discriminations, consistently imposing an active voice interpretation on passive-voice constructions; four elderly from the mild or moderate AD severity category gave one correct response, and 16 subjects gave no correct responses. This inability was demonstrated again on the Chomsky 'Easy to See Test'. Eleven of the 20 AD patients stated that the doll was 'hard to see' because *she* couldn't see with the bandana around her eyes, thus discriminating erroneously in terms of the subject and object of the verb *to see*. Again, there was a direct relationship between poor AD performance and degree of organicity; all 11 incorrect responses were from subjects in either the moderate or severe AD categories.

Further, the AD subjects were not able to process the communications of propositional, logical relations on the TSC; for example not a single AD participant correctly answered the question, 'Mary is paler than Louise who is paler than Judy; who is the palest?' In contrast, most of the responses given to equal sentence-length communications of concrete action events were correct, for example 'John ran to the store and Mary ran to the store; who ran to the store?' The inability of the AD group to process syntactically mediated logical relationships was demonstrated again on tasks requiring comprehension of reversible possessive relationships. Further, several Chomsky sub-tests showed yet another syntactically complex task which the Alzheimer elderly could not do, that of pronomial reference wherein the participant was asked to make subtle syntactic distinctions revolving around the referents of pronouns (see Chomsky 1979 or Emery 1985). The mean scores on the Chomsky Test of Syntax, which has a maximal score of 100, for AD, normal elderly, and normal pre-middle-aged were 13.2, 58.0, and 90.4, respectively. Breaking down the AD sample into mean scores by severity categories of mild, moderate, and severe, respective scores were 31.0, 16.6, and 5.6 out of maximal score of 100. On the Token

Test with a maximal score of 163, mean scores of AD, normal elderly, and pre-middle-aged were 26.4, 129.8, and 159.9, respectively. On the AD breakdown by severity, mild, moderate, and severe AD patients had mean scores of 70.7, 33.6, and 8.1, in turn. Thus the data from all these tests show that the impairment in AD is the greatest but more prominent with increased syntactic complexity. AD patients were unable to process post-stage II syntactic forms (Brown 1973; Chomsky 1979; Dale 1976), with relatively greater preservation of the simpler syntactic forms (Emery 1982, 1985, 1993). The difficulty with post-stage syntactic forms has been found in a series of subsequent studies; the findings described above were essentially replicated, although with minor variations (Emery 1988*a*, 1992, 1994; Emery and Breslau 1987, 1988, 1989).

Further, in the differential diagnosis between AD patients and demographically equivalent normal elderly, complex syntactic forms had the greatest discriminant function, followed by the meta-naming task of generative naming/word fluency and by the semantic task of reading comprehension (Emery 1988*a*, 1992; Emery and Breslau 1988). More specifically, in the study by Emery and Breslau (1988), using the Omega Squared statistic for discriminant function (Hays 1981), it was found that the Test for Syntactic Complexity discriminated best between AD and normal elderly with an Omega Squared value of 0.64; the Omega Squared values for the Western Aphasia Battery (WAB) (Kertesz 1982) sub-tests of Reading Comprehension and Word Fluency showed the next greatest discriminant function with values of 0.51 and 0.43, respectively. Similarly, in another study of discriminant function between AD and normal controls (Emery 1992), greatest discriminant power was attained by the Test for Syntactic Complexity, WAB Word Fluency, and WAB Reading Comprehension, with Omega Squared values of 0.68, 0.61, and 0.57, respectively. Consistent with this, Kemper *et al.* (1993) concluded that 'syntactic simplifications in written language may be an early marker of the onset of Alzheimer's disease' (p. 86 therein). Unlike the foregoing, where the greatest discriminant power between mild AD and normal elderly is obtained with *complex* syntactic, meta-morphologic, and semantic tasks, the greatest discriminant function between moderate Alzheimer patients and patients with depressive pseudodementia is with the *simplest* of naming tasks, such as the WAB Responsive Speech; it is the AD patient who does not know for sure how many days are in a week and who fails to know other overlearned material and/or items' names (Emery 1988*a*, 1994).

In their investigations of language in AD, Kemper and colleagues (1993) present results that lead them to the conclusion that syntactic ability is preserved in the context of impaired semantic ability. In their study they elicited single written sentences from 368 adults undergoing screening for possible AD. Whilst this study can be criticized for not defining the AD patients sufficiently and also biasing the material by only using responses if they were orginal complete sentences, it did indicate a number of additional interesting findings. Demented patients tended to produce sentences containing prepositions, main and secondary verbs, and conjunctions. They were also discriminated from non-demented adults by changes in clause length. These conclusions are consonant with the findings of Emery (1985, 1988*a*, 1993, 1994), Kopelman (1986), Nebes *et al.* (1986), and Patel and Satz (1994).

As with other studies suggesting syntactic preservation in AD, this issue should not be cast into a dichotomous frame which may not reflect the continuous quality of the variable. When syntax is less impaired than is semantics, this indicates only a *relative* preservation of syntax when compared to the greater decrements in semantic processing However, the main conclusion drawn by Kemper *et al.* (1993) as well as by Kempler *et al.* (1987), that semantic processing, overall, is more impaired than syntax in AD finds agreement in the works of others (e.g. Emery 1982, 1985; Irigaray 1973; Schwartz *et al.* 1979; Whitaker 1976).

In conclusion of this section, there is no question that AD patients can produce syntactically acceptable vocalizations, especially of the simple, automatic kind, so long as they can use language. It has been found that language preservation in AD is inversely related to complexity of the language form; this holds true across the semiotic ranks, and also within each semiotic rank (Emery 1982, 1985, 1988*a*, 1994). Accordingly, the simpler the syntactic construction, the more preserved it is in AD; conversely, the more complex the syntactic construction, the more difficulty and decrement are evidenced in AD. It has been suggested that syntactic production in AD consists largely of 'preprogrammed chunks' (Kempler 1984). As with any language form, some are used with greater frequency than others. It is therefore the overlearned, pre-programmed, more automatic syntactic forms that are best preserved in AD. When comprehension of a sentence is contingent on complex syntactic forms in the absence of redundancy and other cues, there is clear impairment in syntactic processing by AD patients.

The data on the comprehension of logical and complex syntactic constructions indicate a clear deficit (Patel and Satz 1994). Data suggest that AD patients show decrement in processing post-stage II syntactic forms, with evidence of regression towards the use of the simpler forms (Emery 1985, 1993). The complex post-stage II syntactic forms that show the greatest decrement in AD are less automatic, lower frequency constructions that developed last in the course of language development (Brown 1973; Chomsky 1979; Dale 1976). Regarding linguistic processing at the different semiotic ranks, AD patients do worse at the syntactic level than at the phonological level; phonological processing is the best preserved (Bayles and Kaszniak 1987; Oxman and Baynes 1994; Whitaker 1976). When tested with post-stage II complex syntactic forms, syntactic processing shows greater decrement than does morphologic processing (Emery 1985, 1993; Emery and Breslau 1988). However, AD patients show greater impairment at the semantic rank than they do at the syntactic rank of the hierarchy (Emery 1985; Irigaray 1973; Kempler *et al.* 1987; Schwartz *et al.* 1979; Whitaker 1976).

Differences pertaining to syntactic decrement found across different studies appear, in large measure, to be a function of dichotomous as against continuity frameworks; differences are also a function of how syntax is defined. Studies defining syntax in its most procedural sense find less decrement than do studies imposing rigorous requirements for meaning on syntactic structures. But, given that phonology is the only semiotic rank that by definition does not involve meaning (Bloomfield 1933; deSaussure 1966; Yngve 1986), it cannot be valid to define syntactic processing without the requirement of meaning. Accordingly, studies that use overlearned, pre-programmed syntactic chunks without regard to meaning as an indicator of syntactic processing and preservation are not really measuring syntax as it is defined; syntax *by definition* includes the factor of meaning (deSaussure 1966; Huck and Ojeda 1987; Yngve 1986). Thus, the use of phonosyntactic constructions without regard to meaning in the presumed measure of syntax in AD is problematic in terms of construct validity. In this light, neurolinguistic theory that posits that syntactic capacity constitutes an independent module dissociable from semantic knowledge (e.g. Benson 1979; Caramazza and Berndt 1982; Kempler *et al.* 1987) is problematic because, by definition, syntax must include the component of meaning, namely semantics.

Semantic decrement in AD

Let us now look at the linguistic level of semantics. Semantics refers to the analysis, organization, and interpretation of meaning. Whereas phonology, morphology, and syntax form a true hierarchy, semantics cross-cuts both morphology and syntax (Yngve 1986). Despite this overlap, semantics constitutes a separate rank because of its specified focus on meaning, and certain emergent qualities of the rank, for instance the organization of meaning. The semantic level involves the integration and organization of meaning with sound. Semantics, as a linguistic dimension, requires that the speaker renders meaningful a string of parts of words/words, phrases, sentences, paragraphs, including the concepts inherent in these linguistic units, through processes of comprehension, analysis, organization, and interpretation. Semantic processing at the level of the part of word/single word is less complex than at the level of larger aggregates of words. Length, namely the number of words, is a dimension of complexity in and of itself (Brown 1973). Accordingly, AD performance is better at the level of parts of words/single words than at the more complex semantic level requiring comprehension of larger groupings of words (Emery 1985, 1993).

In contrast to the debate related to syntactic processing in AD, there is a consensus among investigators that semantic processing is impaired significantly and consistently in AD (e.g. Bayles and Kaszniak 1987; Emery 1985, 1988*a*, 1992, 1993; Irigaray 1973; Kempler 1984; Kempler *et al.* 1987; Kertesz 1994; Kirshner 1994; Light and Burke 1993; Patel and Satz 1994; Schwartz *et al.* 1979; Whitaker 1976). Most studies of semantic processing have been at the level of the single word (see discussion under morphologic decrement in Alzheimer's syndrome). Despite the broad agreement amongst investigators that semantics is substantially impaired in the AD patient, the systematic study of semantic processing at its larger aggregates of words in this disorder is, as yet, in its infancy.

Bayles and Kaszniak (1987) have suggested that 'semantic knowledge is our knowledge of meaning properties and relations, referential properties and relations, and truth properties and relations' (p. 166 therein). In this discussion, Bayles and Kaszniak further stated that, as best they know, no one has studied comprehensively the AD patient's processing of 'meaning, reference, and truth properties and relations' (p. 169 therein). More recently, Oxman and Baynes (1994) came to a similar conclusion; such investigations are just beginning.

At the semantic level, the integration of sound with meaning is, by definition, required, We have pointed out already that the best AD performance at the level of vocabulary occurs under conditions of automatized treatment of lexicon in which integration between meaning and sound—thought and language—need be minimal. At the level of larger aggregates of words, such as the sentence, data indicate that the more abstract, logical, and complex the structure of the sentence, the greater the AD decrement, and the less the decoding of meaning. Maximal semantic processing for people with Alzheimer's syndrome has a direct relationship to simplicity and concreteness in code (Emery 1985, 1993, 1994). There is an inverse relationship between adequate semantic processing and necessity for integration of meaning with sound.

In discussing semantics, Jakobson (1964) stated that there are two basic modes of relation: the internal relation of similarity (equivalence) and the external relation of contiguity. Put another way, the speaker and hearer must have a common denotational and connotational system, a common code and common context in order to understand one another. In an investigation of elderly AD performance at the semantic level, 20 patients' responses were coded for equivalence in code (denotation) and commonality in context, (connotation) with the result that only 6 out of 20 patients showed both consistent equivalence in code and commonality in context; these six were in the mild or moderate severity categories (Emery 1985, 1993). Another three AD patients showed equivalence in code, but consistently shifted the context of discourse through the interjections of highly personal connotations. For example an 85-year-old accountant with AD, who understood quite well all the testing terms, and who had perfect scores on all naming measures, showed idiosyncractic connotation to common coding, for example when he was asked who was the president of the United States; he replied, 'Well, it isn't me . . . it's the one who was straight up'.

From the earliest beginnings of ontogenetic development, a person is socialized (Emery and Csikszentmihalyi 1981*a*, *b*) into the normative use of language; the progressive incapacity of the patient with Alzheimer's syndrome to code and decode within the normative range is akin to a process of desocialization. Language is a system of rule-governed or socialized behaviour; AD appears to be a process which progressively destroys the capacity for participation in rule-governed or socialized behaviour.

Vygotsky (1962) made the original observation that thought and language represent two separate lines of development until around two years of age, after which the two developmental lines intersect and become merged. The results from the research described in this chapter suggest that AD is a process in which the two lines of thought and language, or in our terms, meaning and sound, which were merged at one time in development, once again are separated or are in the process of separating. It is for this reason that semantic performance has a direct relationship to the requirement for integration between meaning or thought with sound. Once it is realized that Alzheimer dementing involves the process of separation of thought or meaning from sound, various symptoms of the disorder become comprehensible, for example vague, stereotyped, and imprecise language with circumlocutory phrases (American Psychiatric Association 1987, 1994). The linguistic forms on which Alzheimer patients do best all require the more minimal integration of thought or meaning with sound, for instance repetition, rote speech, overlearned phrases, automatization, cliches, stereotypes, pre-programmed syntactic chunks, and so forth.

To conclude this discussion of AD language in the context of the semiotic hierarchy, there appears to be an overall relationship between linguistic descrement in AD and linguistic complexity both across the ranks of the semiotic hierarchy, and within each rank. Further, there appears to be a concomitant inverse relationship between sequence in language development and subsequent linguistic deterioration; in other words the later the developmental acquisition of a linguistic form, the greater the linguistic complexity, the earlier the linguistic deterioration. Also, the data suggest there is a fundamental correlation between degree of organic impairment and degree of linguistic decrement (e.g. Emery 1985, 1994; Kemper *et al.* 1993); there appears to be a direct relationship between normative use of language—normative denotation and connotation—and organic intactness. In summary, we would suggest that Alzheimer dementia is inherently a process in which the patient suffers a progressive dedifferentiation and desocialization.

The aphasia profile in AD

There are many systems for the classification of aphasia, indicating a lack of consensus as to the form, content, and boundaries of the problem. Currently, there are eight patterns of aphasia that are well recognized: Broca's, Wernicke's, anomic, conduction, transcortical, global, semantic, and modality-specific aphasia (Kertesz 1979). These classes of aphasia were derived on the basis of sampling from populations of patients with focal lesions, (for instance brain-injured accident, war, stroke, and tumour victims). Patients with AD have not been part of the populations used in developing aphasia typology. For this reason, it should not be surprising that there is a fundamental lack of goodness-of-fit between the structure of language deficits in Alzheimer's syndrome and the focally-defined aphasia types (Emery 1985, 1993). In a detailed study of linguistic decrements in AD in the context of the eight well-defined existent aphasia types, it was found that none of those patterns were valid descriptions of the structure of language decrement which is part of the diffuse organic deterioration of AD (Emery 1985, 1993). Accordingly, I would recommend that an additional pattern of aphasia be defined which is based on the configuration of deficits in AD; further, I suggest that this ninth pattern of aphasia be termed 'Alzheimer aphasia'. For a contrasting and detailed discussion of how the language deficits of AD can be subsumed under existing aphasia typology, see Kertesz (1979, 1994); also, see Appell *et al.* (1982) and Hier *et al.* (1985).

FUTURE DIRECTIONS

This chapter has given an empirical and theoretical overview of the language deficits in Alzheimer's syndrome. Interestingly, further progress in the content domain of language in Alzheimer's syndrome depends as much on nosologic progress as it does on additional research, with which it is interdependent. Greater specificity in knowledge of the pattern of language decrements in Alzheimer's syndrome is, in part, contingent on nosologic clarification and subtyping of AD. Preliminary evidence exists for some linguistic variation on the basic structure and function of language in AD according to subtypes; for discussion see, for example, Blennow *et al.* 1990, 1991, 1994; Emery *et al.* 1994, 1995; Emery and Oxman 1992, 1994*b*; Kirshner 1994; Kirshner *et al.* 1984*b*; Mesulam 1987; Mulsant and Zubenko 1994; Tyrrell *et al.* 1990. Further improved definition and construct validation of Alzheimer subtypes can be facilitated by the careful study and description of language in AD as it differs as a concomitant of different clinical presentations and other clinical variables. It is probably impossible to get a clearer picture of language in AD as long as a construct and nosologic clarification of the overarching disease category with its subtypes is lacking.

In a similar vein, future directions must include greater care in the use of terminology in scientific and other professional communications, whereby the problem of phenomenal identity is averted. Phenomenal identity consists of calling the same disease entity by many different terms, and conversely, using the identical term to describe different disease entities. Further, terms such as 'dementia' and 'Alzheimer-type dementia' should not be used interchangeably; subtypes should not be discussed as if they were identical or co-extensive with overarching classification categories.

Still on the theoretical front, the relationship between semantics as a dimension of language and semantic memory needs to be worked on; some preliminary efforts can be found in Emery (1992, 1994).

Looking at future directions for research, language in AD as a function of stage of illness is, as yet, poorly defined. Understanding the progression of language deterioration in AD can best be achieved by diachronic or longitudinal investigations, of which there are, at present, very few; for preliminary data, see for example, Appell *et al.* (1982); Kaszniak and Wilson (1985); Kertesz (1979, 1994); Kral and Emery (1989); Storandt *et al.* 1992. Many other research needs have been pointed out throughout this chapter.

To conclude, there has been a discussion of AD as a phenotype or endpoint presentation with subtypes, and there has been a discussion of language in AD. This discussion has used broad brush-strokes, cross-cutting possible subtype and stage of progression variations. There has been an attempt to pull together the many disparate findings on language in Alzheimer's syndrome, and to outline a nomological context for these discrete data; the semiotic hierarchical system has been utilized for this purpose. The many deficiencies in our present knowledge about language in Alzheimer's syndrome have been pointed to, and accordingly, some future directions for theory and inquiry have been mentioned.

REFERENCES

Akmajian, A., Demers, R. A., and Harnish, R. M. (1979). *Linguistics: An introduction to language and communication.* MIT Press, Cambridge USA;

Albert, M. L. (1980). Language in normal and dementing elderly. In *Language and communication in the elderly* (ed. L. K. Obler and M. L. Albert), pp. 83–102. D. C. Heath and Company, Boston.

Alexopoulos, G. S. and Nambudiri, D. E. (1994). Depressive dementia: Cognitive and biologic correlates and the course of illness. In *Dementia: Presentations, differential diagnosis, and nosology* (ed. V.O.B. Emery and T. E. Oxman), pp. 321–36. Johns Hopkins University Press, Baltimore.

Alzheimer, A. (1907). On a peculiar disease of the cerebral cortex. *Allgemeine Zeitschrift für Psychiatrie*, **64**, 146–8.

American Psychiatric Association. (1987). *Diagnostic and statistical manual of mental disorders* (3rd edn. revised). American Psychiatric Association, Washington, DC.

American Psychiatric Association (1994). *Diagnostic and statistic manual of mental disorders* (4th edn). American Psychiatric Association, Washington, DC.

Appell, J., Kertesz, A., and Fisman, M. (1982). A study of language functioning in Alzheimer patients. *Brain and Language*, **17**, 73–91.

Arora, R. C., Emery, V. O. B., and Meltzer, H. Y. (1991). Serotonin uptake in the blood platelets of Alzheimer's disease patients. *Neurology*, **41**, 1307–9.

Barker, M. and Lawson, J. (1968). Nominal aphasia in dementia. *British Journal of Psychiatry*, **114**, 1351–6.

Bayles, K. A. (1982). Language function in senile dementia. *Brain and Language*, **16**, 265–80.

Bayles, K. A. (1985). Effects of dementing illness on communicative function. Paper presented at the *International Neuropsychological Society Meeting*, San Diego, California.

Bayles, K. A. (1991). Age-at-onset of Alzheimer's disease: Relation to language dysfunction. *Archives of Neurology*, **48**, 155–9.

Bayles, K. A. and Boone, D. R. (1982). The potential of language tasks for identifying senile dementia. *Journal of Speech and Hearing Disorders*, **47**, 210–17.

Bayles, K. A. and Kaszniak, A. W. (1987). *Communication and cognition in normal aging and dementia.* College-Hill Press, Boston.

Bayles, K. A. and Tomoeda, C. K. (1983). Confrontation naming impairment in dementia. *Brain and Language*, **19**, 98–114.

Blennow, K., Wallin, A., and Gottfries, C. G. (1990). Confusional symptomatology distinguishes early and late onset Alzheimer's disease. *Aging*, **2**, 395–401.

Blennow, K., Wallin, A., and Gottfries, C. G. (1991). Presence of parietal lobe symptomatology distinguishes early and late Alzheimer's disease. *International Journal of Geriatric Psychiatry*, **6**, 147–54.

Blennow, K., Wallin, A., and Gottfries, C. G. (1994). Clinical subgroups of Alzheimer disease. In *Dementia: Presentations, differential diagnosis, and nosology* (ed. V. O. B. Emery and T.E. Oxman), pp. 95–107. Johns Hopkins University Press, Baltimore.

Bloomfield, L. (1933). *Language*. Henry Holt, New York.

Brown, R. (1973). *A first language: The early stages*. Harvard University Press, Cambridge, USA.

Butterworth, B., Howard, D., and McLaughlin, P. (1984). The semantic deficit in aphasia: The relationship between semantic errors in auditory comprehension and picture naming. *Neuropsychologia*, **22**, 409–26.

Caramazza, A. and Berndt, R.S. (1982). Semantic and syntactic processes in aphasia: A review of the literature. *Psychological Bulletin*, **84**, 898–918.

Chomsky, C. (1979). *The acquisition of syntax in children from 5 to 10*. MIT Press, Cambridge, USA.

Critchley, M. (1964). The neurology of psychotic speech. *British Journal of Psychiatry*, **110**, 353–64.

Cummings, J.L., Houlihan, J.P., and Hill, M.A. (1986). The pattern of reading deterioration in dementia of the Alzheimer type: Observations and implications. *Brain and Language*, **29**, 315–23.

Dale, P. (1976). *Language development: Structure and function*. Holt, Rinehart, and Winston, New York.

Darden, W. (1974). Introduction. In *Papers from the parasession on natural* phonology (ed. A. Bruck, R. Fox, and M. LeGaly), pp. ii–xi. Chicago Linguistic Society, Chicago.

DeRenzi, E. and Vignolo, L. (1962). The token test: A sensitive test to detect receptive disturbances in aphasics. *Brain*, **85**, 665–78.

deSaussure, F. (1966). *Course in general linguistics*. McGraw-Hill, New York.

Emery, V. O. B. (1982). Linguistic patterning in the second half of the life cycle. D. Phil. dissertation. The University of Chicago.

Emery, V. O. B. (1985). Language and aging. *Experimental Aging Research Monograph Series* **11**, 1–63.

Emery, V. O. B. (1986). Linguistic decrement in normal aging. *Language and Communication*, **6**, 47–62.

Emery, V. O. B. (1988*a*). *Pseudodementia: A theoretical and empirical discussion*. Western Reserve Geriatric Education Center Interdisciplinary Monograph Series. Case Western Reserve University School of Medicine, Cleveland.

Emery, V. O. B. (1988*b*). The deficit of thought in senile dementia Alzheimer's type. *Psychiatric Journal of the University of Ottawa*, **13**, 2–8.

Emery, V. O. B. (1992). Interaction of language and memory in major depression/unipolar and senile dementia Alzheimer's type. In *Memory functioning in dementia* (ed. L. Backman), pp. 175–204. Elsevier Science Publishers, North Holland.

Emery, V. O. B. (1993). Language and memory processing in senile dementia Alzheimer's type. In *Language, memory, and aging* (ed. L. Light and D. Burke), pp. 221–43. Cambridge University Press, New York.

Emery, V. O. B. (1994). The interaction of memory and language in depressive dementia. In *Dementia: Presentations, differential diagnosis, and nosology* (ed. V. O.

B. Emery and T. E. Oxman), pp. 298–321. Johns Hopkins University Press, Baltimore.

Emery, V. O. B. and Breslau, L. D. (1987*a*). The acceleration process in Alzheimer's disease: Thought dissolution in Alzheimer's disease early onset and senile dementia Alzheimer's type. *American Journal of Alzheimer's Care*, **2**, 24–32.

Emery, V. O. B. and Breslau, L. D. (1987*b*). Linguistic cues in the differential diagnosis of Alzheimer's disease. *Clinical Gerontologist*, **6**, 59–62.

Emery, V. O. B. and Breslau, L. D. (1988). The problem of naming in SDAT: A relative deficit. *Experimental Aging Research*, **14**, 181–93.

Emery, V. O. B. and Breslau, L. D. (1989). Language deficits in depression: Comparisons with SDAT and normal aging. *Journal of Gerontology*, **44**, 85–92.

Emery, V. O. B. and Csikszentmihalyi, M. (1981*a*). The socialization effects of cultural role models in ontogenetic development and upward mobility. *Child Psychiatry and Human Development*, **12** 3–18.

Emery, V. O. B. and Csikszentimihalyi, M. (1981*b*). An epistemological approach to psychiatry: On the psychology/psychopathology of knowledge. *Journal of Mind and Behavior*, **2**, 375–96.

Emery, V.O.B., Gillie, E.X., and Ramdev, P. T. (1993). Spectrum of vascular dementia and the interface with Alzheimer's disease. In *Alzheimer's disease and related disorders* (ed. M. Nicolini, P.F. Zatta, and B. Corain), pp. 13–15. Pergamon Press, Oxford.

Emery, V.O.B., Gillie, E.X., and Ramdev, P. T. (1994). Vascular dementia redefined. In *Dementia: Presentations, differential diagnosis, and nosology* (ed. V. O. B. Emery and T.E. Oxman), pp. 162–95. Johns Hopkins University Press, Baltimore.

Emery, V.O.B., Gillie, E.X., and Ramdev, P.T. (1995). Noninfarct vascular dementia. In *Treating Alzheimer's and other dementias* (ed. M. Bergener and S. Finkel), pp. 184–203. Springer Publishing Company, New York.

Emery, V.O.B., Gillie, E.X., and Smith, J.A. (1996). Reclassification of the vascular dementias: comprising of infarct and non-infarct vascular dementias. *International Psychogeriatrics*, **8**, 33–61.

Emery, V.O.B. and Oxman, T.E. (1992). Update on the dementia spectrum of depression. *American Journal of Psychiatry*, **149**, 305–17.

Emery, V.O.B. and Oxman, T.E. (1994*a*). The spectrum of depressive dementia. In *Dementia: Presentations, differential diagnosis, and nosology* (ed. V.O.B. Emery and T.E. Oxman), pp. 251–77. Johns Hopkins University Press, Baltimore.

Emery, V.O.B. and Oxman, T.E. (1994*b*). The spectra of the dementias. In *Dementia: Presentations, differential diagnosis, and nosology*, (ed. V.O.B. Emery and T.E. Oxman), pp. 384–409. Johns Hopkins University Press, Baltimore.

Faber-Langendoen, K., Morris, J.C., Knesevich, J., LaBarbe, E., Miller, J., and Berg, L. (1988). Aphasia in senile dementia of the Alzheimer type. *Annals of Neurology*, **23**, 365–70.

Ferm, L. (1974). Behavioral activities in demented geriatric patients. *Gerontology Clinics*, **16**, 185–94.

Filley, C.M., Kelly, J., and Heaton, R. (1986). Neuropsychologic features of early-onset and late-onset Alzheimer's disease. *Archives of Neurology*, **43**, 574–6.

Folstein, M.F. and Breitner, J.C. (1982). Language disorder predicts familial Alzheimer's disease. In *Alzheimer's disease: A report of progress* (ed. S. Corkin), pp. 18–27. Raven Press, New York.

Goldstein, K. (1942). *Aftereffects of brain injuries in war.* Grune & Stratton, New York.

Goodglass, H. and Kaplan, E. (1972). *The assessment of aphasia and related disorders.* Lea and Febinger, Philadelphia.

Gottfries, C. G., Blennow, K., Regland, B., and Wallin, A. (1990). Alzheimer's disease—one, two, or several? In *Alzheimer's disease: Epidemiology, neuropathology, neurochemistry, and clinics* (ed. K. Maurer, P. Riederer, and H. Beckman), pp. 342–56. Springer-Verlag, New York.

Haass, C., Hung, A., and Selkoe, D. (1991). Expression of B-amyloid precursor protein (BAPP) in microglial cells and astrocytes. *Journal of Neuropathology and Experimental Neurology*, **50**, 340.

Hart, S. (1988). Language and dementia: A review. *Psychological Medicine,* **18**, 99–112.

Hays, W. (1981). *Statistics.* Holt, Rinehart, and Winston, New York.

Head, H. (1926). *Aphasia and kindred disorders of speech.* Cambridge University Press, Cambridge, England.

Hier, D., Hagenlocker, K., and Shindler, A. (1985). Language and disintegration in dementia: Effects of etiology and severity. *Brain and Language,* **25**, 117–33.

Huck, G. and Ojeda, A. (1987). *Syntax and semantics.* Academic Press, New York.

Huff, J. (1993). The disorder of naming in Alzheimer's disease. In *Language, memory, and aging* (ed. L. Light and D. Burke), pp. 209–21. Cambridge University Press, New York.

Huff, J. Corkin, S., and Growdon, J. H. (1986). Semantic impairment and anomia in Alzheimer's disease. *Brain and Language,* **28**, 235–49.

Irigaray, L. (1967). Approche psycholinguistique du langage des dements. *Neuropsychologia,* **5**, 25–52.

Irigaray, L. (1973). *Le langage de dements.* Mouton, The Hague.

Jackson, H. (1884). Evolution and dissolution of the nervous system. *British Medical Journal,* **660**, 703–22.

Jagust, W. J. (1994). Functional imaging in dementia: An overview. *Journal of Clinical Psychiatry,* **55**, 5–11.

Jakobson, R. (1964). Towards a linguistic typology of aphasic impairments. In *Disorders of language* (ed. A. DeReuck and M. O'Connor), pp. 28–40. Little, Brown, and Company, Boston.

Jobst, K., Hindley, N., King, E., and Smith, A. D. (1994). The diagnosis of Alzheimer's disease: A question of image? *Journal of Clinical Psychiatry,* **55**, 22–31.

Kaszniak, A. W. and Wilson, R. S. (1985). Longitudinal deterioration of language and cognition in dementia of the Alzheimer's type. International Neuropsychological Society, San Diego, California.

Kemper, S., LaBarge, E., Farraro, R., Cheung, H., Cheung, H., and Storandt, M. (1993). On the preservation of syntax in Alzheimer's disease. *Archives of Neurology,* **50**, 81–6.

Kempler, D. (1984). Syntactic and symbolic abilities in Alzheimer's disease. Unpublished Doctoral Dissertation, University of California, Los Angeles.

Kempler, D. (1991). Language changes in dementia of the Alzheimer type. In *Dementia and communication* (ed. R. Lubinski), pp. 98–114. B. C. Decker, Philadelphia.

Kempler, D., Curtiss, S., and Jackson, C. (1987). Syntactic preservation in Alzheimer's disease. *Journal of Speech and Hearing Research,* **30**, 343–50.

Kertesz, A. (1979). *Aphasia and associated disorders.* Grune and Stratton, New York.

Kertesz, A. (1982). *The Western Aphasia Battery.* Grune and Stratton, New York

Kertesz, A. (1994). Language deterioration in dementia. In *Dementia: Presentations, differential diagnosis, and nosology* (ed. V.O.B. Emery and T.E. Oxman), pp. 123–38. Johns Hopkins University Press, Baltimore.

Kertesz, A., Appell, J., and Fisman, M. (1986). The dissolution of language in Alzheimer's disease. *Canadian Journal of Neurological Sciences,* **13**, 415–18.

Kirshner, H.S., Webb, W.G., and Kelly, M. (1984*a*). The naming disorder of dementia. *Neuropsychologia,* **22**, 23–30.

Kirshner, H.S., Webb, W.G., Kelly, M., and Wells, C. E. (1984*b*). Language disturbance: An initial symptom of cortical degeneration and dementia. *Archives of Neurology,* **41**, 491–6.

Kral, V. (1983). The relationship between senile dementia (Alzheimer type) and depression. *Canadian Journal of Psychiatry,* **28**, 304–6.

Kral, V. and Emery, V.O.B. (1989). Long-term follow-up of depressive pseudodementia. *Canadian Journal of Psychiatry,* **35**, 445–7.

Lederer, R. (1980). *English word making.* University of New Hampshire Press, Durham.

Lederer, R. (1984). Rhyme with reason. *Verbatim,* **15**, 3–10.

Light, L. and Burke, D. (1993). Patterns of language and memory in old age. In *Language, memory, and aging* (ed. L. Light and D. Burke), pp. 244–71. Cambridge University Press, New York,

Luria, A. (1973). *The working brain.* Basic Books, New York.

Luria, A. (1980). *Higher cortical functions in man.* Basic Books, New York.

Massman, P.J., Butters, N., and Delis, D. (1994). Some comparisons of the verbal learning deficits in Alzheimer dementia, Huntington disease, and depression. In *Dementia: Presentations, differential diagnosis, and nosology* (ed. V.O.B. Emery and T.E. Oxman), pp. 232–48. Johns Hopkins University Press, Baltimore.

Mathews, P. J., Obler, L.K., and Albert, M.L. (1994). Wernicke and Alzheimer on the language disturbances of dementia and aphasia. *Brain and Language,* **46**, 439–62.

Mesulam, M.M. (1987). Slowly progressive aphasia without generalized dementia. *Annals of Neurology,* **11**, 592–8.

Mesulam, M.M. (1987). Primary progressive aphasia: Differentiation from Alzheimer's disease. *Annals of Neurology,* **22**, 533–4.

Miller, E. (1977). *Abnormal ageing.* John Wiley and Sons, London.

Miller, E. and Hague, F. (1975). Some statistical characteristics of speech in presenile dementia. *Psychological Medicine,* **5**, 255–9.

Monakow, C. (1914). *Die lokalisation in grosshirn and der abbau der funktionen durch corticale herde.* Bergmann, Weisbaden, Germany.

Morris, R.G. (1987). Articulatory rehearsal in Alzheimer type dementia. *Brain and Language,* **30** 351–62.

Morris, J.C., Cole, M., Banker, B.Q., and Wright, D. (1984). Hereditary dysphasic dementia and the Pick–Alzheimer spectrum, *Annals of Neurology,* **16**, 455–66.

Moss, M. and Albert, M.S. (1988). Alzheimer's disease and other dementing disorders. In *Geriatric neuropsychology* (ed. M.S. Albert and M. Moss), pp. 145–78. Guilford Press, New York.

Mulsant, B.H. and Zubenko, G.S. (1994). Clinical, neuropathologic, and neurochemical correlates of depression and psychosis in primary dementia. In *Dementia:*

Presentations, differential diagnosis, and nosology (ed. V.O.B. Emery and T.E. Oxman), pp. 336–53. Johns Hopkins University Press. Baltimore.

National Institute on Aging. (1995). Update on Alzheimer's disease. *The Harvard Mental Health Letter*, **11** (8), 1–4.

Newmeyer, F. (1980). *Linguistic theory in America.* Academic Press, New York.

Nicholas, M., Obler, L.K., Albert, M.L., and Helm-Estabrook, N. (1985). Empty speech in Alzheimer's disease and fluent aphasia. *Journal of Speech and Hearing Research*, **28**, 4–5–10.

Oxman, T.E. and Baynes, K. (1994). Boundaries between normal aging and dementia. In *Dementia: Presentations, differential diagnosis, and nosology* (ed. V.O.B. Emery and T.E. Oxman), pp. 3–19. Johns Hopkins University Press, Baltimore.

Patel, P.G. and Satz, P. (1994). The language production system and senile dementia of Alzheimer's type: Neuropathological implications. *Aphasiology*, **8**, 1–18.

Pearce, J. and Miller, E. (1973). *Clinical aspects of dementia.* Williams and Wilkins, Baltimore.

Piaget, J. (1952). *The origins of intelligence in children.* International Universities Press, New York.

Price, B., Gurvit, H., Weintraub, S., Geula C., Leimkuhler, E., and Mesulam, M. (1993). Neuropsychological patterns and language deficits in 20 consecutive cases of autopsy-confirmed Alzheimer's disease. *Archives of Neurology*, **50**, 931–7.

Roth, M., Tomlinson, B., and Blessed, G. (1966). Correlations between scores for dementia and counts of senile plaques in cerebral gray matter of elderly subjects. *Nature*, **209**, 109–10.

Schwartz, M., Marin, O., and Saffran, E. (1979). Dissociations of language function in dementia: A case study. *Brain and Language*, **7**, 277–306.

Selkoe, D.J., Abraham, C., Rasool, C.G., McClusky, A., Kosik, K., and Duffy, L.K. (1985). Paired helical filaments in human neurons: Relationship to neurofilaments. *Annals of the New York Academy of Science*, **455**, 583–96.

Selnes, O.A., Carson, K., Rovner, B., and Gordon, B. (1988). Language dysfunction in early- and late-onset possible Alzheimer's disease. *Neurology*, **38**, 1053–6.

Seltzer, B. and Sherwin, I. (1983). A comparison of clinical features in early- and late-onset primary degenerative dementia. *Archives of Neurology*, **40**, 143–6.

Skelton-Robinson, M. and Jones, S. (1984). Nominal dysphasia and the severity of senile dementia. *British Journal of Psychiatry*, **145**, 168–171.

Slobin, D. (1970). Universals of grammatical development in children. In *Advances in psycholinguistics* (ed. G. d'Arcais and W. Levelt), pp. 55–68. North Holland Publishing Company, Amsterdam.

Sourander, P. and Sjogren, H. (1970). The concept of Alzheimer's disease and its clinical implications. In *Alzheimer's disease* (ed. G.E.W. Wolstenholme and M. O'Connors), pp. 11–36. Churchill Livingstone, London.

Spreen, O. and Benton, A. (1969). *The Token Test.* University of Victoria, BC, Canada.

Stevens, S.J. (1992). Differentiating the language disorder in dementia from dysphasia—the potential of a screening test. *European Journal of Disorders of Communication*, **27**, 275–88.

Storandt, M., Morris, J.C., Rubin, E.H., Cohen, L.A., and Berg, L. (1992). Progression of senile dementia of the Alzheimer type on a battery of psychometric tests. In *Memory functioning in dementia* (ed. L. Backman), pp. 207–26. Elsevier Science Publishers, North Holland.

Svedelius, C. (1897). *L'analyse du langage.* Almqvist and Wiksell, Upsala, Sweden.

Tyrrell, P.J., Warrington, E.K., Frackowiak, R.S.J., and Rossor, M.N. (1990). Heterogeneity in progressive aphasia due to focal cortical atrophy. *Brain,* **113**, 1321–36.

Vygotsky, L. (1962). *Thought and language.* MIT Press, Cambridge, USA.

Wechsler, D. and Stone, C. (1979). *Wechsler Memory Scale.* The Psychological Corporation, New York.

Wegiel, J. and Wisniewski, H.M. (1990). The complex of microglial cells and amyloid star in three-dimensional reconstruction. *Acta Neuropathologica* (Berlin), **81**, 116–24.

Whitaker, H. (1976). A case of isolation of language function. In *Studies in neurolinguistics* (ed. H. Whitaker and H.A. Whitaker), pp. 1–58. Academic Press, New York.

Wisniewski, H.M., Wegiel, J., Morys, J., and Bobinski, M. (1994). Alzheimer dementia neuropathology. In *Dementia: Presentations, differential diagnosis, and nosology* (ed. V.O.B. Emery and T.E. Oxman), pp. 79–94. Johns Hopkins University Press, Baltimore.

Wisniewski, H.M., Wegiel, J., Wang, K.C., and Lach, B. (1992). Ultrastructural studies of the cells forming amyloid in the vessel wall in Alzheimer disease. *Acta Neuropathologica* (Berlin), **84**, 117–27.

Yngve, V. (1986). *Linguistics as a science.* Indiana University Press, Bloomington, Indiana.

ELEVEN

Visuospatial functioning

H. Branch Coslett and Eleanor M. Saffran

INTRODUCTION

Though long thought to be associated with deficits spanning the entire range of cognitive faculties, recent research has demonstrated that Alzheimer-type dementia may selectively impair specific mental capacities such as memory, language, or semantics. A subset of AD cases has also been identified in which visuoperceptual processes are disproportionately impaired relative to other cognitive functions; in such patients, visual or spatial difficulties are generally noted to be the earliest symptom of cognitive decline, although verbal IQ can remain fairly well preserved at a point where performance IQ is virtually untestable (De Renzi 1986; Martin *et al.* 1986; Saffran *et al.*, 1990; Thaiss and De Blesser 1992). These patients are of particular interest for several reasons. First, the investigation of these patients may be expected to contribute substantially to the ongoing effort to generate a behaviourally meaningful typology of patients with AD. Second, as we shall attempt to demonstrate below, the distinct patterns of deficits observed in these patients may be attributable to disruption of specific visual processing mechanisms and may therefore contribute to the understanding of normal visual processing. Finally, there is precedent for believing that theoretically motivated investigations of neuropsychological deficits can provide the basis for the development of more adequate therapeutic approaches to these disorders (see, for example, Schwartz *et al.* 1994)

In this chapter we will briefly describe our working model of normal visual processing. Subsequently, we will review the reports of patients with AD (or other dementing disorders; see Ross *et al.* 1990) exhibiting selective deficits in visuospatial processing. Three major types of processing deficits may be identified, each implicating a distinct level of processing or representation postulated in the model described below. The majority of AD patients who exhibit prominent but selective visual impairments appear to have deficits in visual selective attention. In a smaller number of patients, the deficits seem to involve processes that mediate object recognition—that is, the 'what' system—or those that support object location—that is, the egocentric map of space mediated by the 'where' system.

A MODEL OF VISUAL PROCESSING

Our model postulates the following stages and processes. First, the account assumes that basic attributes of the visual array, such as colour and line orientation, are registered effortlessly and in parallel in separate retinotopically organized maps. While this stage of representation is of short duration, it encodes complete information about the visual display, as indicated by the fact that information at a particular locus is fully recoverable if probed within 100 ms of presentation (e.g. DiLollo and Dixon 1988; Phillips 1974).

Although these visual feature maps collectively provide sufficient data to assemble a veridical image of the visual environment, 'seeing' requires the integration of information from each of these maps. Visual feature information is assumed to be integrated by a limited-capacity, effort-requiring process, that is, 'visual selective attention'. Visual attention has been likened to a 'spotlight' (James 1950; Umilta, 1988) or 'zoom lens' (Eriksen and Eriksen 1974; Eriksen and Murphy 1987; Eriksen and St James 1986); implicit in this metaphor is the assumption that there is an inverse relationship between the size of the region to which attention can be deployed and the 'intensity' or resolution of the attentional spotlight (Eriksen and St James 1986; Henderson 1991). From this account, a limitation in the capacity of the spotlight of visual attention may be expected to be associated with a restriction in the domain from which visual feature information can be integrated. As will be demonstrated below, a number of AD patients with significant visual deficits have exhibited such a phenomenon.

The model incorporates the basic distinction between systems mediating the processing of 'what' and 'where' (or in some cases, 'how to'). Thus, we postulate that the 'spatial map' represents the most abstract level at which visual information is represented. The spatial map is assumed to provide an *egocentric* or viewer-centred representation of the surrounding environment, in which objects or sites of relevance are registered by the creation of a 'token' or 'marker' which specifies object location in relation to the observer and, indirectly, with respect to other objects in the environment. Information in the spatial map persists over seconds (Irwin 1991; Irwin and Yeomans 1986; Kroll *et al.* 1970; Phillips 1974), accumulates over several fixations and is, at least in part, responsible for the phenomenon of perceptual constancy. Although the spatial map does not represent information about object identity *per se*, we assume that it does encode information about object dimensions. Thus, information represented on the spatial map may be sufficient to support reaching movements to a location as well as the object-appropriate shaping of the hand (that is, prehension) (Goodale and Milner 1992; Goodale and 1991 Milner *et al.* 1991).

Impairment of the spatial map may be expected to be associated with an inability to compute the location of visual and auditory, and, perhaps, tactile stimuli in relation to one's body. Object recognition should, however, remain intact. A patient with presumed AD who exhibited this pattern of performance will be described below.

Visual object recognition, we assume, requires that integrated visual feature information contact abstract, stored representations of words ('Visual word forms') and objects ('structural descriptions'), respectively. Whether the process by which the integrated visual feature information contacts these representations involves 'template' (e.g. Ullman 1989) or feature (e.g. Hummel and Biederman 1992) matching is, at present, unresolved. Our analysis shows that deficits at this level of representation may be responsible for (at least some forms of) object agnosia (Humphreys and Riddoch 1987). Under normal circumstances, this process culminates in access to appropriate semantic representations.

We hypothesize that conscious perception of the visual environment normally involves articulation of integrated feature information with the corresponding location in the spatial map and with stored information in the visual word form/structural description systems. It is the binding of information in the spatial map to the appropriate stored information about stimulus identity that enables conscious awareness of the stimulus and permits interpretation of the visual input. We assume that the capacity to maintain the linkages between tokens at the spatial map and stored descriptions is limited; we have suggested that, at least for some patients, the clinical syndrome of simultanagnosia is, in fact, attributable to a pathologic reduction in this capacity (Coslett and Saffran 1991). Viewed in this context, then, the binding operation may be regarded as a second, distinct attentional operation necessary for normal vision.

DISORDERS OF VISUAL SELECTIVE ATTENTION

Though there is variability from patient to patient, the descriptions of most of the patients with progressive visual disorders point to an underlying deficit in visual attention. Indeed, Pick, in the first report of such a case in 1908, characterized the deficit as an attentional disorder. His patient had difficulty recognizing larger objects, often identifying a part rather than the whole; the size effect also emerged with letters and digits. Pick concluded that the patient suffered from a reduction in the attentional field, in consequence of which the possibility of 'consciously taking in at a glance the separate parts of the whole in its total spatial relation is missing' (p. 48 therein).

Although patients with prominent visual deficits in the context of dementia were infrequently reported in the decades following Pick's (1908) original description, recently there have been a number of studies of patients with progressive visual deficits out of proportion to other types of cognitive, language, or mnemonic disturbance (Benson *et al.* 1988; Cogan 1985; 1983; Levine *et al.* 1993; 1988; Nissen *et al.*; Thaiss and De Blesser 1992, 1985). Cogan (patient 1, 1985), for example, described a patient with presumed AD who, despite normal visual acuity (20/25 ou) and apparently full visual fields was unable to locate objects placed in front of her except by touch; she lost her place on the page while reading and, under some circumstances, was unable to fix her gaze on an object held directly in front of her. In the later stages of her illness she exhibited increasing difficulties identifying objects and faces. Saffran, *et al.* (1990) reported two patients with presumed AD who exhibited visual deficits out of proportion to their memory and other cognitive deficits. One patient, 'Marie', although exhibiting normal visual acuity, visual fields, and eye movements, behaved as if she were blind in many settings. Thus, she was unable to find the handle to a door and was unable to locate an item in a busy array even after her finger was placed on the item by the examiner. She was usually unable to identify the words placed directly in front of her, frequently failing to direct her gaze to the stimuli. Her ability to identify single letters was a function of their size; like Pick's (1908) patient, she was able to identify small letters, but not large ones. In contrast, on occasion she quickly and accurately read signs at a distance from the car in which she was riding. Saffran *et al.* (1990) concluded that Marie's deficits were attributable to a deficit in visual attention.

Deficits of a similar nature have been reported by Bender and Feldman (1972), Cogan (1985), De Renzi (1986), Nissen *et al.* (1985), and Thaiss and De Blesser (1992). Prominent among the symptoms exhibited by these patients are impairment in reading—characterized by a tendency to lose one's place on a page, difficulty driving—attributable to a failure to perceive traffic signals, other cars, and pedestrians, and a tendency to get lost in familiar places. A number of patients with particular difficulties in the processing of complicated arrays, described as simultanagnosic (Graff-Radford *et al.* 1994) or having, in addition, the ocular motility problems characteristic of Balint's syndrome (Benson *et al.* 1988; Hof *et al.* 1990), have also been described. Many of these patients have also exhibited piecemeal processing of single stimuli resulting in letter-by-letter reading (Thaiss and De Blesser 1992; Price and Humphreys 1994) and object recognition deficits (DeRenzi 1986; Levine *et al.* 1993; Thaiss and De Blesser 1992).

Though differences in the extent and nature of the clinical and experimental investigations performed with these patients hinder attempts to establish the nature of the processing deficits underlying their symptoms, a number of investigators have suggested that the symptoms reflect a deficit in visual attention. We have recently completed detailed investigations of two subjects, with prominent visual processing deficits in the context of presumed AD, whose performance is consistent with this account (Coslett *et al.* 1995).

HW is a 57-year-old right-handed, college-educated engineer who, at the age of 55 began to lose his place on the page while reading. Approximately one year later, HW began to have difficulty driving; he stated that when concentrating on the road in front of the car, he often failed to see traffic lights as well as cars and other stationary and moving objects located to either the right or left of the car. At this point he also began to complain of difficulty finding his way around familiar environments, such as his place of work and the neighbourhood in which he had lived for many years. As these problems worsened, HW also began to experience word-finding and short-term memory deficits. Personality and interpersonal interactions appeared to be unaffected; he was unfailingly congenial and cooperative during the testing described below. Neurologic examination demonstrated mental status abnormalities, but was otherwise normal. Note that low-level visual processes, including visual acuity, visual fields, ocular motility flicker fusion, and the ability to perceive form from motion (Siegel and Andersen 1991), were normal.

RC is a 60-year-old right-handed, labourer with a high school education who, at age 54, first noted difficulty locating tools on his cluttered workbench. At approximately the same time he also noted difficulties reading text which he attributed to 'getting lost' on the page. Over the ensuing five years, his difficulties in reading and in locating objects in an array slowly progressed. At the time of the evaluation reported here, for example, he stated that he could not visually locate items in the refrigerator but identified them by palpation; thus, for example, when attempting to find the ketchup he was forced to rely on the feel of the bottle cap as the other bottles, jars, and cans 'confused' him. In the two years prior to these investigations he began to notice difficulties in recognizing some objects, particularly large ones. He experienced less trouble with small objects and, for example, routinely assisted his wife by threading her needles. Neurologic examination was normal except for visual and cognitive deficits as described below. Visual acuity was 20/25 ou with correction; colour naming was normal. Ocular movements were normal except for a modest reduction in upgaze. Visual field examination to confrontation revealed that he detected finger movements in both visual fields quickly and accurately; responses were asymmetric, however, in that he required movements of greater amplitude on the left. He exhibited a Riddoch phenomenon bilaterally; that is, previously visualized objects faded from view when stationary but were quickly detected once again when moved.

Evidence supporting the hypothesis that the patients' visual symptoms were attributable to an impairment in visual attention came from a number of investigations. First, an experiment assessing visual selective attention (Treisman and Souther 1985, Experiment 1) was performed. In this task subjects are simply required to discriminate between circles (hereafter designated 'O's) and circles of the same size with an intersecting vertical line at the six o'clock position (hereafter designated 'Q's). In the pre-attentive condition, the task is to detect a 'Q' in an array of 'O's; detection is normally rapid, effortless, and independent of the size of the array. In the attentive condition, the task is to detect an 'O' in an array of 'Q's; normal subjects do show an effect of array size in this condition, presumably reflecting the need to carry out a serial search of the array. Both subjects demonstrated significant deficits on this task; RC, in fact, performed at chance.

Having demonstrated with these (and other) data that HW and RC exhibited deficits in visual attention, we sought to test the more specific hypothesis that the patients' deficits were attributable to a reduction in the *capacity* of the spotlight of attention, such that the domain over which visual feature information could be integrated was reduced. We reasoned that if the patients' deficit is attributable to a restricted 'spotlight', the subjects would be impaired in the identification of large stimuli such as words or line drawings which extended beyond the region encompassed by the spotlight of attention compared to small stimuli which were fully encompassed by the attentional spotlight. To test this hypothesis the subjects were asked to name line drawings and words which were presented on different occasions in different sizes. Consistent with the hypothesis that the patients' visual deficit is attributable primarily to a reduced attentional capacity, HW and RC identified smaller words significantly more reliably than their large counterparts; RC showed a similar effect with line drawings.

A final point about the subgroup of AD patients with visual attentional disorders concerns the pathologic substrate of this disorder. Hof *et al.* (1990) reported eight patients with AD who, on the basis of the limited clinical data available in a retrospective chart review, appeared to show deficits similar to those described above. (The patients were said to have exhibited Balint's syndrome, a disorder which may be attributable to a visual attentional deficit.) In comparison to the brains of patients with AD without prominent visual deficit, those of the patients with AD and Balint's sydrome exhibited significantly greater numbers of neuritic plaques and neurofibrillary tangles in visual association cortex including areas 18 and 19, as well as the posterior parietal cortex. As several lines of evidence suggest that the latter region provides, at least in part, the neural substrate for selective attention, these data support the contention that the visual deficits in these patients reflect a disturbance in visual attention.

DISORDERS OF VISUAL OBJECT RECOGNITION

Although impairments in visual object, word, and face recognition were encountered in our patients as well as in others described above (Cogan 1985; DeRenzi 1986; Hof *et al.* 1990; Levine *et al.* 1993; Thaiss and De Blesser 1992), these patients were at least relatively good at identifying small stimuli. As the recognition of words and objects is not typically influenced by stimulus dimensions, this size effect suggests that these recognition deficits may be attributable to a reduction in the domain from which subjects are able to integrate visual feature information rather than to an impairment in the stored representations accessed in object and word recognition. In Lissauer's classical terminology, then, these patients may be said to exhibit an 'apperceptive agnosia'[1] (Lissauer 1889).

Disorders of visual object recognition in the absence of significant attentional or early visual deficits—that is, an associative agnosia—have, however, been reported in demented patients with progressive visual disorders. We are aware of two such reports. Taylor and Warrington (1971) described a 65-year-old, right-handed man with a progressive dementia who exhibited considerable deficits in object recognition in the context of largely preserved low-level visual processing. The patient exhibited a substantial impairment in object recognition, both in activities of daily living as well as in more formal testing situations. For example after stating that his tea needed more sugar, he failed to recognize the lumps of sugar placed before him; on another occasion, he attempted to cut paper with a screwdriver. He recognized only 8 out of 30 line drawings of common objects. He also exhibited an impairment of facial recognition, failing to recognize the photographed faces of famous people as well as the faces of hospital personnel with whom he had had extensive contact.

In contrast to his seriously impaired object and face recognition abilities, the patient performed well on a variety of tests of low-level *visual processing*. Thus, he performed normally on tasks requiring shape,

[1] In the context of the model described above, a deficit prior to or at the level at which visual feature information is integrated would constitute an appreceptive agnosia, whereas a disruption of stored information about word or object form or a failure to contact these structural descriptions would constitute an associative agnosia.

length, and figure-ground discriminations and performed well on the Block Design sub-test from the WAIS. Finally, although his drawings of common objects from memory were distorted and bereft of detail, he produced precise, detailed copies of line drawings. This pattern of performance is, of course, consistent with the claim that he exhibits a disruption of or failure to access structural descriptions.

Although the paucity of behavioural data precludes a definitive determination, a patient with autopsy-proven AD reported by Hof and Bouras (1991) may also have exhibited object agnosia. When initially evaluated for 'slight memory problems and disorientation', this patient was able to name objects by touch, but not by sight. Subsequently, he developed prosopagnosia. Elementary visual processes including visual acuity, visual fields, and ocular motility were normal, as was language.

Pathologic data reported by Hof and Bouras (1991) were at least consistent with current claims regarding the pathologic basis of impaired object recognition. In comparison to the brains of six patients with AD, quantitative neuropathological analysis of the brain of this patient revealed a dramatic increase in lesion counts in the occipitotemporal visual pathways—that is, the 'what' processing stream—whereas the patient's occipitoparietal visual pathway was less affected than that of AD control patients.

DISORDERS OF SPATIAL REPRESENTATION

As previously noted, our working model of high-level visual processing postulates that visual processing culminates in the creation of a 'spatial map' on which the location of perceived stimuli is marked in an egocentric coordinate frame. We have recently described a patient (GW) with presumed AD whose processing deficit appeared to be restricted to this level of representation (Stark *et al.*, in press).

The patient first began, in her early sixties, to experience difficulty driving. She was involved in five accidents over the course of approximately one year, all of which she attributed to an inability to determine the spatial relationships between her car and other cars or objects. Over the ensuing years she experienced increasing difficulty in navigating through familiar areas such as her town and home; despite having clearly seen and identified objects around her, she tended to bump into things on either side of her. She also began to have difficulty sitting down in chairs and positioning herself to lie in bed; for example early in the course of her illness she attempted to take her seat in a restaurant only to miss the chair and find herself sprawled on the floor. GW also noted that she was unable to localize sounds. While crossing a street, for example, she was unable to determine if the sound of a horn honking emanated from a car to her left or right. Similarly, it was observed that she often turned in the wrong direction when greeted by someone who was out of her line of vision.

In contrast to her profound spatial deficits, she reported no difficulties recognizing people or objects. She also denied problems with language or memory, and stated that she continued to enjoy reading although she admitted to losing her place on the page. Unlike the patients with visual attentional deficits described above, however, she experienced no problems in dealing with large, complex arrays such as the shelves in a grocery store.

Neurologic evaluation demonstrated myoclonic jerks in the left and, occasionally, the right arm. GW exhibited normal visual acuity, visual fields, and ocular motility. Although vibratory and movement detection thresholds were normal, she was unable to indicate the direction in which her extermities were moved. MRI scan revealed focal cortical atrophy involving the posterior superior parietal lobes bilaterally (Brodmann's area 7).

Neuropsychological evaluation revealed a verbal IQ of 99, whereas performance IQ was unmeasurable. Confrontation naming was normal, as indicated by a score of 83/85 correct on the Boston Naming Test (Kaplan *et al.* 1976). Memory was normal. Although her scores on these and other measures probably reflect some decline from her premorbid level of functioning, her non-spatial abilities appear well preserved relative to her capacity to deal with spatial material.

In contrast to her relatively good performance on the above tasks, GW was profoundly impaired on all spatial tasks. For example she performed abnormally on all subtests of the Visual Object and Space Perception Test (Warrington and James 1991).

A variety of experimental tasks were performed to establish the nature of the processing deficit. GW performed well on the task described above assessing pre-attentive and attention requiring visual processing as well as on a task evaluating the ability to shift attention. She also performed well on tasks assessing object and word recognition. GW was significantly impaired in judging the spatial location of stimuli in her environment. Thus, relative to age-matched normal controls as well as to other patients with presumed AD, she was grossly impaired in judging whether two 'X's presented in rapid succession on a computer screen occupied the same or different locations. The deficit in stimulus localization was not restricted to visual input; she performed at chance on a task in which she was asked to identify the speaker from which a 1000-Hz tone was presented. Finally, she was unable to compute the position of her body relative to objects in the environment; for example she was often unable to orient her head to her pillow or to sit on a chair without assistance.

These data are consistent with the claim that GW suffers from an impairment of the spatial map which provides an egocentric, modality-independent spatial representation.

MULTICOMPONENT DEFICITS

Although we have argued that AD (and other progressive disorders) may selectively disrupt distinct components of the visual system including the visual attention system, the spatial map, and systems mediating object recognition, we do not suggest that all—or even most—patients with AD exhibit visual processing deficits selectively involving a single component of the visual system. Indeed, patients who appear to exhibit deficits involving a number of visual processing modules have been reported. Thus, Levine *et al.* (1993), for example, described a man with AD who exhibited deficits which appeared to implicate visual selective attention as well as systems mediating object recognition. This patient exhibited difficulties driving and reading early in the course of his illness. Unable to 'see' whole words, he reported seeing only one letter at a time; when attempting to read he felt as though he were looking 'through a drinking straw'. These deficits are reminiscent of those described in patients with visual attentional deficits.

Additionally, however, as the patient's symptoms progressed, he became increasingly impaired in identifying words, line drawings, and photographs of faces; visual identification of real objects was relatively preserved, but ultimately became unreliable. The latter deficits were interpreted by the authors as evidence of disruption of the systems mediating object, word, and face recognition. The distribution of the pathologic markers of AD was consistent with this claim. Thus, Levine *et al.* (1993) found that nerve cell loss, neurofibrillary tangles, and senile plaques did not preferentially disrupt either the 'what' or 'where' pathways, but were unusually prominent in both the ventral and dorsal portions of areas 18 and 19.

CONCLUSIONS

We have reviewed case reports and single subject investigations demonstrating that AD may selectively disrupt specific visuospatial processing mechanisms, including visual selective attention, processes mediating object recognition, and the spatial representation system or 'spatial map'. We hope that these data serve to illustrate the manner in which cognitive analyses of AD may serve both to develop a more sophisticated behavioural typology of AD and to contribute to the understanding of normal cognitive and perceptual operations.

ACKNOWLEDGEMENT

Supported, in part, by grant RO1 AG08870 awarded to H.B.C. by the National Institute on Aging.

REFERENCES

Bender, M.B. and Feldman, M. (1972). The so-called 'visual agnosias.' *Brain* **95**, 173–86.

Benson, D.F., Davis, J., and Snyder, B.D. (1988). Posterior cortical atrophy. *Archives of Neurology*, **45**, 789–93.

Cogan, D.G. (1985) Visual disturbances with focal progressive dementing disease. *American Journal of Ophthalmology*, **100**, 68–72.

Coslett, H.B. and Saffran, E.M. (1991). To see but not two see. *Brain,* **114**, 1523–45.

Coslett, H.B., Stark, M., Rajaram, S., and Saffran, E.M. (1995). Narrowing the spotlight: a visual attentional disorder in presumed Alzheimer's Disease. *Neurocase,* **1**, 305–18.

DeRenzi, E. (1986). Slowly progressive visual agnosia or apraxia without dementia. *Cortex,* **22**, 171–80.

DiLollo, V. and Dixon, P. (1988). Two forms of persistence in visual information processing. *Journal of Experimental Psychology: Human Perception and Performance,* **14**, 671–81.

Eriksen, B.A. and Eriksen, C.W. (1974). Effects of noise letters upon the identification of target letter in a non-search task. *Perception and Psychophysiology,* **16**, 143–9.

Eriksen, C.W. and Murphy, T.D. (1987). Movement of attentional focus across the visual field: A critical look at the evidence. *Perception and Psychophysiology,* **42**, 299–305.

Eriksen, C.W. and St James, J.D. (1986). Visual attention within and around the field of focal attention: A zoom lens model. *Perception and Psychophysiology,* **40**, 225–40.

Goodale, M.A. and Milner, A.D. (1992). Separate visual pathways for perception and action. *Trends in Neuroscience,* **15** 20–5.

Graff-Radford, N.R., Bolling, J.P., Earnest, F., Shuster, E.A., Caselli, R.J., and Brazis, P.W. (1993). Simultanagnosia as the initial sign of degernerative dementia. *Mayo Clinic Proceedings,* **68**, 955–64.

Henderson, J.M. (1991). Stimulus discrimination following covert attentional orienting to an exogenous cue. *Journal of Experimental Psychology: Human Perception and Performance,* **17**, 91–106.

Hof, P.R., and Bouras, C. (1991). Object recognition deficit in Alzheimer's disease: Probable disconnection of the occipito-temporal component of the visual system. *Neurscience Newsletter*, **122**, 53–6.

Hof, P.R. Constantin, B., Constantinidis, J., and Morrison, J.H. (1990). Selective disconnection of specific visual association pathways in case of Alzheimer's disease presenting with Balint's syndrome. *Journal of Neuropathology and Experimental Neurology*, **49**, 168–84.

Hummel, J.E. and Biederman, I. (1992). Dynamic binding in a neural network for shape recognition. *Psychological Review*, **99**, 480–517.

Humphreys, G.W. and Price, C.J. (1994). Visual feature discrimination in simultanagnosia: A study of two cases. *Cognitive Neuropsychology*, **11**, 393–434.

Humphreys, G.W. and Riddoch, M.J. (1987). *To see but not to see.* Erlbaum, London.

Irwin, D.E. (1991). Information integration across saccadic eye movements. *Cognitive Psychology*, **23**, 420–56.

Irwin, D.E. and Yeomans, J.M. (1986). Sensory registration and informational persistence. *Journal of Experimental Psychology: Human Perception and Performance*, **12**, 343–60.

James, W. (1950). *The principals of psychology*. Dover Press, New York.

Kaplan, E., Goodglass, H., and Weintraub, S. (1976). *The Boston Naming Test.* Veteran's Administration, Boston.

Kroll, N.E.A., Parks, T.E., Parkinson, S.R., Bieber, S.L., and Johnson, A.L. (1970). Short-term memory while shadowing: Recall of visually and aurally presented letters. *Journal of Experimental Psychology*, **85**, 220–4.

Levine, D.N., Lee, J.M., and Fisher, C.M. (1993). The visual variant of Alzheimer's disease: A clinicopathologic case study. *Neurology*, **43**, 305–13.

Lissauer, H. (1889). Ein Fall von Seelenblindheit nebst conem Beitrage zur Theorie derselben. *Archiv Psychiatrie*, **21**, 222–70.

Martin, A., Brouwers, P., Lalonde, F., Cox, C., Teleska, P., and Fedio, P. (1986). Towards a behavioral typology of Alzheimer's patients. *Journal of clinical and Experimental Neurpsychology*, **8**, 594–610.

Milner, A.D., Perrett, D.I., Johnston, R.S., Benson, P.J., Jordan, T.R., Heeley, D.W., *et al.* (1991). Perception and action in 'visual form agnosia'. *Brain*, **114**, 405–28.

Nissen, M.J., Corkin, S., Buonanno, F.S., Growdon, J.H., Wray, S.H., and Bauer, J. (1985). Spatial vision in Alzheimer's Disease: General findings and a case report. *Archives of Neurology*, **42**, 667–71.

Pick, A. (1908). Zur Symptomatologie des Atrophischen Hinterhauptslappens. Studien zur Hirnpathologie and Psychologie. *Sonderabdruck aus der Deutschen Psychiatrischen Universitätsklinik.*

Phillips, W.A. (1974). On the distinction between sensory storage and short-term visual memory. *Perception and Psychophysiology*, **16**, 283–90.

Ross, G.W., Benson, D.F., Verity, A.M., and Victoroff J.I. (1990). Posterior cortical atrophy: Neuropathological correlations. *Neurology*, **40**, 200.

Saffran, E., Fitzpatrick-DeSalme, E.J., and Coslett, H.B., (1990). In *Modular deficits in Alzheimer-type dementia* (ed. M.F. Schwartz), pp. 297–328. MIT Press, Cambridge, MA.

Schwartz, M.F., Saffran, E.M., Fink, R.B., Myers, J.L., and Martin, N. (1994). Mapping therapy: A treatment program for agrammatism. *Aphasiology*, **8**, 19–54.

Siegel, R.M. and Andersen, R.A. (1991). The perception of structure from visual motion in monkey and man. *Journal of Congnitive Neuroscience*, **2** 306–19.

Stark, M., Coslett, H.B., and Saffran, E.M. Navigating without a map: A case study. *Cognitive Neuropsychology* (in press.)

Taylor, A. and Warrington, E.K. (1971). Visual agnosia: A single case report. *Cortex* **7**, 152–61.

Thaiss, L. and De Blesser, R. (1992). Visual agnosia: A case of reduced attentional 'spotlight'? *Cortex*, **28**, 601–21.

Treisman, A. and Souther, J. (1985) Search asymmetry: A diagnostic for preattentive processing of separable features. *Journal of Experimental Psychology*, **114**, 285–310.

Ullman, S. (1989) Aligning pictorial descriptions: An approach to object recognition. Cog. **32**, 193–254.

Umilta, C. (198?). In *Handbook of neuropsychology* (ed. F. Boller and J. Grafman), pp. 175–93. Elsevier, Amsterdam.

Warrington, E.K. and James, M. (1991) *The visual object and space perception battery.* Thames Valley Test Co., Bury St Edmunds, England.

TWELVE

Motor functioning

Daphne Kidron and Morris Freedman

INTRODUCTION

It has become increasingly evident that motor features are not only common in patients with Alzheimer-type dementia (AD) but that their presence may also provide insight into the natural course and possible heterogeneity of this disease (Table 12.1). Included among the motor findings in AD are extrapyramidal signs such as bradykinesia, rigidity and tremor, myoclonus, seizures, primitive reflexes such as the grasp, suck, snout, glabellar and palmomental reflexes, ideational and ideomotor apraxia, motor impersistence, motor perseveration, and utilization behaviour. Pyramidal signs such as hyperreflexia and extensor plantar responses have also been associated with AD (Franssen *et al.* 1993; Golaz *et al.* 1992). Although the NINCDS–ADRDA criteria explicitly incorporate the motor features of increased muscle tone, gait disorder, myoclonus, and seizures into the profile of 'probable AD' (McKhann *et al.* 1984), this spectrum of motor deficits in AD should probably be expanded to reflect many of the features described above.

Not all patients exhibit the full spectrum of motor deficits that have been described in AD. For example, according to a study by Förstl *et al.* (1992), which examined neurological signs and their neuropathological correlates in a sample of 56 patients with autopsy-vertified AD, rigidity was present in 35.7%, myoclonus in 21.4%, and generalized motor seizures in 10.7%. A grasp reflex was present in 33.9% of patients and 44.6% had a snout reflex. This variability raises the question of whether motor signs represent variation that may be seen across individuals with any disease or whether they carry specific significance with respect to subtypes of AD (Mayeux *et al.* 1992). This question, however, is a controversial one and requires further study. Nevertheless, motor findings may play an important role.

EXTRAPYRAMIDAL SIGNS

Extrapyramidal signs have been well documented in AD (Chui *et al.* 1985; Funkenstein *et al.* 1993; Huff *et al.* 1987; Mayeux *et al.*

TABLE 12.1 Motor symptoms in AD

Extrapyramidal signs
Tremor
Rigidity
Motor retardation (bradykinesia)
Gait disturbance
Role of medication
Myoclonus and seizures
Pyramidal signs
Hyperreflexia
Plantar responses
Primitive reflexes
Apraxia
Ideational
Ideomotor
Motor impersistence and motor persistence
Utilization behaviour

1985; Mölsa *et al.* 1984; Pearce 1974). The most common signs are bradykinesia (slowness of movement) and rigidity (increased resitance to passive movement) Tremor is relatively infrequent (Mayeux *et al.* 1985; Mölsa *et al.* 1984; Morris *et al.* 1989; Pearce 1974). Depending on patient samples, diagnostic criteria, clinical evaluation, and stage of disease, extrapyramindal signs have been described in 9–100% of patients with AD (Koller *et al.* 1984; Mölsa, *et al.* 1984; Morris *et al.* 1989; Sjögren *et al.* 1952; Thal *et al.* 1988). Extrapyramidal signs are more common in patients who have taken neuroleptic drugs, but also appear in 12–28% of patients who are drug-free (Burns *et al.* 1991*a*: Girling and Berrios 1990; Mayeux *et al.* 1985). The extrapyramidal signs frequently occur within the first few years of disease. Mayeux *et al.* (1992) estimate that the initial prevalence of extrapyramidal signs is 25–28% and the cumulative risk of developing them later is 32.7%. Soininen *et al.* (1992) followed 32 patients with probable AD for 3 years and observed, at entry, bradykinesia and rigidity in 39% and 11% of the neuroleptic-free patients, respectively. At year 3, bradykinesia was present in 72% and rigidity in 61%. Of the neuroleptic treated patients, 75–100% showed bradykinesia, rigidity, or orofacial dyskinesia. Tremor was not a prominent feature and its occurrence had not increased with time. Kischka *et al.* (1993), using quantitative neurophysiologic measures, studied 50 patients with probable AD who did not display extrapyramidal signs on conventional clinical testing.

They found that these patients had greater rigidity and bradykinesia compared to age-matched control subjects. Both features, especially the rigidity, occurred early in many patients with AD, and correlated positively with the severity of dementia. Measures of tremor frequency and amplitude did not differ between patients with AD and control subjects.

The term bradykinesia also encompasses the common gait abnormalities seen in advanced AD. The patients display slowness in walking, decreased step length, increased step-to-step variability, paucity of arm swing, and stooped posture, characteristics which are reminiscent of the parkinsonian gait. None the less, tremor, shuffling, and festination of gait, common in advanced parkinsonism, are seen less frequently (Franssen *et al.* 1993; Morris *et al.* 1989; Visser 1983). Sudden loss of ambulation in late-stage AD has also been described (Sjögren, *et al.* 1952), but the underlying mechanism is unclear. Another manifestation of AD, which is reflected in the gait, relates to increased daily locomotor activity (pacing behaviour). The patients exhibit almost constant walking and an inability to remain seated unless restrained. Satlin *et al.* (1991) suggested that the disturbed locomotor activity in such patients is compatible with reports of altered circadian rhythms of endocrine and other physiologic parameters.

Although the presence of extrapyramidal signs may relate to subtypes of AD (Chui *et al.* 1985; Mayeux, *et al.* 1985, 1992), many studies have suggested that their presence as well as myoclonus and psychosis, may be markers of disease progression, signifying greater disease severity at any given stage and a more rapid course of the disease over time (Burns *et al.* 1991*b*; Chen *et al.* 1991; Miller *et al.* 1991; Soininen *et al.* 1992; Wallin and Blennow 1992). The multicentre 'Predictors Study' (Richards *et al.* 1993; Stern *et al.* 1993), conducted on a cohort of 224 mild AD patients, is part of the attempt to determine the usefulness of abnormal neurological findings as potential markers of disease by trying to develop a model that can predict the disease course of individual patients and to identify milestones in disease progression. So far, only baseline measures have been published. It is of interest that the extrapyramidal signs (hypomimia, tremor, rigidity, stooped posture, bradykinesia, and gait abnormality) were found to be common at entry, but myoclonus was rarely observed.

Franssen *et al.* (1991, 1993) have studied advanced AD patients to examine relationships between neurological signs and functional capacity. A longitudinal study on 56 severely demented AD patients, showed a significant association between certain extrapyramidal signs (bradykinesia, rigidity, hypomimia, stooped posture), frontal release signs (paratonia, the tactile sucking reflex, and the grasp reflexes of the hands and feet), pyramidal signs (extensor plantar reflexes, hyperactive jaw jerk reflex, ankle clonus), and the magnitude of functional impairment. Signs that did not show any significant increments with continuing functional decline included hyperreflexia, the palmomental reflex, cogwheeling, resting tremor, shuffling gait, and festination. The glabellar blink reflex decreased in prevalence with more severe functional impairment. The findings of a relatively low incidence of tremor, cogwheeling, and festination differs from what is usually seen in the advanced stage of classical Parkinson's disease (Hoehn and Yahr 1967). Some PET studies support these observations, finding no significant difference in fluoro-18-dopa uptake in the caudate and putamen of patients with AD and in extrapyramidal signs, whereas patients with Parkinson's disease have shown marked reduction in fluoro-18-uptake in the putamen (Smith *et al.* 1992; Tyrrell *et al.* 1990).

MYOCLONUS AND SEIZURES

Myoclonus and major motor seizures may both appear during the natural course of AD (Clark *et al.* 1991; Romanelli *et al.* 1990). However, the frequency of occurrence of these problems, separately or in combination, and their relationship to the duration or severity of the disease is unclear. The prevalence of myoclonus in studies based on clinical observations varies between 4.3% and 19% (Chui *et al.* 1985; Heyman *et al.* 1987; Mayeux *et al.* 1985; Stern *et al.* 1987). In studies of autopsy-verified AD the variation is even greater and ranges from 9.8% to 62% (Bird *et al.* 1983; Duffy *et al.* 1988; Hauser *et al.* 1986; Risse *et al.* 1990). Similarly, the frequency of major motor seizures varies between 0.2% and 12.7% in clinical studies (Chandra *et al.* 1986; Seltzer and Sherwin 1983), and 9.8% to 64% in autopsy-verified AD studies (Hauser *et al.* 1986; Neary *et al.* 1986; Risse *et al.* 1990). Precise seizure classification in patients with AD is difficult since seizures may go unnoticed or unrecognized. In most case reports of seizures in AD, the seizures are described as generalized without specific mention whether these were primary generalized or focal seizures with rapid secondary generalization (Hauser *et al.* 1986; Romanelli *et al.* 1990). The correlation of seizures with EEG abnormalities in AD has yet to be determined, but it has been shown that seizures are not always evident in AD patients with epileptiform EEG activity (Rae-Grant *et al.* 1987).

In many of the above studies, myoclonus and seizures were reported to be a late manifestation in the course of the illness. However, Mayeux *et al.* (1985) reported a 10% prevalence of myoclonus in the early stages of AD. It is of note that those patients with myoclonus had a significantly earlier onset of dementia. Kaye *et al.* (1988) also observed a relationship between myoclonus and earlier age of onset. In addition, patients with myoclonus had more severe disease. In a longitudinal study of 93 patients, Clark *et al.* (1991) found a 5.4% cumulative rate of myoclonus five years after the onset of AD which had increased to 18.4% by the tenth year. The myoclonus appeared to be associated with an earlier onset of AD, but did not seem to indicate a worse prognosis. The cumulative rates of major motor seizures were 1.2% and 15.6% five and ten years, respectively, after the onset of AD. Whereas myoclonus could be observed either early or late in the course of disease, generalized seizures were usually associated with the late stages of illness and they also indicated a poorer prognosis. As many as 72% of the patients who developed multifocal myoclonus, later developed seizures. A cross-sectional study by the same authors (Clark *et al.* 1991) found no significant differences in age, gender, or duration of disease between AD patients with and without myoclonus.

PYRAMIDAL SIGNS

Evidence from neuropathologic studies and neuromaging studies generally indicates that the primary motor cortex is relatively spared in AD. Several studies, however, suggest that this is not invariably the case (Burns *et al.* 1991*a*; Franssen *et al.*, 1991, 1993; Golaz *et al.* 1992). For example Franssen *et al.* (1991, 1993) report a significant prevalence of hyperreflexia, extensor plantar responses, hyperactive jaw jerk reflex, and ankle clonus in AD, increasing with the severity of dementia. The mechanisms underlying the pyramidal signs are, however, unclear, but they may be related to diffuse white matter changes in AD (Bennett *et al.* 1992; Brun and Eglund 1986) or associated vascular dementia (Burns *et al.* 1991*a*). Jenkyn and Reeves (1981) suggest pyramidal signs can even accompany the process of uncomplicated ageing.

PRIMITIVE REFLEXES

Primitive reflexes, also referred to as release signs, developmental/neonatal reflexes, cortical or frontal disinhibition signs, include prehensile reflexes such as grasping, sucking, and rooting, and nociceptive reflexes such as the snout reflex, the glabellar blink reflex, and the palmomental reflex. The nociceptive reflexes occur in approximately 20% of normal elderley subjects (Jacobs and Gossman 1980; Jenkyn and Reeves 1981, 1983; Jenkyn *et al.* 1985; Paulson and Gottlieb 1968; Tweedy *et al.* 1982; Villeneuve *et al.* 1974). All the primitive reflexes, however, are more commonly associated with diffuse cerebral dysfunction (Basavaraju *et al.* 1981; Crichton and McDonald 1991; Franssen *et al.* 1993; Girling and Berrios 1990; Huff *et al.* 1987; Jenkyn and Reeves 1977). In AD, the frequency of nociceptive reflexes is 20–50%, the snout and the palmomental reflexes being the most common. They can appear early in the disease and do not correlate tightly to the severity of disease. The prehensile reflexes are less frequent (10–20%) but are distinctly associated with late-stage dementia. Among this group of reflexes, the grasp reflex is the most significant in terms of indicating pathology (Burns and Levy 1991*a*; Crichton and McDonald 1991; Franssen *et al.* 1991; Galasko *et al.* 1990; Girling and Berrios 1990; Huff *et al.* 1987; Molloy *et al.* 1991; Paulson and Gottlieb 1968; Tweedy *et al.* 1982). As yet, the clinical significance of the primitive reflexes is uncertain.

APRAXIA

Geschwind (1975), has defined apraxia as a failure to produce a learned movement in the absence of weakness, sensory loss, incoordination, incomprehension of or inattention to commands. With time and use by different health-care disciplines, the term apraxia has expanded to include numerous behaviours, often very different from each other. Due to this diverse use, there is some ambiguity concerning the prevalence, prognostic value, and localizing value of apraxia. Operationally, apraxia has been defined by Heilman and Rothi (1993) 'by exclusion, as a disorder of skilled movement not caused by weakness, akinesia, deafferentation, abnormal tone or posture, movement disorders, intellectual deterioration, poor comprehension, or uncooperativeness'. The same authors also point out the frequent association between apraxia and aphasia which can result in an erroneous diagnosis of either.

The common types of apraxia associated with AD are the ideomotor and ideational apraxias (De Renzi 1989; Della Sala *et al.* 1987; Lucchelli *et al.* 1993). Edwards *et al.* (1991), in a study of 142 patients with AD who fell into four stages of dementia severity, reported the combined presence of ideomotor and ideational apraxia in 35% of patients with mild AD, 58% of patients with moderate AD and 98% of patients with severe AD. Yesavage *et al.* (1993), who studied two separate cohorts of AD patients also found that the presence of apraxia or aphasia was associated with accelerated decline. In contrast, Burns and colleagues (1991*b*), found that the presence or absence of apraxia (or aphasia) had no influence on the rate of progression of AD. This group, however, found apraxia to be a stronger predictor of early death than aphasia or memory loss (Burns *et al.* 1991*c*).

In ideomotor apraxia there is an impairment in the selection of the elements that constitute a movement. The errors that are made are spatial and temporal. The patients have the greatest difficulty when they are asked to gesture to command (Goodglass and Kaplan 1963) but their performance may improve by imitating a movement or when using an actual object. Ideational apraxia has been defined as an inability to perform a correct sequence of acts. Patients with ideational apraxia perform poorly even with the use of actual objects (De Renzi *et al.* 1968; Pick 1905). Some authors prefer the use of conceptual apraxia to signify errors in content (De Renzi and Luccheli 1988; Ochipa *et al.* 1989) where patients may not recall the types of action associated with specific tools or objects or may have difficulty associating tools with objects (Heilman and Rothi 1993). Ideomotor apraxia can be seen with either focal or bilateral brain damage but ideational apraxia is seen only when both hemispheres are involved.

It has been shown that in demented patients apraxia of one type is not necessarily related directly to another type. The reports regarding the relationships between the different apraxias and the onset of disease are, however, conflicting. In a study of 32 patients with probable AD, all patients were found to have some degree of conceptual apraxia, but not all displayed ideomotor apraxia (Ochipa *et al.* 1992). In contrast, Edwards *et al.* (1991) reported that when ideomotor and ideational apraxia were considered separately, ideomotor apraxia was apparent in mild dementia, whereas ideational apraxia was found only in moderate and severe apraxia. Travniczek-Marterer *et al.* (1993) have also shown significant ideomotor apraxia in mild AD, which was significantly correlated with aphasia. Predictably, ideomotor apraxia has been shown to deteriorate with the course of disease (Della Sala *et al.* 1987).

There are several other behaviours associated with motor dysfunction to which the term apraxia has been applied. These include dressing apraxia, gait apraxia, gaze apraxia, eye-lid closing/opening apraxia, speech apraxia, and constructional apraxia. The use of the term apraxia is controversial in many of these cases (Poeck 1985), since they each refer to separate clinical phenomena that bear little relation to each other or to the basic concepts underlying ideomotor apraxia as defined by Geschwind (1975), Heilman and Rothi (1993), and Liepmann (1920).

MOTOR IMPERSISTENCE AND MOTOR PERSISTENCE

Motor impersistence refers to the inability to sustain a voluntary movement such as keeping the eyes closed, the tongue protruded, or the mouth open, making a prolonged 'ah' sound, fixating gaze, holding a deep breath, exerting steady hand-grip pressure, or keeping the head turned away during sensory testing of the hands (Benton *et al.* 1983); Berlin 1955; Fisher 1956; Joynt *et al.* 1962; Kertesz *et al.* 1985; Stuss *et al.* 1987). It is not an apraxia, as suggested at one time (Atack and Suranyi 1975; Fisher 1956), since patients can perform the movement and can also maintain it with proper verbal regulation. The impairment is of regulation of activity. Currently, motor impersistence is considered a disorder of sustained attention and is strongly associated with frontal system involvement (Stuss *et al.* 1987). Motor impersistence is most commonly reported after focal right hemisphere pathology, but may be found after diffuse or bilateral brain damage. Lopez *et al.* (1991), in a study of 166 patients with probable AD, observed motor impersistence in 10% of the cases, all of which were moderately or severely demented. The presence of motor impersistence was not associated with any specific neuropsychological impairment.

Motor persistence (namely perseveration) can also be observed in frontal system involvement (reviewed in Sandson and Albert 1984). It can be observed during reproduction of rhythmic structures, such as multiple loops, alternating squares and triangles (ramparts), or Ms and Ns, drawing of simple geometric shapes (for instance a circle) or when performing a movement to command (Nitrini 1987).

Luria (1965) proposed two types of motor perseveration, one characterized by unchecked repetition of a movement and the other manifested as a difficulty in switching from one activity to the next. The first type, which Luria termed 'efferent motor' perseveration, is compatible with the 'clonic' perseveration of Liepmann (1905), the 'compulsive repetition' of Freeman and Gathercole (1966), and the 'continuous' perseveration of Helmick and Berg (1976) and Sandson and Albert (1984). The second type, which Luria called 'perseveration due to impairment in the program of action' is equivalent to the 'impairment of switching' of Freeman and Gathercole (1966) and the 'stuck-in-set' perseveration of Sandson and Albert (1984). Sandson and Albert have suggested that continuous perseveration involves a disturbance in motor output characterized by post-facilitation of motor impulses, and that the stuck-in-set perseveration involves a breakdown between intent and action. Furthermore, they suggest a third type of perseveration called 'recurrent' perseveration, in which there is 'unintentional repetition, after cessation, of a previously emitted response to a subsequent stimulus'. The recurrent perseveration can be immediate or delayed. The process deficit in this case is hypothesized to be a failure of the usual inhibition of memory traces.

In AD the most common type of perseveration reported, whether motor or verbal, is the recurrent perseveration (Bayles *et al.* 1985; Fuld *et al.* 1982; Shindler *et al.* 1984). Fuld *et al.* (1982) reported that as many as 88% of patients with AD produced at least one delayed perseveration (namely intrusion) on a neuropsychological battery.

UTILIZATION BEHAVIOUR

Utilization behaviour is characterized by disinhibited, exaggerated dependency on objects in the environment for response cues (Eslinger *et al.* 1991; Lhermitte 1983; Lhermitte *et al.* 1986). The patients seem to be impelled to grasp and use objects within reach. Lhermitte *et al.* (1986) consider imitation to be a related behaviour, in which patients imitate the examiner's gestures and behaviour without being prompted to do so. Utilization behaviour is a less studied phenomenon and, as yet, little is known regarding its prevalence and prognostic importance in a clinical setting. It was found to be associated with grasp reflexes (Bindschaedler and Assal 1992; Fukui *et al.* 1993) and restlessness (Gustafson 1993) and has been described as occurring predominantly with frontal lobe damage, usually bilateral (Eslinger *et al.* 1991; Fukui *et al.* 1993; Gustafson 1993; Lhermitte 1983; Lhermitte *et al.* 1986). As yet, it is a motor behaviour which has not been studied extensively in AD.

Utilization behaviour and environmental dependency, as well as capture errors on a sequencing task (that is to say, invalid associations that are not broken in completing the task), are thought to be 'action lapses' (Norman 1981; Reason 1979; Shallice 1982). Subjects perform automatic routine actions which in the course of normal selection of behaviour should have been efficiently overriden and inhibited. They experience these difficulties in overcoming habitual responses, presumably due to inadequate control from the frontal systems (Della Malva *et al.* 1993; Norman and Shallice 1986; Reason 1979; Shallice 1982, 1988).

CONCLUSIONS

Motor symptoms and signs clearly comprise an important feature of AD. These symptoms and signs are varied and include different manifestations, such as extrapyramidal signs, myoclonus and seizures, pyramidal signs, primitive reflexes, apraxia, motor impersistence, perseverations, and utilization behaviour. Whether these features reflect markers for subgroups of AD or have prognostic significance, remains an open question. Additional studies are required to address these issues.

ACKNOWLEDGEMENTS

During the preparation of this manuscript, Dr Freedman's ongoing research was supported by grants from the Medical Research Council of Canada and the Ontario Mental Health Foundation.

REFERENCES

Atack, E. A. and Suranyi, L. (1975). Respiratory inhibitory apraxia. *Canadian Journal of Neurological Sciences*, **2**, 37–43.

Basavaraju, N. G., Silverstone, F., Libow, L., and Paraskeros, K. (1981). Primitive reflexes and perceptual sensory tests in the elderly: Their usefulness in dementia. *Journal of Chronic Diseases*, **34**, 367–77.

Bayles, K. A., Tomoeda, C. K., Kaszniak, A. W., Stern, L. Z., and Eagans, K.K. (1985). Verbal perseveration of dementia patients. *Brain and Language*, **25** 102–16.

Bennett, D. A., Gilley, D. W., Wilson, R. S., Huckman, M. S., and Fox, J.H. (1992). Clinical correlates of high signal lesions on magnetic resonance imaging in Alzheimer's disease. *Journal of Neurology*, **239**, 186–90.

Benton, A. L., Hamsher, K. deS., Varney, N. R., and Spreen, O. (1983). Motor impersistence. In *Contributions to neuropsychological assessment: A clinical manual*, pp. 126–37. Oxford University Press, New York.

Berlin, L. (1955). Compulsive eye opening and associated phenomena. *Archives of Neurology and Psychiatry*, **73**, 597–601.

Bindschaedler, C. and Assal, G. (1992). Environmental dependence in brain lesions: Imitative behavior, prehension and utilization (in French). *Schweizer Archiv für Neurologie und Psychiatrie*, **143** 175–87.

Bird, T. D., Stranahan, S., Sumi, M., and Raskind, M. A. (1983). Alzheimer's disease choline acetyltransferase activity in brain tissue from clinical and pathological subgroups. *Annals of Neurology*, **14**, 284–93

Brun, A. and Eglund E. (1986). A white matter disorder in dementia of the Alzheimer type: A pathoanatomical study. *Annals of Neurology*, **19**, 253–62.

Burns, A., Jacoby, R., and Levy, R. (1991*a*). Neurological signs in Alzheimer's disease. *Age and Ageing*, **20**, 45–51.

Burns, A., Jacoby, R., and Levy, R. (1991*b*). Progression of cognitive impairment in Alzheimer's disease. *Journal of the American Geriatric Society*, **39**, 39–45.

Burns, A., Lewis, G., Jacoby, R., and Levy, R. (1991*c*). Factors affecting survival in Alzheimer's disease. *Psychological Medicine*, **21**, 363–70.

Chandra, V., Bharucha, N. E., and Schoenberg, B. S. (1986). Conditions associated with Alzheimer's disease at death: Case-control studies. *Neurology*, **36**, 209–11.

Chen, J. Y., Stern, Y., Sano, M., and Mayeux, R. (1991). Cumulative risks of developing extrapyramidal signs, psychosis, or myoclonus in the course of Alzheimer's disease. *Archives of Neurology*, **48**, 1141–3.

Chui, H., Teng, E. L., Henderson, V. W., and Moy, A. C. (1985). Clinical subtypes of dementia of the Alzheimer type. *Neurology*, **35**, 1544–50.

Clark, C., Heyman, A., Earl, N., Utley, C., and Haynes, C. (1991). Myoclonus in Alzheimer's disease. In *Alzheimer's disease: Basic mechanisms, diagnosis and therapeutic strategies* (ed. K. Iqbal, D. R. C. McLachlan, B. Winblad, and H.M. Wisniewski), pp. 35–40. John Wiley & Sons, New York.

Crichton, P. and McDonald, C. (1991). Primitive reflexes in Alzheimer's disease (letter). *British Journal of Psychiatry*, **158**, 436.

Della Malva, C. L., Stuss, D. T., D'Alton, J., and Willmer, J. (1993). Capture errors and sequencing after frontal brain lesions. *Neuropsychologia*, **31**, 363–72.

Della Sala, S., Lucchelli, F., and Spinnler, H. (1987). Ideomotor apraxia in patients with dementia of Alzheimer type. *Journal of Neurology*, **234**, 91–3.

De Renzi, E. (1989). Apraxia. In *Handbook of neuropsychology*, Vol. 2 (ed. F. Boller and J. Grafman), pp. 245–63. Elsevier Science Publishers B. V., North Holland.

De Renzi, E. and Lucchelli, F. (1988). Ideational apraxia. *Brain*, **113**, 1173–88.

De Renzi, E., Pieczuro, A., and Vignolo, L. (1968). Ideational apraxia: A quantitative study. *Neuropsychologia*, **6**, 41–52.

Duffy, P., Mayeux, R., and Kupsky, W. (1988). Familial Alzheimer's disease with myoclonus and 'spongy changes'. *Archives of Neurology*, **45**, 1097–100.

Edwards, D. F., Deuel, R. K., Baum, C. M., and Morris, J. C. (1991). A quantitative analysis of apraxia in senile dementia of the Alzheimer type: Stage-related differences in prevalence and type. *Dementia*, **2**, 142–9.

Eslinger, P. J., Warner, G. C., Grattan, L. M., and Easton, J. D. (1991). 'Frontal lobe' utilization behavior associated with paramedian thalamic infarction. *Neurology*, **41**, 450–2.

Fisher, M. (1956). Left hemiplegia and motor impersistence. *Journal of Nervous and Mental Diseases*, **123**, 201–18.

Förstl, H., Burns, A., Levy, R., Cairns, N., Luthert, P., and Lantos, P. (1992). Neurologic signs in Alzheimer's disease. Results of a prospective clinical and neuropathologic study. *Archives of Neurology*, **49**, 1038–42.

Franssen, E. H., Reisberg, B., Kluger, A., Sinaiko, E., and Boja, C. (1991). Cognition-independent neurologic symptoms in normal aging and probable Alzheimer's disease. *Archives of Neurology*, **48**, 148–54.

Franssen, E. H., Kluger, A., Torossian, C. L., and Reisberg, B. (1993). The neurologic syndrome of severe Alzheimer's disease: Relationship to functional decline. *Archives of Neurology*, **50**, 1029–39.

Freeman, T. and Gathercole, C. (1966). Perseveration—the clinical symptoms—in chronic schizophrenia and organic dementia. *British Journal of Psychiatry*, **112**, 27–32.

Fukui, T., Hasegawa, Y., Sugita, K., and Tsukagoshi, H. (1993). Utilization behavior and concomitant motor neglect by bilateral frontal lobe damage. *European Neurology*, **33**, 325–30.

Fuld, P., Katzman, R., Davies, P., and Terry, R. (1982). Intrusions as a sign of Alzheimer's dementia: Chemical and pathological verification. *Annals of Neurology*, **11**, 155–9.

Funkenstein, H., Albert, M., Cook, N., West, C., Scherr, P., Chown, M., *et al.* (1993). Extrapyramidal signs and other neurologic findings in clinically diagnosed Alzheimer's disease: A community-based study. *Archives of Neurology*, **50** 51–6.

Galasko, D., Kwo-on-Yuen, P. F., Klauber, M. R., and Thal, L. J. (1990). Neurological findings in Alzheimer's disease and normal aging. *Archives of Neurology*, **47**, 625–7.

Geschwind, N. (1975). The apraxias: Neural mechanisms of disorders of learned movement. *American Scientist*, **63**, 188–95.

Girling, D. and Berrios, G. (1990). Extrapyramidal signs, primitive reflexes and frontal lobe function in senile dementia of the Alzheimer type. *British Journal of Psychiatry*, **157**, 888–93.

Golaz, J., Bouras, C., and Hof, P. R. (1992). Motor cortex involvement in presenile dementia: Report of a case. *Journal of Geriatric Psychiatry and Neurology*, **5**, 85–92.

Goodglass, H. and Kaplan, E. (1963). Disturbance of gesture and pantomime in aphasia. *Brain*, **86**, 703–20.

Gustafson, L. (1993). Clinical picture of frontal lobe degeneration of non-Alzheimer type. *Dementia*, **4**, 143–8.

Hauser, W. A., Morris, M. L., Heston, L. L., and Anderson, V. E. (1986). Seizures and myoclonus in patients with Alzheimer's disease. *Neurology*, **36**, 1226–30.

Heilman, K. M. and Rothi, L. J. G. (1993). Apraxia. In *Clinical neuropsychology* (3rd edn) (ed. K. M. Heilman and E. Valenstein), pp. 141–63. Oxford University Press, New York.

Helmick, J. and Berg, C. (1976). Perseveration in brain-injured adults. *Journal of Communicable Diseases*, **9**, 571–82.

Heyman, A., Wilkinson, W. E., Hurwitz, B. J., Helms, M. J., Haynes, C. S., Utley, C. M., *et al.* (1987). Early-onset Alzheimer's disease. *Neurology*, **37**, 980–4.

Hoehn, M. H., and Yahr, M. D. (1967). Parkinsonism: Onset, progression and mortality. *Neurology*, **17**, 427–42.

Huff, F. J., Boller, F., Lucchelli, F., Querriera, R., Beyer, J., and Belle, S. (1987). The neurological examination in patients with probable Alzheimer's disease. *Archives of Neurology*, **44**, 929–33.

Jacobs, L. and Gossman, M. D. (1980). Three primitive reflexes in normal adults. *Neurology*, **30**, 184–8.

Jenkyn, L. R. and Reeves, A. G. (1977). Clinical signs in diffuse cerebral dysfunction. *Journal of Neurology, Neurosurgery and Psychiatry*, **41**, 956–66.

Jenkyn, L. R. and Reeves, A. G. (1981). Neurologic signs in uncomplicated aging (senescence). *Seminars in Neurology*, **1**, 21–30.

Jenkyn, L. R. and Reeves, A. G. (1983). Evaluating cortical disinhibition signs. *Neurology*, **33**, 957.

Jenkyn, L. R., Reeves, A. G., Warren, T., Whiting, R. K., Clayton, R. J., Moore, W. W., *et al.* (1985). Neurologic signs in senescence. *Archives of Neurology*, **42**, 1154–7.

Joynt, R. J., Benton, A. L., and Fogel, M. L. (1962). Behavioral and pathological correlates of motor impersistence. *Neurology*, **12**, 867–81.

Kaye, J. A., Moore, A. M., Friedland, R. F., and Rapoport, S. I. (1988). Distinctive features of patients with dementia of the Alzheimer type and myoclonus. *Annals of Neurology*, **24**, 132.

Kertesz, A., Nicholson, I., Cancelliere, A., Kassa, K., and Black, S. E. (1985). Motor impersistence: A right-hemisphere syndrome. *Neurology*, **34**, 662–6.

Kischka, U., Mandir, A. S., Ghika, J., and Growdon, J. H. (1993). Electrophysiologic detection of extrapyramidal motor signs in Alzheimer's disease. *Neurology*, **43**, 500–5.

Koller, W. C., Wilson, R. S., Glatt, S. F., and Fox, J. H. (1984). Motor signs are infrequent in dementia of the Alzheimer type. *Annals of Neurology*, **16**, 514–15.

Lhermitte, F. (1983). 'Utilization behaviour' and its relation to lesions of the frontal lobes. *Brain*, **106**, 237–55.

Lhermitte, F., Pillon, B., and Serdaru, M. (1986). Human autonomy and the frontal lobes. Part I: Imitation and utilization behavior: A neuropsychological study of 75 patients. *Annals of Neurology*, **19**, 326–34.

Liepmann, H. (1905). *Über storungen des handlens bei gehirnkranken.* Karger, Berlin. Referenced in Sandson, J. and Albert, M. L. (1984). Varieties of perseveration. *Neuropsychologia*, **22**, 715–32.

Liepmann, H. (1920). Apraxia. *Ergebnisse der Gesamten Medizin*, **1**, 516–43. Referenced in Heilman, K. M. and Rothi, L. J. G. (1993). Apraxia. In *Clinical neuropsychology* (3rd edn) (ed. K. M. Heilman and E. Valenstein), pp. 141–63. Oxford University Press, New York.

Lopez, O. L., Becker, J. T., and Boller, F. (1991). Motor impersistence in Alzheimer's disease. *Cortex*, **27**, 93–9.

Lucchelli, F., Lopez, O. L., Faglioni, P., and Boller, F. (1993). Ideomotor and ideational apraxia in Alzheimer's disease. *International Journal of Geriatric Psychiatry*, **8**, 413–17.

Luria, A. (1965). Two kinds of motor perseveration in massive injury of the frontal lobes. *Brain*, **88**, 1–10.

Mayeux, R., Stern, Y., and Spanton, S. (1985). Heterogeneity in dementia of the Alzheimer type: Evidence of subgroups. *Neurology*, **35**, 453–61.

McKhann, G., Drachman, D., Folstein, M., Katzman, R., Price, D., and Stadlan, E. (1984). Clinical diagnosis of Alzheimer's disease: Report of the NINCDS-ADRDA Work Group under the auspices of the Department of Health and Human Services Task Force on Alzheimer's disease. *Neurology*, **34**, 939–44.

Mayeux, R., Stern, Y., and Sano, M. (1992). A comparison of clinical outcome and survival in various forms of Alzheimer's disease. In *Heterogeneity of Alzheimer's disease* (ed. F. Boller, F. Forette, Z. Khachaturian, M. Poncet, and Y. Christen), pp. 4–11. Springer-Verlag, Berlin.

Miller, T. P., Tinklenberg, J. R., Brooks, J. O., and Yesavage, J. A. (1991). Cognitive decline in patients with Alzheimer's disease: Differences in patients with and without extrapyramidal signs. *Alzheimer Disease and Associated Disorders*, **5**, 251–6.

Molloy, D. W., Clarnette, R. M., McIlroy, W. E., Guyatt, G., Rees, L., and Lever, J. (1991). Clinical significance of primitive reflexes in Alzheimer's disease. *Journal of the American Geriatric Society*, **39**, 1160–3.

Mölsa, P. K., Marttila, R. J., and Rinne, U. K. (1984). Extrapyramidal signs in Alzheimer's disease. *Neurology*, **34**, 1114–16.

Morris, J. C., Drazner, M., Fulling, K., Grant, E. A., and Goldring, J. (1989). Clinical and pathological aspects of parkinsonism in Alzheimer's disease. A role for extranigral factors? *Archives of Neurology*, **46**, 651–7.

Neary, D., Snowden, J. S., Bowen, D. M., Sims, N. R., Mann, D. M., Yates, P. O., *et al.* (1986). Cerebral biopsy in the investigation of presenile dementia due to cerebral atrophy. *Journal of Neurology, Neurosurgery and Psychiatry*, **49**, 157–62.

Nitrini, R. (1987). Elementary motor perseveration in early diagnosis of progressive supranuclear palsy. *Arquivos de Neuro-Psiquiatria*, **45**, 29–32.

Norman, D. A. (1981). Categorization of action slips. *Psychological Review*, **88**, 1–15.

Norman, D. A. and Shallice, T. (1986). Attention to action: Willed and automatic control of behavior. In *Consciousness and self-regulation: Advances in research and theory*, Vol. 4 (ed. R. J. Davidson, G. E. Schwartz and D. Shapiro), pp. 1–18. Plenum Press, New York.

Ochipa, C., Rothi, L. J. G., and Heilman, K. M. (1989). Ideational apraxia: A deficit in tool selection and use. *Annals of Neurology*, **25**, 190–3.

Ochipa, C., Rothi, L. J. G., and Heilman, K. M. (1992). Conceptual apraxia in Alzheimer's disease. *Brain*, **115**, 1061–71.

Paulson, G. and Gottlieb, G. (1968). Developmental reflexes: The reappearance of foetal and neonatal reflexes in aged patients. *Brain*, **91**, 37–52.

Pearce, J. (1974). The extrapyramidal disorder of Alzheimer's disease. *European Neurology*, **12**, 94–103.

Pick, A. (1905). *Studien über motorische apraxie and ihre nahesthende erscheinungen: Ihre bedeutung in der symptomatologie psychopathologischer symptomenkomplexe.* Deuticke, Leipzig. Referenced in De Renzi, E. (1989). Apraxia. In *Handbook of neuropsychology*, Vol. 2 (ed. F. Boller, and J. Grafman), pp. 245–63. Elsevier Science Publishers B. V., North Holland.

Poeck, K. (1985). Clues to the nature of disruptions to limb praxis. In *Neuropsychological studies of apraxia and related disorders* (ed. E. A. Roy), pp. 99–109. Elsevier Science Publishers B. V., North Holland.

Rae-Grant, A., Blume, W., Lau, C., Hachinski, V., Fishman, M., and Mersky, H. (1987). The electroencephalogram in Alzheimer-type dementia: A sequential study correlating the electroencephalogram with psychometric and quantitative pathologic data. *Archives of Neurology*, **44**, 50–4.

Reason, J. T. (1979). Action not as planned. In *Aspects of consciousness* (ed. G. Underwood and R. Stevens), pp. 67–88. Academic Press, London.

Richards, M., Folstein, M., Albert, M., Miller, L., Bylsma, F., Lafleche, G., *et al.* (1993). Multicenter study of predictors of disease course in Alzheimer's disease (the 'Predictors Study'). II. Neurological, psychiatric and demographic influences on baseline measures of disease severity. *Alzheimer Disease and Associated Disorders*, **7**, 22–32.

Risse, S. C., Lampe, T. H., Bird, T. D., Nochlin, D., Sumi, S. M., Keenan, T., *et al.* (1990). Myoclonus, seizures and paratonia in Alzheimer's disease. *Alzheimer Disease and Associated Disorders*, **4** 217–25.

Romanelli, M. F., Morris, J. C., Ashkin, K., and Coben, L. A. (1990). Advanced Alzheimer's disease is a risk factor for late-onset seizures. *Archives of Neurology*, **47**, 847–50.

Sandson, J. and Albert, M. L. (1984). Varieties of perseveration. *Neuropsychologia*, **22**, 715–32.

Satlin, A., Teicher, M. H., Lieberman, H. R., Baldessarini, R. J., Volicer, L., and Rheaume, Y. (1991). Circadian locomotor activity rhythms in Alzheimer's disease. *Neuropsychopharmacology*, **5**, 115–26.

Seltzer, B. and Sherwin, I. (1983). A comparison of clinical features in early and late-onset primary degenerative dementia. *Archives of Neurology*, **40**, 143–6.

Shallice, T. (1982). Specific impairements of planning. In *The neuropsychology of cognitive function* (ed. D. E. Broadbent and L. Weiskrantz), pp. 199–209. The Royal Society, London.

Shallice, T. (1988). *From neuropsychology to mental structure.* Cambridge University Press.

Shindler, A. G., Caplan, L. R., and Hier, D. B. (1984). Intrusions and perseverations. *Brain and Language*, **23**, 148–58.

Sjögren, T., Sjögren, H., and Lindgren, A. G. H. (1952). Morbus Alzheimer and morbus Pick: A genetic, clinical and patho-anatomical study. *Acta Psychiatrica et Neurologica Scandinavica*, **82**, (Suppl.), 1–152.

Smith, G. S., de Leon, M. J., George, A. E., Kluger, A., Volkow, N. D., McRae, T., *et al.* (1992). Topography of cross-sectional and longitudinal glucose metabolic deficits in Alzheimer's disease: Pathophysiologic implications. *Archives of Neurology*, **49**, 1142–50.

Soininen, H., Laulumaa, V., Helkala, E. L., Hartikainen, P., and Riekkinen, P.J. (1992). Extrapyramidal signs in Alzheimer's disease: A 3-year follow-up study. *Journal of Neural Transmission*, **4**, 107–19.

Stern, Y., Mayeux, R., Sano, M., Hauser, W. A., and Bush, T. (1987). Predictors of disease course in patients with probable Alzheimer's disease. *Neurology*, **37**, 1649–53.

Stern, Y., Folstein, M., Albert, M., Richards, M., Miller, L., Bylsma, F., *et al.* (1993). Multicenter study of predictors of disease course in Alzheimer's disease (the 'Predictors Study'). I. Study design, cohort description and intersite comparisons. *Alzheimer Disease and Associated Disorders*, **7**, 3–21.

Stuss, D. T., Delgado, M., and Guzman, D. A. (1987). Verbal regulation in the control of motor impersistence: A proposed rehabilitation procedure. *Journal of Neurologic Rehabilitation*, **1**, 19–24.

Thal, L. J., Grundman, M., and Klauber, M. R. (1988). Dementia: Characteristics of a referral population and factors associated with progression. *Neurology*, **38**, 1083–90.

Travniczek-Marterer, A., Danielczyk, W., Simanyi, M., and Fischer, P. (1993). Ideomotor apraxia in Alzheimer's disease. *Acta Neurologica Scandinavica*, **88**, 1–4.

Tweedy, J., Reding, M., Garcia, C., Schulman, P., Deutsch, G., and Antin, S. (1982). Significance of cortical disinhibition signs. *Neurology*, **32**, 169–73.

Tyrrell, P. J., Sawle, G. V., Ibanez, V., Bloomfield, P. M., Leenders, K. L., Frackowiak, R. S., *et al.* (1990). Clinical and PET studies in the 'extrapyramidal syndrome' of dementia of the Alzheimer type. *Archives of Neurology*, **47**, 1318–23.

Villeneuve, A., Turcotte, J., Bouchard, M., Cote, J. M., and Jus, A. (1974). Release phenomena and iterative activities in psychiatric geriatric patients. *Canadian Medical Association Journal*, **19**, 147–53.

Visser, H. (1983). Gait and balance in senile dementia of Alzheimer's type. *Age and Ageing*, **12**, 296–301.

Wallin, A. and Blennow, K. (1992). Neurologic motor signs in early and late onset Alzheimer's disease. *Dementia*, **3**, 314–19.

Yesavage, J. A., Brooks, J. O., Taylor, J., and Tinkelberg, J. (1993). Development of aphasia, apraxia and agnosia and decline in Alzheimer's disease. *American Journal of Psychiatry*, **150**, 742–7.

III. Neurobiology

THIRTEEN

Neurobiological correlates of cognitive dysfunction

Robin G. Morris

INTRODUCTION

In 1906, Alöis Alzheimer presented the famous case of what has now come to be called Alzheimer disease (AD), producing a further short publication in 1907 and a subsequent paper in 1911 (see Förstl and Levy 1991). In doing so he had identified the main neuropathological markers associated with AD, the so-called neuritic plaques and neurofibrillary tangles, his neuropathological descriptions containing many important points that have subsequently been 'rediscovered'. The neurohistological features he described are complex and variable, but in essence became the main defining neuropathological characteristics when AD was established as the main cause of dementia in old age during the 1950s and 1960s (Tomlinson *et al.* 1970). A range of neurochemical, neurophysiological, and neuroimaging investigations has in followed in recent years. This chapter focuses on these different aspects, with the exception of the neurochemistry (dealt with in Chapter 14), and, in keeping with the theme of the book, how they relate specifically to cognitive impairment in AD.

MACROSCOPIC PATHOLOGY

The gross features of the brain of an AD patient are well known. These include cerebral atrophy, with widened sulci and narrow convolutions, decreased white matter, and ventricular enlargement, particularly the size of the lateral ventricles. Brain atrophy is associated with a reduction in weight, the greatest occuring in the cerebral hemispheres. Although there is much overlap in individual cases within the normal range, figures of approximately 7–8% reduction in brain weight have been described (Esiri 1990). Even on gross pathology, the frontoparietal region and the temporal lobes may be more severely affected than the rest of the brain (Lantos and Cairns 1994). 'Pitting' of the parahippocampal gyrus has been observed, indicating the substantial neuronal damage to this structure (Hyman *et al.* 1990). The decrement in the mesiotemporal lobe region is reflected in additional space between the hippocampus and walls of the temporal horns. Of note, a reduction in the cortical length rather than width suggests a loss of columns of cells and their interconnections in a perpendicular fashion. Indeed, there is evidence for a specific association between the length of the cortical ribbon and cognitive impairment measured crudely using a dementia rating scale (Duyckaerts *et al.* 1985). In general, however, these changes are variable and it is possible to find patients with grossly reduced intellectual function whose brain weight are 'normal' and vice versa (Terry 1990).

There is good agreement between neuropathological and *in vivo* neuroimaging studies, starting with computerized axial tomography (CT) scanning in the early 1980s (Jacoby and Levy 1980). More recent structural magnetic resonance imaging (MRI) has demonstrated changes with more precision. As well as measurements of whole brain volume, MR images can be used to measure the volume of particular structures, including, for example, the hippocampal formation (see below). Seab *et al.* (1988), using this method, have shown a mean reduction of 40% in hippocampal volume, compared to controls. The measure also discriminated much more powerfully than an estimate of overall brain atrophy using changes in ventricular size and generalized brain atrophy. Of note, changes in overall brain atrophy correlated best with the severity of dementia. Nevertheless, in a subsequent study, by Kesslak *et al.* (1991), using a similar method, changes in hippocampal and parahippocampal volume correlated best with the Mini-Mental State score, a general measure of cognitive functioning.

MICROSCOPIC CHANGES

AD may be caused by a specific neuronal disease, but the neurohistological features are complex and variable and, at present, the pathology defies precise definition. This is partly because of the considerable overlap with the neuropathological markers that occur with normal ageing and no universally accepted quantitative distinction between the two has been drawn (Khachaturian 1985; Mirra *et al.* 1991). Nevertheless, the salient neuronal changes have been well described and investigated in terms of how they relate to cognitive changes. Here, cognitive dysfunction tends to be considered in a rudimentary fashion, measured using brief cognitive rating scales such as the Clinical Dementia Rating scale (CDR) (Hughes *et al.* 1982) or the Blessed Dementia Scale (Blessed *et al.* 1988).

A prominent feature of AD is the presences of senile or neuritic plaques (SPs). These are recognized microscopically as abnormal tissue or neuropil consisting of an amyloid core surrounded by argyrophilic axonal and dendritic processes (Lantos and Cairns 1994). This core contains a fibrillary amyloid protein, beta/A4 (Masters *et al.* 1985), the identification of which has revealed the more widespread distribution of amyloid than originally established by traditional staining methods (Majocha *et al.* 1988). SPs are present in variable numbers in elderly non-demented or mildly demented individuals, but are more uniformally present in moderately or severely demented patients (Mirra *et al.* 1991). They are generally widely distributed in AD, to be found in numerous quantities in cerebral cortex, hippocampus, and certain subcortical nuclei, including the putamen, locus coerulus, and hypothalamus. They tend to be more numerous in association than in sensory areas of the neocortex and also in laminae containing large pyramidal cells. Although they are used in neuropathological diagnosis, in which the density of SPs contributes to defining AD, recent carefully controlled studies (excluding non-dementing individuals) have tended to show little or no association with the extent of cognitive decline, with a lack of correlation between amyloid deposition and dementia (Dickson *et al.* 1992). Studies also show that SPs tend to occur first in neocortical areas other than the hippocampal formation, and doubt is expressed as to whether they are necessarily involved in the development of clinical symptoms of cognitive impairment (Arriagada *et al.* 1992; Bierer *et al.* 1995; Braak and Braak 1991).

More closely related to cognitive dysfunction in AD are the so-called neurofibrillary tangles (NFT). They consist of abnormal, helically wound, paired filaments, a major component being a phosphorylated isoform of tau, a microtubule associated glycoprotein (Goedert *et al.* 1988). Whilst still not specific to AD, they are clearly more numerous than in normal ageing and affect different regions of the brain more extensively than SPs. The main regions not only include extensive neocortical involvement, the medial temporal structures, including the hippocampus, amygdala, and parahippocampal gyri, but also subcortical regions, including the thalamus and mammillary bodies, the nucleus basalis of Meynert, substantia nigra, and locus coerulus, all structures implicated in cognitive or memory function. The density of NFTs in neocortical structures, including frontal, parietal, and temporal regions, have been found to correlate well with the level of dementia in several studies, including the finding that the strongest association is found in relation to the superior temporal cortex (Arriagada *et al.* 1992; Bierer *et al.* 1995; Wilcock and Esiri 1982). Although correlations between NFTs and dementia have not always been reported in relation to the hippocampal formation, they are found in large quantities in the entorhinal cortex, principally affecting layers II and IV (Arriagada *et al.* 1992; Esiri 1991). Other neuropathological changes include granulovacuolar degeneration and Hirano bodies. The former consist of abnormal cytoplasmic structures found in pyramidal neurones. They are virtually restricted to the hippocampus and are found in high densities in severe cases (Lantos and Cairns 1994). Hirano bodies are rod- or carrot-shaped structures, again found in the pyramidal cells of the hippocampus, or close to these cells.

The additional factor of neuronal loss is more difficult to establish than the other histopathological markers, partly because of the technical difficulties relating to counting cells. However, accompanying the neuropathological markers is a substantial loss of nerve cells. For example, within neocortical areas where NFTs are prominent, such as the neocortex and hippocampus, cell loss is estimated at approximately 30% or more. Within the neocortex, the loss appears to be greatest in the frontal and temporal lobes, with the parietal and occipital regions relatively spared (Mountjoy *et al.* 1982). Substantial decreases are also seen in the large neurones within layers III and V of the neocortex (Terry and Katzman 1983). Within the mesiotemporal region, the hippocampus is more severely affected, with a reported 40% reduction in area H1 (Mann *et al.* 1985). Perhaps because it is easier to quantify, cell loss has been measured more reliably in more discrete subcortical nuclei. Substantial loss has been found in nuclei from which diffuse neocortical projections originate. These include the nucleus basalis of Meynert (cholinergic) (Whitehouse *et al.* 1981), the locus coerulus (noradrenergic) (Marcyniuk *et al.* 1986), and raphe nuclei (serotonergic) (Yamamoto and Hirano 1985), all of which are implicated in attentional mechanisms (see Chapter 14).

FUNCTIONAL CHANGES

In theory, structural and histopathological changes in AD should have a direct correlate in functional changes. In other words, the neurobiological lesions in AD will be reflected in measurable changes in neuronal activity, in turn predicting the pattern of cognitive deficits. This section reviews studies that have explored these relationships, using electrophysiological and radiological approaches.

EEG correlates

In a relatively crude form, functional changes have been observed using electroencephalography (EEG), a technique which has the advantage of good temporal resolution, in the order or milliseconds. Patients with AD typically show a slowing in the alpha rhythm and amplitude, and an increase in diffuse and symmetrical theta and alpha waves in the posterior regions (Visser 1985). The advent of quantitative techniques has increased the sophistication of measurement and these have been used to show a correlation with cerebral blood flow changes Gustafson *et al.* 1987; Marc-Vergnes *et al.* 1986). One recent area of investigation has been the degree of 'coherence' between activity in different brain regions. The structural connectivity between brain areas is reflected in the degree of shared electrical activity, as found in normal subjects. For example 'coherence' can be computed for anterior lobe versus posterior electrode sites, indicating the degree to which frontal and parietal cortical functioning is synchronized. In normal subjects, this coherence is established developmentally and can be readily measured (Tucker *et al.* 1986). In AD there is evidence for a breakdown of anterior–posterior cortical coherence (Leuchter *et al.* 1987, 1992; O'Connor *et al.* 1979) which distinguishes AD from multi-infarct dementia (MID) patients, the latter showing a reduction in coherence either within the anterior or posterior cortex, but not between these regions (Leuchter *et al.* 1992) (see below for further discussion of this finding).

An alternative use of EEG is to measure evoked potentials (EP), EEG changes recorded following sensory stimulation. Visual potentials (VEPs) are evoked using either flashes of lights (FVEP recording) or reverse checkerboard presentation (PRVEP recording), reflecting, respectively, striate cortical and visual association area activation (Whittaker and Siegfried 1983). These techniques have shown equivocal evidence for alterations of activity in AD. Some studies report an increased latency of components of FVEPs, whilst others have failed to do so (see Philpot 1994 for a review). The differences between the latencies of the major components of the FVEP and the PRVEP has been found to show abnormalities in AD (Wright *et al.* 1984), and may indicate an impairment in passage of visual information from the striate cortex to sensory association areas. However, studies have shown that the changes are not specific to AD, and are found to the same extent in multi-infarct dementia (MID) (Wright and Furlong 1988). Little systematic research has been carried out using auditory or somatosensory evoked potentials in AD, but delays in the major peaks of the EP traces have been observed in both cases (Hendrickson *et al.* 1979; Huisman *et al.* 1985).

In contrast to EPs another technique is to present a subject with a stimulus which needs some decision to be made, thus requiring active cognitive participation. This produces what are termed event-related potentials (ERPs), the most common technique being to distinguish between high and low tones, producing auditory event-related potentials (AERPs). The most characteristic component of the EEG trace occurs at about 250 ms and is the P3 or P300. Several studies have shown a delay in the latency of P3 in AD in comparison to normal controls (most recently, see for example, Williams *et al.* 1991), but again this has been equivocal (Kraiuhin *et al.* 1990; Ruessman *et al* 1990). Attempts to correlate changes with neuropsychological functioning have been few, but Blackwood *et al.* (1987) reports that the reduction in P3 latency and amplitude in AD correlates with the severity of language impairment and visual memory. Changes in P3 following a period of one year also corresponded to a more general intellectual deterioration. AERPs, however, have not been found to differentiate well between different patient groups, including the study by Filipovic *et al.* (1990) which compared AD, Huntington's chorea, and Parkinson's disease.

Neuroimaging

Functional brain imaging provides greater regional specificity than EEG, in terms of detecting loss of brain functioning *in vivo*. Throughout the last 15 years, the two main methods have been based on detecting regional cerebral blood flow (rCBF), namely single photon emission computed tomography (SPECT) and positron emission tomography (PET) (Moseley 1993). More recently functional magnetic resonance imaging (fMRI) has been available, having the advantage of not requiring the injection of radioactive substances, combined with a greater spatial resolution. It also has the potential to improve on the poor temporal resolution of radionucleotide approaches (1–2 minutes). This technique is at an early stage and studies using it with AD have only just begun.

Within SPET and PET a wide range of different methodologies exist, but their application has tended to produce consistent findings with AD (Geaney 1994; Kennedy and Frackowiak 1994). First, SPET studies, including those using the more recently available [23I]IMP (nosine monophosphate) and [99mTc]HMPAO (hexamethyl propylene amine oxine) radiotracers, have tended to show maximal changes in perfusion within the parietal or temporal region (Gemmell *et al.* 1990, Jagust *et al.* 1987; Kuwabara *et al.* 1990). Changes are also found in the frontal cortex, but these are less consistent and are found to be associated with more severe cases of presenile onset (Habert *et al.* 1991; Jagust *et al.* 1990; Montaldi *et al.* 1990). In addition, several studies report negative correlations between rCBF and neuropsychological functioning, the most consistent concerning left temporal and parietal regions (Burns *et al.* Burns *et al.* 1989; Hunter *et al.* 1989; Montaldi *et al.* 1990). These associations can be quite specific, for example language dysfunction associated with left parietal and temporal changes, versus praxic disturbances associated with reduced rCBF in bilateral and parietal lobes (Burns *et al.* 1989; Hunter *et al.* 1989; Montaldi *et al.* 1990).

A similar pattern has emerged from studies using PET, the main techniques based on measuring either cerebral oxygen metabolism using ^{15}O as the radioactive tracer, or cerebral glucose metabolism using the radioactive isotope [18F]deoxyglucose (FDG). One of the main early studies was conducted by Frackowiak *et al.* (1981), using the oxygen method, which showed a substantial reduction in resting activity in the parietal lobes, with the lowest reduction in the occipital lobes. There was a trend towards significant correlation between both praxis and speech with reductions in metabolism overall. Frontal hypometabolism was found with the greater severity of dementia, similar to the SPECT findings, but not in comparative vascular cases. Other notable studies have used the FDG method, producing findings that are broadly consistent, with prominent changes in the temporal and parietal lobes, additional, but less consistent changes in the frontal lobes, with the least in the visual and motor cortex (see, for example, Chase *et al.* 1984; Farakas *et al.* 1982; Ferris *et al.* 1980; Friedland *et al.* 1983; Haxby *et al.* 1986, 1990). Longitudinal studies show that the decline in metabolism is also greatest in the regions impaired early on in AD. For example the greatest decline has been observed in the middle temporal, inferior temporal, angular, and superior parietal gyri (McGeer *et al.* 1990).

Taking these studies together there is the suggestion of maximal reduction in brain activity within the temporal or parietal lobes, with later involvement of the frontal cortex. An important issue is the extent to which changes in glucose or oxygen metabolism represent *real* changes in neuronal tissue, or merely a reduction in volume. Atrophy of cortical tissue gives rise to enlarged cerebrospinal fluid spaces, resulting in falsely lower values (Kennedy and Frackowiak 1984). In other words, are the putative activity reductions a reflection of loss of brain tissue volume, a reduction in physiological activity, or a combination of both? There are techniques for solving this partial volume artefact (e.g. Bullmore *et al.* 1995), and some of these have been tried in relation to AD. For example Chawluk *et al.* (1987) combined PET scanning of AD patients with structural neuroimaging, using CT. The degree of atrophy, estimated from CT images, was used to compute a correction factor when analysing the FDG PET data. Their conclusion was that a proportion of the loss of metabolic activity can be accounted for directly by the loss of neuronal tissue. More recent approaches to neuroimaging, particularly the advent of functional MRI, may enable these distinctions to be made with greater sophistication.

FUNCTIONAL NEUROIMAGING

SPET, PET, and now functional MRI, have the capacity to measure brain activity during cognitive activation. In relation to AD, studies have been few because of the practical difficulties of ensuring that a patient complies with the procedures. For example it is difficult to distinguish between whether nonactivation of brain regions is due to poor compliance with a task, or real depletion in brain activity.

Despite this, a few studies have been reported, including that of Kessler *et al.* (1991), who used a continuous visual recognition memory task combined with FDG PET. The task involves continuous presentation of items, including in this case words, letters, and drawings of objects. After a while, items are repeated and the subject has to decide whether they have been seen before. The task is predicted to activate widespread regions of the brain, involving visual perception, language, and memory functioning. Brain activation during this task was compared to a resting FDG PET condition. The latter produced, as perhaps expected, the most substantial degree of impairment within the temporoparietal region. In the cognitive activation condition, robust increases in activity were seen throughout the association cortices in control subjects, but this was much less in the AD patients.

Of note, in the Kessler *et al.* (1991) study there was also a shift in activation to more widespread cortical regions. This has also been observed in other studies, for example one by Grady *et al.* (1990) and, more recently, by Becker *et al.* (1994) (see also Becker *et al.* Chapter 5). In the study by Becker and colleagues, which compared single- and three-word repetition and eight-word free recall, and comparisons of these as well as a rest condition both produced a characteristic pattern of brain activation, which in AD showed greater spatial distribution.

There are various explanations for this finding, which has been replicated in kind across studies. One is that inhibitory processes that produce more tightly focused activation associated with normal efficient cognitive activity are impaired. This produces an abnormal spread of activation and would predict interference between domains of cognitive activity which share proximal neuronal substrates (not necessarily *spatially* proximal within the cortex, but related as well to the topographical organization of neural networks). Another is that neurobiological deterioration makes cognitive processing generally less efficient. To compensate for this, the information processing system has to recruit more widespread cognitive modules or systems, thus bringing into play wider regions of the brain. For example a task that would hitherto be carried out relatively 'automatically' in a normal subject may need to be conducted using alternative and more 'effortful' cognitive operations as a means of compensation.

Some hint of this is seen in the Becker *et al.* (1994; Chapter 5) study, where a comparison of the eight-word and free recall and three-word rehearsal produced activation primarily in the middle frontal gyrus bilaterally in the controls. In the AD patients this also extended to the dorsolateral prefrontal cortex, Brodmann's areas 8 BA9 and BA10. The more widespread recruitment of prefrontal cortical neuronal systems might relate to the greater involvement of control processes needed to perform the free recall task for the AD patients.

COGNITION AND NEUROBIOLOGY

The finding of 'core' neurobiological changes within posterior bilateral association cortex is remarkably consistent across different methods of investigation, including histological and neuroradiological (as summarized in Fig. 13.1). This figure is based on histological changes, but is very similar in pattern to the known areas of hypoperfusion identified using SPET and PET. To what extent can these changes be related to the breakdown in specific areas of cognitive functioning? The remainder of this chapter takes a more theoretical approach and attempts to draw links with what is known about the neurobiology of AD and impairment in different domains of cognition.

METABOLIC ASYMMETRIES, LANGUAGE, AND VISUOSPATIAL FUNCTIONING

The finding of specific regions of hypometabolism using SPET or PET have direct correlates with impaired 'focal' neuropsychological dysfunction. One main division is the difference in metabolic functioning of the two cerebral hemispheres. Left versus right brain asymmetries in function are expressed in terms of ratios, which have the advantage of incorporating a within-subject comparison, thereby reducing the degree of variance in the data produced by more random changes in brain functioning. Ratios also exploit the hemispheric differences in cognition that occur in normal subjects and, in particular, the language dominance of the left hemisphere. Foster *et al.* (1983) was the first to report language dysfunction associated with left frontotemporoparietal changes in AD and spatial dysfunction with right parietal hypometabolism. Subsequent studies additionally showed that AD patients with more right angular gyrus hypometabolism tended to be dyscalculic, whilst those with left frontal hypometabolism had

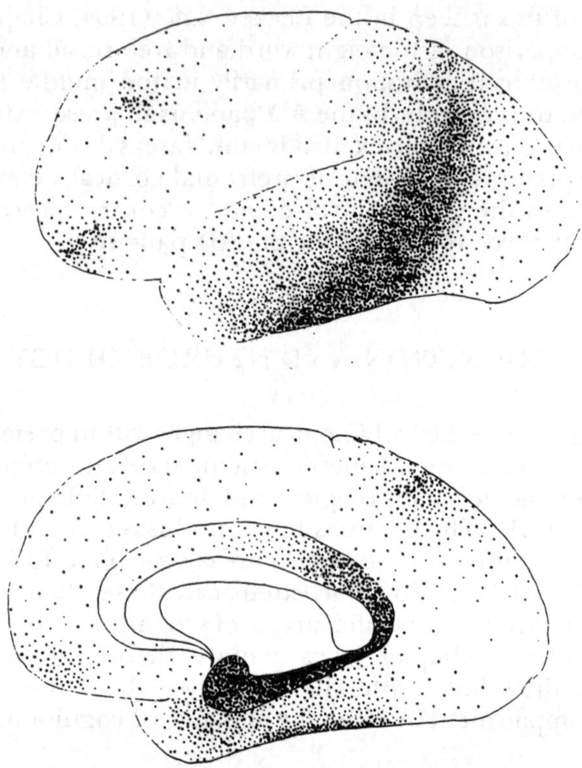

FIG. 13.1 A schematic representation of the regional distribution and severity of neuropathological changes in Alzheimer's disease. More dense shading indicates more pronounced degeneration. The mesial view is shown at the top, illustrating substantial neurodegeneration within the mesiotemporal lobe. The lateral view illustrates the parietal–temporal changes. (Taken from A. Brun (1983). An overview of light and election microscope. In *Alzheimer's disease: the standard reference* (ed. B. Reisberg), Free Press, New York. Copyright 1983 by Arne Brune. Also reproduced in Parasuraman and Haxby (1993).

sensory dysphasias (Chase *et al.* 1984; Foster *et al.* 1984). In contrast, McGeer *et al.* (1990) report that their neuropsychological profiles correlate only with changes in multiple cortical regions, reflecting perhaps the fact that neuropsychological functioning tends to be reliant on neuronal networks involving more than one focus.

Metabolic asymmetries have been detected using PET early on in the time course of AD, and may even precede marked neuropsychological impairment. For example Haxby *et al.* (1986) found asymmetries in early AD uncorrelated with neuropsychological discrepancies. Longitudinal studies have revealed that as dementia progresses, hypoperfusion asymmetries are accentuated and begin to correlate with neuropsychological functioning in an expected fashion (right changes associated with visuospatial disturbance and left with verbal impairment) (Haxby *et al.* 1990). In general, the metabolic asymmetries are much more pronounced in the association cortices than in the primary cortices, in keeping with neuropathological findings (see above). Haxby *et al.* (1990) also noted that in the severe stages of dementia the asymmetries decreased again, in keeping with the notion that the disease process 'catches' up with all associative regions of the cortex 'eventually'.

Recently and in a more experimental vein, Penniello *et al.* (1995). have used metabolic asymmetry analyses in relation to spelling in AD, patients. They explored the functional anatomy of writing, and how this breaks down in AD. Neuropsychological investigation has revealed two distinct routes for spelling under dictation; a phonological route based on processing the 'sound form' of words, linked neurologically with the anterior–inferior part of the left supramarginal gyrus, and a lexical–semantic route associated with the posterior–superior part of the angular gyrus. Damage to the phonological route gives rise to impaired spelling of non-words, but preserves spelling of lexical material regardless of word regularity (Shallice 1981). An impairment in the lexical–semantic route results in spelling errors for orthographically ambiguous and irregular words (Beauvois and Derouesne 1981). Penniello *et al.* (1995) analysed these two types of spelling errors in AD patients and also measured cerebral glucose utilization with FDG PET in the resting state. Similar to the technique used by Haxby and colleagues (Haxby 1990), they computed ratios between left supramarginal and angular gyri metabolic activity. A further ratio was computed between 'phonological' and 'lexical' errors. In a sample of 11 patients, these two ratios were found to be highly correlated. This particular finding further supports the role of focal, in addition to diffuse brain damage, in producing a breakdown of cognitive functioning in AD.

EXECUTIVE FUNCTIONING

The ability to coordinate mental processes, to process several types of information at once, possibly from a variety of sources, and to sequence and execute a series of responses are key components of executive functioning. As discussed in Chapter 4, this function is severely impaired in AD, leading, for example, to substantial difficulties on tasks which require divided attention (see also, Morris, 1994*a*,*b*; Morris and

Baddeley 1988). In summary, neuropsychological studies point towards the control mechanisms of cognitive functioning being impaired in AD, with some preservation of more 'automatic' forms of processing. The extent to which the neurobiological changes in AD explain this pattern of impairment is discussed below. Various explanations have been considered before (e.g. Morris 1994*a,b*; Parasuraman and Haxby 1993) and these are discussed in turn.

Frontal lobe dysfunction

One possible cause of executive dysfunction in AD is focal frontal lobe neurodegeneration. This would be consistent with a localizationist view in executive functioning, in general, espoused by many researchers (Baddeley *et al.* 1991; Shallice 1988; Stuss and Benson 1987). For example Baddeley *et al.* (1991) link executive functioning to the prefrontal cortex, drawing upon the Norman and Shallice (1986) model of attentional control. The model assumes that most actions are controlled by established routines or 'schemas'. These are mutually inhibitory, the most active schema preventing others from being activated. These schemas cope with routine activity in a more or less 'automatic' fashion. They are triggered by environmental events or stimuli which have formed pre-existing associations. For novel events, however, triggering routine activity is not sufficient and problem-solving activity is necessary. For this, a higher level system, termed the Supervisory Attentional System (SAS) comes into play and triggers the appropriate schema. Shallice (1988) relates an impairment in the SAS to difficulties patients with prefrontal cortical impairment have in problem solving. The link between the SAS and the Central Executive System (CES) has been introduced by Baddeley *et al.* (1991), who suggest that an SAS impairment also results in the reduced capacity to direct and control attentional resources.

An impairment in frontal lobe dysfunction would provide a ready explanation for the executive impairments in AD, but this notion does have a number of difficulties. As indicated in Fig. 13.1, frontal lobe dysfunction is not a prominent feature of AD, particularly in the early stages, and is reflected in low levels of hypometabolism (Habert *et al.* 1991; Jagust *et al.* 1990; Montaldi *et al.* 1990). Becker *et al.* (1992) have examined the neurological and behavioural characteristics of AD patients who show pronounced executive functioning impairment. These patients showed none of the prominent neurological signs of frontal lobe dysfunction, including primitive reflex or release signs. In addition, the behavioural syndromes (for example, apathy, disinhibition, and distractibility), were absent. Conversely, patients with known focal prefrontal lesions have not been shown to be impaired on tests of divided attention, which would 'stress' the CES (Frisk and Milner 1990).

Neural network dysfunction

Alternative explanations are couched in terms of a neural network encompassing executive functioning. According to this notion, the CES is the 'emergent property of different association regions within the cortex acting together in an integrative fashion' (Morris 1994*c*). Particular executive functions (for example response inhibition or selective attention) may have a more localized neurobiological basis, but the overall system is distributed throughout the neocortex. This concept is consistent with the view of the CES relying on a network of interactive systems, rather than one focused cognitive module (Barnard 1985; Shallice 1988). It also leads to several ways of explaining the executive impairment in AD other than a localizationalist account.

Mass action

One such way is the application of the theory of 'mass action' to AD. Originally, this theory, introduced by Lashley (1950) proposes that the whole brain participates in every behaviour and that any deficit is proportional to the amount of tissue removed. Whilst more or less disproved in relation to human cognition, because of the clear localization of function in the brain, it can be readily applied to a function considered to be distributed throughout a neural network, such as executive functioning. In AD, non-focal dysfunction involving multiple areas would reduce the efficiency of the CES. Principally, in AD the damage would be to parietal and temporal contributions, but additional impairment in the frontal cortex would play an increasing role later on in the course of AD.

Functional distance

Against this theory is the lack of specificity about the mechanisms of executive functions and a degree of circularity in the argument. Using the same overall framework, Morris (1992) has applied the notion of functional distance to AD, first proposed by Kinsbourne (1980). According to this notion, neurologically, one of the difficulties of coordinating mental activity is to maintain separateness of cognitive operations. Interference occurs not only because of competition for the same physiological substrate, but because adjacent physiological activity sets up mutual interference. Shallice (1988) approaches this problem, albeit at a cognitive level of description, by proposing a contention scheduling system in which various schema act in a mutually inhibitory fashion to ensure one activity at a time. However, the nature of many tasks is to maintain more than one activity, with the CES in a coordinating role. According to Kinsbourne (1980) a functional distance is normally kept between operations, particularly if they are different in nature, such as visual versus verbal processing.

Morris (1992) has proposed that the breakdown of the physiological functioning of association areas effectively reduces this functional distance at a physiological level, the result being that cognitive operations literally 'run into' each other. Additionally, there may be some breakdown in the mechanisms that keep the cognitive operations apart. Some support for this finding comes from the functional neuroimaging studies cited above, in which it has been observed that, in AD, the same tasks recruit greater areas of cortex and additional regions (Becker *et al.* 1994; Kessler *et al.* 1991). Against this is the possibility, raised above, that this reflects compensatory strategies rather than a lack of neuronal specificity in processing. Nevertheless, this notion still stands as a possible candidate for explaining the marked difficulties that AD patients have when dividing attention between more than one mental operation.

A concept of a loss in 'functional distance' is, in reality, very similar to that of declining processing resources. The latter relates to a pool of general purpose cognitive resources which can be allocated to different types of cognitive functions (Kahneman 1973; Norman and Bobrow 1975). These resources have a finite capacity, such that the more is required of information processing, the more they are used up, again explaining dual-task interference. The neurobiological correlate of finite processing resources is presumably the neuronal network, which is limited in the amount of cognitive activity it can support. In AD, the degradation of neuronal structures would reduce this resource and so account for the apparent executive functioning impairment. Indeed, it has been suggested that a processing resource may account, in part, for many of the cognitive deficits in AD. Nevertheless, the concept of unitary processing capacity, although neurobiologically plausible, has poor explanatory power in general and is difficult to prove.

Alzheimer's disease—dysconnection syndrome *par excellence*?

More recently, Morris (1994*a*, *b*, *c*) has suggested that rather than cognitive processes running into each other, they become more loosely connected (Morris 1994*c*). The concept of a dysconnection was revived by Geschwind in the 1960s (Geschwind 1965) to explain certain forms of focal neuropsychological impairment, for example

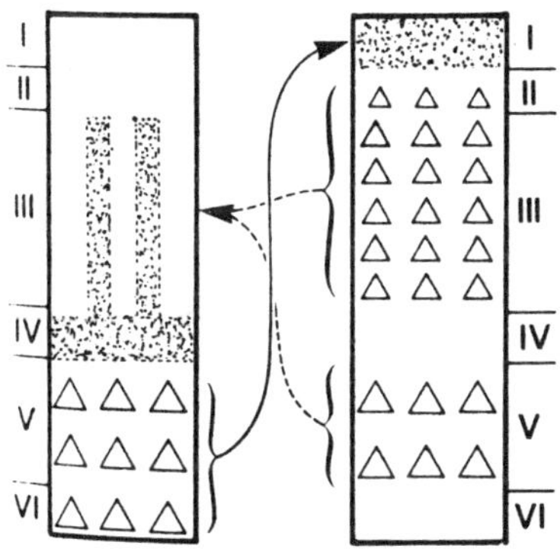

FIG. 13.2 The feedback and feedforward corticocortical neural systems connecting the posterior and anterior cortex. The figure shows the lawinar distribution of the neuronal terminals within the cortex (dots). (Taken from Van Hoesen (1990), with permission.)

apraxia and agnosia. The notion is that one or more pathways between key neuronal processing modules are lesioned, producing a neuropsychological deficit. In AD, there is strong evidence for a breakdown in connections between the main cortical association areas (De Lacoste and White 1993; Morrison *et al.* 1986).

The secondary and tertiary association areas of the brain which support higher level cognition are joined by long bands of fibres, the corticocortical association fibres of the brain. The available evidence suggests a network of corticocortical links with laminar specificity as shown in Fig. 13.2, connecting specifically the parietal and frontal regions of the cortex (Fuster 1989, 1993; Goldman-Rakic 1987, 1988; Van Hoesen 1990). A feedforward system, stems from the posterior association cortex, involved in processing higher level sensory information, projecting to the anterior hemisphere. The projections arise from both the supragranular (layers II and III) as shown in Fig. 13.2. A feedback system originates largely from layers 5 and 6.

In AD there is evidence for substantial neuronal damage to both these pathways. (Morrison *et al.* 1986; Pearson *et al.* 1985; Rogers and Morrison 1985). Layers 2 and 3 have been shown to have some of the greatest numbers of SPs, particularly within the pyramidal cells (Lewis *et al.* 1987). There is also evidence of a severe loss of synapses in those lamina regions innervated by corticocortical fibres (De Kosky and Scheffe 1990; Masliah *et al.* 1991; Terry *et al.* 1990). The selective vulnerability of these pathways has even led to the suggestion that

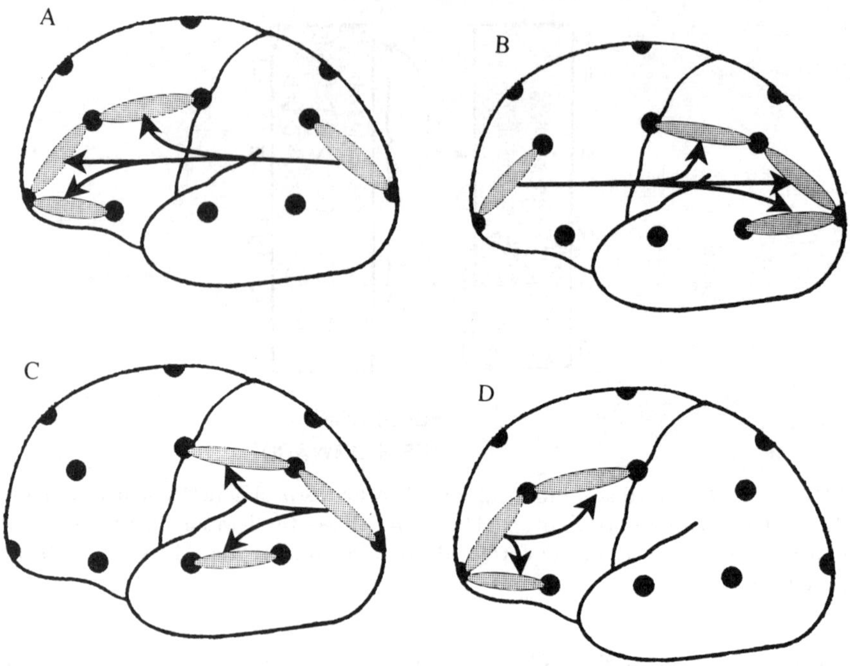

FIG. 13.3 Electrode sites for measures of brain coherence in AD according to Leuchter *et al.* (1992). Coherence variables were grouped in four combinations. A is postero–anterior coherence transmitted via the superior longitudinal fasciculus. B represents transmission in the antero–posterior direction. C and D show connectivity within either the anterior or posterior brain. The AD patients had systematic decreases in coherence with the anterior and posterior linkage (reproduced with permission).

Alzheimer's disease spreads throughout the brain via these pathways, therefore affecting them more substantially (Saper 1986).

The anatomical loss of connectivity has been shown to have a direct parallel in terms of the degree to which anterior and posterior brain areas act in synchrony. This synchronous activity, termed coherence, can be determined by exploring the correlation between changes in activity of different brain regions, using either EEG or functional neuroimaging systems. Leuchter *et al.* (1992) used EEG to measure coherence of activity between different brain regions as shown in Fig. 13.3. By combining electrode measurements, comparisons can be made between posterior and anterior cortical sites (crossing the Rolandic fissure) and within either the prefrontal or posterior regions. In AD, maximal loss of coherence was found across the Rolandic fissure, as predicted from the histological studies. This finding cannot be simply explained by a generalized loss of brain functioning, since in multi-infarct dementia, Leuchter *et al.* (1992) found the opposite pattern of results with maximal loss of coherence within the anterior or posterior regions. Loss of coherence can also be investigated using PET, where interregional correlations between brain activity can be explored when the subject is in a resting state. Studies by Horwitz *et al.* (1987) and by Azari *et al.* (1992) indicate generally lower correlational levels, but the most marked decrease between the frontal and parietal regions.

Synchronizing mental activity

These findings have been taken to support a specific dysconnection syndrome in AD (Leuchter *et al.* 1992). Their implication for cognition is more speculative, but Morris (1994*a, b, c*) has taken the view that they explain the marked breakdown in executive functioning, and, in particular, the difficulties that AD patients have in performing simultaneous mental activities.

A breakdown in coherence would disrupt the ability of the information processing system to direct and coordinate the cognitive components of complex tasks efficiently, particularly those involving divided attention. An example is the combination of tracking and digit span which was used to highlight executive impairments in AD by Baddeley *et al.* (1986, 1991). In this task, explained in more detail in Chapter 4, the patient simultaneously tracks a moving stimulus on a computer screen and repeats back strings of digits. Patients with AD show a much greater deficit when these two tasks are combined than when they are presented individually. Neurologically, these tasks require the synchronous activity of widely distributed brain regions. For example keeping in mind a string of digits is thought to require the activity of both anterior (Broca's area) and posterior (supramarginal gyrus) regions (Shallice and Vallar 1990; Paulescu *et al.* 1993). Tracking a moving object may require right parietal activation, in addition to perceptual and motor output regions of the cortex.

If the neuronal transmission between the different centres involved becomes less efficient, then there might be an escalating negative effect on the coordination of mental activity. In contrast, more localized neuronal networks might not be so vulnerable to the effects of loss of coherence. For example, in digit span alone, the main supporting cognitive system employed has a relatively restricted neural network. In this case, as indicated by Morris in Chapter 4, maintenance of digits in short-term memory is achieved largely by the articulatory loop system, which relies on specific language centres in the dominant hemisphere.

Breaking the perception–action cycle

Of note, very few attempts have been made to develop models of executive functioning that reflect the notion of integrative activity across different regions of the brain. This may be because of the known involvement of the frontal lobes in aspects of executive activity such as sequencing, initiation, and response inhibition, which has tended to focus theorizing on this structure (Kolb and Whishaw 1990). One approach, for example, is the hierarchical model proposed by Fuster (1989, 1993) which incorporates the notion of a perceptual hierarchy of neuronal processes linking at each level to the successive stages of motor output. The interconnections between the hierarchies (perceptual and motor) form the basis for coordinated action. Thus a perception–action cycle integrating input to the organism and motor output is hypothesized. Previous theorizing by Morris (1994) has suggested that this perception–action cycle is specifically disrupted in AD.

A neuronal system involved in executive system is proposed in Fig. 13.4 based on what is known about intra- and intercortical connections relating to sensory input and motor output (Pandya and Barnes 1987).

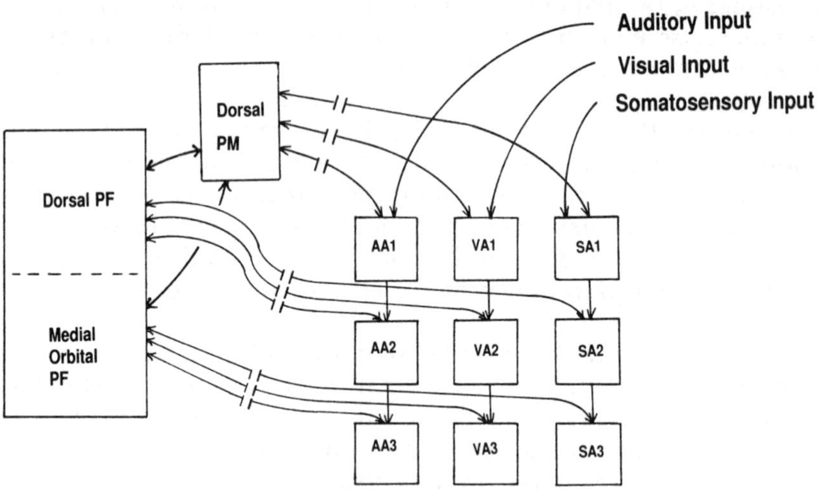

FIG. 13.4 A summary of main connections linking up the main sensory pathways and the frontal cortex. Three main subdivisions of the frontal lobe are shown (dorsal premotor (PM), dorsal prefrontal (PF), and medial orbital prefrontal (PF)) and their interconnections with the three main sensory systems. The breaks in connections represents loss in anterior–posterior connectivity in AD.

For each type of sensory input (for example somatosensory, auditory, and visual) there are separate hierarchical networks. For example, for visual processing, the processing modules are chained together in an orderly sequences of connections from areas VA1, VA2, to VA3 (Jones and Powell 1970; Kuypers *et al.* 1965). Each of these has differential projections to the frontal cortex, VA1 (first order) projecting to dorsal and ventral regions of area 8 (premotor), VA2 (second order) to area 46, and VA3 to area 11 (orbitofrontal cortex). This pattern of connections may form the basis for coordinating the flow of sensory processing and subsequent integration with motor output, involving the premotor cortex.

In AD, a disruption of the posterior/anterior flow of information would disconnect the sensory hierarchies from the functioning of the prefrontal cortex. Loss of coherence between the sensory and motor hierarchy in AD would disrupt this cycle, with the prediction of a breakdown in the ability to control and sequence cognitive operations responsive to visual input and involving motor output. Of note, the reiterative nature of the cycle means that lack of coordination should escalate as cognitive activity proceeds, leading perhaps to a catastrophic effect on the ability to carry out complex tasks. Indeed, it has been observed that even during the early stages of, AD patients can be completely unable to perform more complex reaction time tasks that involve simultaneously viewing visual arrays and responding using choice response keys, unless the task is kept very simple (Morris 1984).

In summary, distributed capacity models, such as the one described above, provide a framework for understanding the executive functioning impairment in AD. The paucity of hypotheses in this area, however, precludes more detailed analysis, but as neurocomputational approaches are developed it may be possible to model the executive impairment in AD.

Selective attention

A more specific component of executive processes is selective attention, investigated most extensively in relation to attentional shifts in spatial tasks (see also Chapter 4). Posner *et al.* (1984*a*) has distinguished between the three components that underlie attentional shifting, namely engaging or focusing, shifting, and disengagement of attention. There is substantial evidence that *shifting* of attention is controlled, in part, by the posterior parietal region of the brain (LaBerge 1990; Posner *et al.* 1984*b*). Because of the substantial functional impairment in the posterior parietal cortex in AD, a specific attentional deficit would be predicted (Haxby *et al.* 1986; Horwitz *et al.* 1987; Petersen *et al.* 1988).

A study by Parasuraman *et al.* (1992) suggests this is the case. As part of a larger study, they used a selective attention task in which subjects observed a central fixation point and were required to decide whether a letter presented to the left or right of this point was a vowel or a consonant (more highly educated patients were included, who knew what this distinction meant). A 'location' cue preceded each letter in the form of an arrow, which could either point towards or away from the subsequent position of the letter. When the cue is presented centrally, and between 500 and 2000 ms, AD patients show a marked reduction in their speed of response compared to age-matched healthy elderly controls in the condition where the invalid cue is presented. This suggests difficulties in switching attention away from the invalid cue. Parasuraman *et al.* (1992) computed measurements relating to speed of switching attention, expressed in what is termed 'reaction time (RT) costs plus benefits.' They also measured resting levels of glucose metabolism using PET and used this to produce a right versus left parietal lobe asymmetry index. Of note, the RT costs and benefits in the AD group were negatively correlated with the right-left asymmetry, indicating that difficulties in switching attention in AD were associated with relative hypometabolism in the right posterior lobe, known to have a dominant role in spatial attention (Weintraub and Mesulam 1987).

MEMORY

A repeated clinical observation is that memory impairment is the most noticeable cognitive deficit during the early stages of AD. Usually, this relates to remembering things that have happened to the person, perhaps conversations or events, or memorizing important pieces of information. This type of memory has been referred to as *episodic* memory functioning and relates to memory for personally experience information, retained over a period of minutes, days, or weeks (Tulving 1983). Formal testing of memory functioning has revealed substantial impairment on a range of tasks, including free recall of word lists, sentences, stories and recognition memory for words, faces, and pictures (Becker *et al.* 1993; Corkin 1982; Grosse *et al.* 1991; Hart *et al.* 1988; Morris 1991).

The episodic memory deficit in AD has been characterized as an amnesic syndrome which is overlaid by various processing deficits, which, in turn, contribute to memory impairment (Morris 1991; Morris and Kopelman 1986). Thus the primary neuronal circuitry involved in supporting memory functioning is heavily implicated in AD. Neuropsychological studies in humans and lesion studies in animals

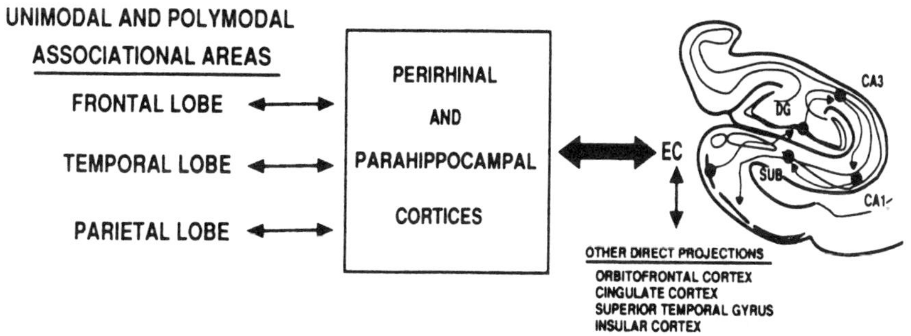

FIG. 13.5 Schematic representations of the connectivity of the mesiotemporal memory circuitry. The width of the arrows corresponds to the relative proportion of inputs arising form the areas indicated. EC, entorhinal cortex; DG, dentate gyrus; SUB, subicular complex; CA3 and CA1 are fields of the hippocampus proper (from Squire *et al.* 1990, reproduced with permission).

suggest this network includes, for example, the hippocampal formation, and perirhinal cortices within the temporal lobe, and anterior thalamus and mammillary bodies within the diencephalon. In AD, there is substantial evidence for damage to the hippocampal formation, in turn producing the marked memory impairment.

The structure of the hippocampal formation is illustrated in Fig. 13.5. A key component of this system is the entorhinal cortex (EC). This is thought to act as a means of channelling information to and from the hippocampus, connecting up the memory system to the rest of cognition. It receives projections from the perirhinal and parahippocampal cortices, which, in turn, are connected to cortical unimodal and polymodal (tertiary) cortical association areas. The role of the hippocampus in memory has long been known, with evidence to support this in patients with selective hippocampal lesions, for example due to mesiotemporal lobe sclerosis or ischaemia (Squire 1992). In addition, there is evidence that the adjacent cortical structures, the perirhinal and parahippocampal cortices, play an important role.

In AD there is evidence for damage both to the input system of the hippocampal formation and fields of the hippocampus proper. Damage to the entorhinal cortex is apparent even at the early stages, effectively lesioning the rest of the cortex from the memory system (Hyman *et al.* 1990). Specifically, neurofibrillary tangles (NFT) are seen in large quantities in the entorhinal cortex and tends to be formed in advance of other brain regions (Arriagada *et al.*, 1992; Esiri 1991). Fig. 13.6 illustrates the development of NFT changes, throughout a series of stages as identified by Braak and Braak (1991). Principally, they are found to affect layers 2 and 4. NFT changes can also be identified in the CA1 field of the hippocampus proper. A hierarchical

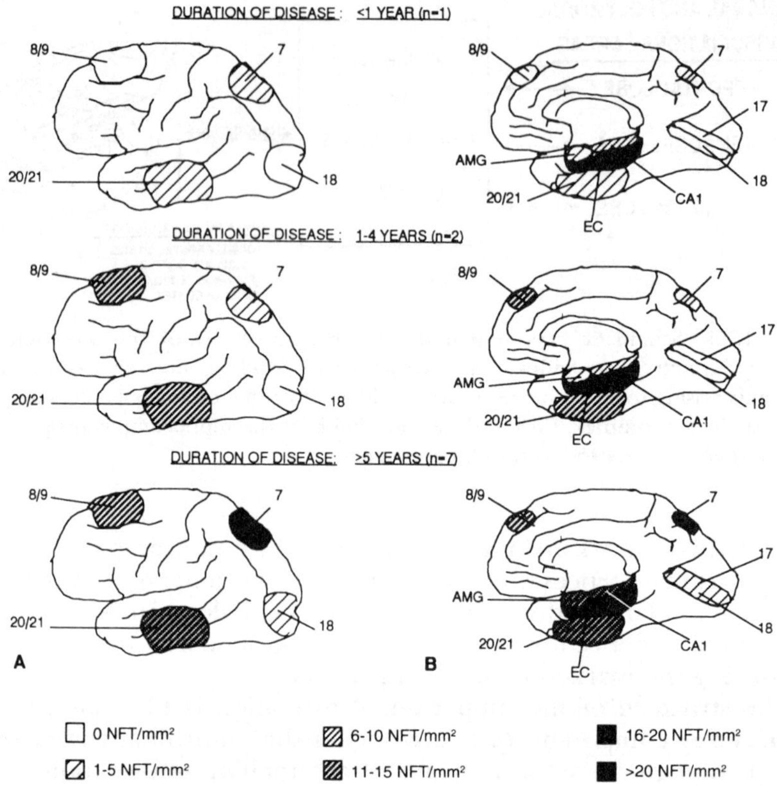

FIG. 13.6 Schematic representation of the relation between density and distribution of neurofibrillary tangles (NFT) and duration of AD (A, lateral view; B, medial view), taken from Arriagada *et al.* (1992). On the right is the legend which gives the density in number of NFTs per millimetre squared represented by the different shading (EC, entorhinal cortex; AMG, amagdala; numbers refer to Brodman map areas of the neocortex). (reproduced from Arriagada *et al.* 1992; reproduced with permission).

progression of vulnerability has been identified in which individual cytoarchitectural fields, such as impairment in the entorhinal cortex, occur first followed by the CA1 field, the amygdala, the association, and then sensory cortics (Arriagada *et al.* 1992). There is also evidence that the numbers of NFT, rather than neuritic plaques correlate with global ratings of dementia (which are more heavily weighted towards memory) (Arriagda *et al.* 1992).

Damage to the CA1 field of the hippocampus may, however, be an equally important determinant of memory impairment in AD, and this has been found to be severe. A major output route exists from this hippocampal field via the subiculum (Amaral 1993). Indeed, damage to the CA1 field has been observed in patients with bilateral selective damage to this field due to ischaemia (Zola-Morgan *et al.* 1986), and lesioning of this region in animal models produces substantial memory impairment (Zola-Morgan and Squire 1990). It can be proposed that the combined severe lesioning of the entorhinal cortex and the CA1 field has the dual effect of cutting off the memory system from the rest of cognition and destroying the neural substrate for memory.

As indicated above, the memory system is supported by a widely distributed network in the brain. Damage to specific memory circuitry outside the mesiotemporal lobes has also been implicated in AD. For example AD patients have been shown to have significant changes in the diencephalon, including the thalamus (Jernigan *et al.* 1991). Indeed, similarities between the episodic memory disturbances in AD and Wernicke–Korsakoff's (WKS) syndrome have been noted, where the primary neuronal damage associated with amnesia is thought to include the dorsomedial nucleus of the thalamus. WKS patients show particular difficulties in encoding material within a temporal context, for example indicating 'when' an item has been encountered, rather than 'what' (Parkin *et al.* 1990). Recently, Becker *et al.* (1993) explored contextual memory in these two groups of patients by presenting four objects to learn in a 2 × 2 array. The patients had then to select from a 4 × 4 array, filled with additional distracter items. The test was repeated several times until the patients had learned which were the target items. On subsequent trials, some of the distracter items then became the context and the patient had to select these as targets. In other words, the patient had to remember in which context they had seen an item, either as a target or distracter item. Both AD and WKS patients showed a substantial deficit on this task, contrasting with elderly controls and amnesic patients with temporal lobe damage. It should be noted, however, that this contextual memory deficit was additional to an underlying memory difficulty, since the AD patients need many more trials in which the original four objects are re-presented to obtain the same level of accuracy as the controls.

DISCUSSION

In summary, the cognitive changes that occur in AD are widespread and affect almost all cognitive functions, including language executive function and memory. A careful dissection of these changes show, however, that they can be related to underlying neurobiological changes, including structural and functional changes in the brains of AD patients. Various theories can be advanced concerning the ways these factors relate. They include a simple notion of a focal lesion leading to a particular cognitive deficit, and also the breakdown of neural networks supporting cognition. The links between the neurobiology of AD and cognition indicate that, in contrast to certain forms of focal brain damage, there is no single neurobiological explanation of dementia.

A common theme is the convergence of neuropathological, neuroradiological, and neuropsychological approaches, such as seen in the studies of attention and executive dysfunction. As neuroradiological techniques continue to be developed, for example the recent advent of fMRI, this coming together of information is likely to increase, producing a more detailed account of the cause of cognitive changes in AD.

REFERENCES

Amaral, D. G. (1993). Emerging principles of intrinsic hippocampal organisation. *Current Opinions in Neurobiology*, **3**, 225–9.

Arriagada, P. V., Growdon, J. H., Hedley-Whyte, T., and Human, B. T. (1992). Neurofibrillary tangles but not senile plaques parallel duration and severity of Alzheimer's disease. *Neurology*, **42**, 631–9.

Azari, N. P., Rapoport, S. I., Grady, C. L., Shapiro, J. A., Salerno, A., Gonzalez-Aviles, B. *et al.* (1992). Patterns of interregional correlation of cerebral glucose metabolic rates in patients with dementia of the Alzheimer's type. *Neurodegeneration*, **1**, 101–11.

Baddeley, A. D. (1992). Working memory. *Science*, **255**, 556–9.

Baddeley, A. D., Logie, R., Bressi, S., Della Sala, S., and Spinnler, H. (1986). Dementia and working memory. *Quarterly Journal of Experimental Psychology*, **38**A, 603–18.

Baddeley, A. D., Bressi, S., Della Sala, S., Logie, R., and Spinnler, H. (1991). The decline of working memory in Alzheimer's disease. *Brain*, **114**, 2521–42.

Barnard, P. (1985). Interacting cognitive subsystems: A psycholinguistic approach to short-term memory. In *Progress in the psychology of language*, Vol. 2 (ed. A. Ellis). Erlbaum, Hillsdale, NJ.

Beauvois, M. F. and Derouesne, J. (1981). Lexical or orthographic agraphia. *Brain*, **104**, 21–49.

Becker, J. T., Bajulaiye, O., and Smith, C. (1992). Longitudinal analysis of a two-component model of the memory deficit in Alzheimer's disease. *Psychological Medicine*, **22**, 437–45.

Becker, J. T., Wess, J., Hunkin, N. M., and Parkin, A. J. (1993). Use of temporal context information in Alzheimer's disease. *Neuropsychologia*, **31**, 137–43.

Becker, J. T., Mintum, M. A., Lopez, O., and De Kosky, T. (1994). Regional brain activity during free recall in probable Alzheimer's disease. *International Conference on Working Memory*, July Magdelene College, Cambridge.

Bierer, L. M., Hof, P. R., Purohi, D. P., Carlin, L., Schmeidler, J., Davis, K. L., *et al.* (1995). Neocortical neurofibrillary tangle correlate with dementia severity in Alzheimer's disease. *Archives of Neurology*, **52**, 81–8.

Blackwood, D. H. R., St Clair, D. M., Blackburn, I. M., and Tyrer, G. M. B. (1987). Cognitive brain potentials and psychological deficits in Alzheimer's dementia and Korsakoff's amnesic syndrome. *Psychological Medicine*, **17**, 349–58.

Blessed, G., Tomlinson, B. E., and Roth, M. (1988). Blessed-Roth dementia scale (DS). *Psychopharmacological Bulletin*, **24**, 705–8.

Braak, H. and Braak, E. (1991). Neuropathological staging of Alzheimer-related changes. *Acta Neuropathologica*, **82**, 239–59.

Bullmore, E., Brammer, M., Rouleua, G., Everitt, B., Simmons, A., Sharma, T., *et al.* (1995). Computational brain tissue classification of magnetic resonance images: a new approach to the problem of partial volume artifact. *Neuroimaging*, **2**, 133–47.

Brian, A. (1983). An overview of light and electron microscope changes. In *Alzheimer's disease: the standard reference*, (ed. B. Reisberg), pp. 37–47, Free Press, New York.

Chase, T., Foster, N., Fedio, P. *et al.* (1984). Regional cortical dysfunction in Alzheimer's disease as determined by positron emission tomography. *Annals of Neurology*, **15**, S170–4.

Burns, A., Philpot, M., Costa, D., *et al.* (1989). The investigation of Alzheimer's disease with single photon emission tomography. *Journal of Neurology, Neurosurgery and Psychiatry*, **52**, 248–53.

Burns, A. and Levy, R. (1994). *Dementia*. Chapman and Hall, London.

Chase, T. N., Foster, N., Fedio, P., *et al.* (1984). Regional cortical dysfunction in Alzheimer's disease as determined by positron emission tomography. *Annals of Neurology*, **15**, S170–4.

Chawluk, J. B. Alzvi, A., Dann, R., *et al.* (1987). Positron emission tomography in aging and dementia: effect of cerebral atrophy. *Journal of Nuclear Medicine*, **28**, 431–7.

Corkin, S. (1982). Some relationships between global amnesias and the memory impairment in Alzheimer's disease. In *Alzheimer's disease: A report of research in progress* (ed. S. Corkin, K. L. Davis, J. H. Growdon, E. Usdin, and R. J. Wurtman), pp. 149–64. Raven Press, New York.

De Kosky, S. T. and Scheffe, S. W. (1990). Synapse loss in frontal cortex biopsies in Alzheimer's disease: correlations with cognitive severity. *Annals of Neurology*, **27**, 457–64.

De Lacoste, M. and White, C. L. (1993). The role of cortical connectivity in Alzheimer's disease pathogenesis: A review and model system. *Neurobiology of Aging*, **14**, 1–16.

Dickson, D. W., Crystal, H.A., Mattiace, L. A., *et al.* (1992). Identification of normal and pathological aging in prospectively studied nondemented elderly humans. *Neurobiology of Aging*, **13**, 179–89.

Duyckearts, C., Delaere, P., Poulain, V; *et al.* (1985). Cortical atrophy in senile dementia of the Alzheimer type is mainly due to a decrease in cortical length. *Acta Neuropathologica (Berlin)*, **66** 72–4.

Esiri, M. (1991). Neuropathology. In *Psychiatry in the elderly* (ed. R. Jacoby and C. Oppenheimer), pp. 113–47. Oxford University Press Oxford.

Farakas, T. Ferris, S., Wolf, A., *et al.* (1982). [^{18}F] F2-deoxy-2-fluoro-D-glucose as a tracer in positron emission tomographic study of senile dementia. *American Journal of Psychiatry*, **139**, 352–3.

Ferris, S., de Leon, M., and Wolf, A. P. (1980). Positron emission tomography in the study of aging and senile dementia. *Neurobiology of Aging*, **1**, 127–31.

Filipovic, S., Kostic, V. S., Sternic, N; *et al* (1990). Auditory event-related potentials in different types of dementia. *European Journal of Neurology*, **30**, 189–93.

Foster, N. L., Chase, T. N., Fedio, P., Patronas, N. J., Brooks, R. A., and DiChiro, G. (1983). Alzheimer's disease: Focal cortical changes shown by positron emission tomography. *Neurology*, **33**, 961–5.

Foster, N. L., Chase, T. N., Mansi, L., *et al.* (1984). Cortical abnormalities in Alzheimer's disease. *Annals of Neurology*, **16**, 649–54.

Förstl, H. and Levy, R. (1991). Forward to the translation of 'On certain peculiar diseases of old age' (by Alöis Alzheimer). *History of Psychiatry*, **ii**, 71–4.

Frackowiak, R. S. J., Pozzili, C., Legg, N. J., Du Boulay, G. H., Marshall, J., Lenzi, G. L., *et al.* (1981). Regional cerebral oxygen supply and utilization in dementia. A clinical and physiological study with oxygen-15 and positron tomography. *Brain*, **104**, 753–88.

Friedland, R. P., Budinger, T. F., Koss, B., and Ober, A. B. (1985). Alzheimer's disease: Anterior-posterior and lateral hemisphere alterations in cortical glucose utilization. *Neuroscience Letters*, **53**, 235–40.

Frisk, V. and Milner, B. (1990). The relationship of working memory to the immediate recall of stones following unilateral temporal or frontal lobectomy. *Neuropsychologia*, **28**, 121–35.

Fuster, J. M. (1989). *The prefrontal cortex: Anatomy, physiology and neuropsychology of the frontal lobe.* Raven Press, New York.

Fuster, J. M. (1993). Frontal lobes. *Current Opinions in Neurobiology*, **3**, 160–5.

Geaney, D. P. (1994). Single photon emission tomography. In *Dementia* (ed. A. Burns and R. Levy), pp. 436–56. Chapman & Hall, London.

Geaney, D., Soper, N., Shepstone, B., and Cowen, P. (1990). Effect of central cholinergic stimulation on regional blood flow agent 99m TCHMPAO: a SPECT study. *Journal of Cerebral Blood Flow and Metabolism*, **11**, 398–402.

Gemmell, H., Evans, N., Besson, J., *et al.* (1990). Regional cerebral blood flow imaging: a quantitative comparison of technetium-99m-HMPAO SPECT with C1502 PET. *Journal of Nuclear Medicine*, **31**, 1595–1600.

Geschwind, N. (1965). Disconnection syndrome in animals and man: Part 1. *Brain*, **88**, 237–94.

Goedert, M., Wischik, C. M., Crowther, R. A., *et al.* (1988). Cloning and sequencing of the cDNA encoding a core protein of the paired helical filament of Alzheimer's disease: identification as the microtubule-associated protein tau. *Proceedings of the National Academy of Sciences, USA*, **85**, 4051–5.

Goldman-Rakic, P. S. (1987). Circuitry of primate prefrontal cortex and regulation of behavior by representational memory. In *Handbook of physiology: The nervous system.* Vol. 5 (ed. F. Plum), pp. 373–417. American Physiology Society, Bethesda.

Goldman-Rakic, P. S. (1988). Topography of cognition: parallel distributed network in primate association cortex. *Annual Review of Neuroscience*, **11**, 137–56.

Grady, C. L., Haxby, J. V., Schapiro, M. B., Gonzales-Aviles, A., Kumar, A., Ball, M. J., *et al.* (1990). Subgroups in dementia of the Alzheimer type identification using positron emission tomography. *Journal of Neuropsychiatry and Clinical Neuroscience*, **2**, 373–84.

Grosse, D. A., Gilley, D. W., and Wilson, R. S. (1991). Episodic and semantic memory in early versus late onset Alzheimer's disease. *Brain and Language*, **41**, 531–7.

Gustafson, L., Edivinsson, L., Dahlgren, N., *et al.* (1987). Intravenous physostigmine treatment of Alzheimer's disease evaluated by psychometric testing, regional cerebral blood flow (RCBF) measurement and EEG. *Psychopharmacology*, **93**, 31–5.

Habert, M., Spampinato, U., Mas, J., *et al.* (1991). A comparative technetium 99m hexamethyl-propylene amine oxime SPET study in different types of dementia. *European Journal of Nuclear Medicine*, **18**, 3–11.

Hart, R. P., Kwentus, J. A., Harkins, S. W., and Taylor, J. R. (1988). Rate of forgetting in mild Alzheimer-type dementia. *Brain and Cognition*, **7**, 31–8.

Haxby, J., Grady, C., Duara, R., *et al.* (1986). Neocortical metabolic abnormalities precede non memory cognitive defects in early Alzheimer-type dementia. *Archives of Neurology*, **43**, 882–5.

Haxby, J. V., Grady, C. L., Koss, E., Horwitz, B., Heston, L., Shapiro, M., *et al.* (1990). Longitudinal study of cerebral metabolic asymmetries and associated neuropsychological patterns in early dementia of the Alzheimer Type. *Archives of Neurology*, **47**, 753–60.

Hendrickson, E., Levy, R., and Post, F. (1979). Averaged evoked responses in relation to cognitive and affective state of elderly psychiatric patients. *British Journal of Psychiatry*, **34**, 494–501.

Horwitz, B., Grady, C. L., Schlageter, N. L., Duara, R., and Rapaport, S. I. (1987). Intercorrelations of regional cerebral glucose metabolic rates in Alzheimer's disease. *Brain Research*, **407**, 294–306.

Hughes, C. P., Berg, L., Danziger, W. L., Coben, L. A., and Martin, R. L. (1982). A new clinical scale for the staging of dementia. *British Journal of Psychiatry*, **140**, 566–72.

Huisman, U. W., Posthuman, J., Hooijer, V., *et al.* (1985). Somatosensory evoked potentials in healthy volunteers and patients with dementia. *Clinical Neurology and Neurosurgery*, **87**, 11–16.

Hunter, R., McLuskie, R., Wyper, D., *et al.* (1989). The pattern of function related cerebral blood flow investigated by single photon emission tomography with 99mTc-HMPAO in patients with presenile Alzheimer's disease and Korsakoff's psychosis. *Psychological Medicine*, **19**, 847–55.

Hyman, B. T., Van Hoesen, G. W., Kromer, L. J., and Damasio, A. R. (1990). Memory-related neuronal systems in Alzheimer's disease: An anatomic study. *Neurology*, **40**, 472–81.

Jacoby, R. and Levy, R. (1980). Computed tomography in the elderly. 2. Senile dementia: diagnosis in functional impairment. *British Journal of Psychiatry*, **136**, 270–5.

Jagust, W., Budinger, T., and Reed, B. (1987). The diagnosis of dementia with single photon emission tomography. *Archives of Neurology*, **44**, 258–62.

Jagust, W., Reed, B., Seab, J., and Budinger, T. (1990). Alzheimer's disease: Age of onset and single-photon emission computed tomographic patterns of regional cerebral blood flow. *Archives of Neurology*, **47**, 626–33.

Jernigan, T. L., Salmon, D. P., Butters, N., and Hesseline, J. R. (1991). Cerebral structures on MRI, Part 2: Specific changes in Alzheimer's and Huntington's diseases. *Biological Psychiatry*, **29**, 68–81.

Jones, E. and Powell, T. P. S. (1970). An anatomical study of converging sensory pathways within the cerebral cortex of the monkey. *Brain*, **93**, 793–820.

Kahneman, D. (1973). *Attention and effort.* Prentice Hall, Englewood Cliffs, NJ.

Kennedy, A. M. and Frackowiak, R. S. J. (1994). Positron emission tomography. In *Dementia* (ed. A. Burns and R. Levy, pp. 457–74. Chapman & Hall, London.

Kesslak, J. P., Nalcioglu, O., and Cotman, C. W. (1991). Quantification of magnetic resonance scans for hippocampal and parahippocampal atrophy in Alzheimer's disease. *Neurology*, **44**, 51–4.

Kessler, J., Herhoz, K., Grond, M., and Heiss, W. D. (1991). Impaired metabolic activation in Alzheimer's disease: A PET study during continuous visual recognition. *Neuropsychologia*, **29**, 229–43.

Khachaturian, (1985). Diagnosis of Alzheimer's disease. *Archives of Neurology*, **42**, 1097–104.

Kinsbourne, M. (1980). Attentional dysfunction in the elderly: Theoretical models and research perspectives. In *New directions in memory and aging*, (ed. L. W. Poon, J. L. Fozard, L. S. Cermak, D. Arenberg, and L. W. Thompson), pp. 112–20. Erlbaum, Hillsdale, NJ.

Kolb, B. and Whishaw, I. Q. (1990). *Fundamentals of human neuropsychology* 3rd edn. W. H. Freeman & Company, New York.

Kraiuhin, C., Gordon, E., Coyle, S., *et al.* (1990). Normal latency of the P300 event-related potential in mild-to-moderate Alzheimer's disease and depression. *Biological Psychiatry*, **28**, 372–86.

Kuwabara, Y., Ichiya, Y., Otsuka, M., *et al.* (1990). Comparison of I–123 ImP and Tc-99m HMPAO SPECT studies with PET in dementia. *Annals of Nuclear Medicine*, **4**, 75–82.

Kuypers, H. G. J. M., Szwarcbart, M. K., Mishkin, M., and Rosvold, H. E. (1965). Occipitotemporal corticocortical connections in the Rhesus monkey. *Experimental Neurology*, **11**, 245–62.

LaBerge, D. (1990). Thalamic and cortical mechanisms of attention suggested by recent positron emission tomographic experiments. *Journal of Neuroscience*, **2**, 358–72.

Lantos, P. L. and Cairns, N. J. (1994). The neuropathology of Alzheimer's disease. In *Dementia*, (ed. A. Burns and R. Levy), pp. 185–207. Chapman & Hall, London.

Lashley, K. S. (1950). Functional determinants of cerebral localisation. In *The neuropsychology of Lashley* (ed. F.A. Beach, D. O. Hebb, C. T. Morgan and, H. W. Nisen), pp. 454–82. McGraw-Hill Book Co., New York.

Leuchter, A. F., Spar, J. E., Walter, D. O. and Weiner, H. (1987). Electroencephalographic spectra and coherence in the diagnosis of Alzhemier-type and multi-infarct dementia: A pilot study. *Archives of General Psychiatry*, **44**, 993–8.

Leuchter, A. F., Newton, T. F., Cook, I.A., Walter, D. O., Rosenberg-Thompson, S., and Lachenbruch, P. A. (1992). Changes in brain functional connectivity in Alzheimer-type and multi-infarct dementia. *Brain*, **115**, 1543–61.

Lewis, D. A., Campbell, M. J., Terry, R. D., and Morrison, J. H. (1987). Laminar and regional distribution of neurofibrillary tangles and neuritic plaques in Alzheimer's disease: A quantitative study of visual and auditory cortices. *Journal of Neuroscience*, **7** 1799–1808.

McGeer, E., Peppard, R., McGeer, P., *et al.* (1990). 18-Fluorodeoxyglucose positron emission tomography studies in presumed Alzheimer cases, including 13 serial scans. *Le Journal Canadien des Sciences Neurologiques*, **36** 1569–74.

Majocha, R. E., Benes, F. M., Reifel, J. L. *et al.* (1988). Laminar-specific distribution and infrastructural detail of amyloid in Alzheimer's disease cortex visualised by computer-enhanced imaging of epitopes recognised by monoclonal antibodies. *Proceedings of the National Academy of Sciences, USA*, **85**, 6182–6.

Mann, D. M. A., Yates, P.O., and Marcyniuk, B. (1985). Some morphometric observations in the cerebral cortex and hippocampus in presenile Alzheimer's disease, senile dementia of the Alzheimer's type and Down's syndrome in middle age. *Journal of Neurological Science*, **69**, 139–59.

Marc-Vergnes, J. P., Le Tinnier, A., Celsis, P., *et al.* (1986). SPECT, computerised EEG and neuropsychological assessment of hemispheric asymmetries in the early stages of DAT. In *Dementia: Early detection* (ed. A. Bes), pp. 144–51. John Libby Eurotext, London.

Marcyniuk, B., Mann, D. M. A., and Yates, P.O. (1986). The topography of cell loss from locus coeruleus in Alzheimer's disease. *Journal of Neurological Science*, **76**, 335–45.

Masliah, E., Terry, R. D., Alford, H., De Teresa., R., and Hansen, L. A. (1991). Cortical and subcortical patterns of synaptophysin-like immunoreactivity in Alzheimer's disease. *American Journal of Pathology*, **138**, 235–46.

Masters, C. L., Multhaup, G., Simms, G., *et al.* (1985). Neuronal origin of a cerebral amyloid: neurofibrillary tangles of Alzheimer's disease contain the same protein as the amyloid of plaque cores and blood vessels. *EMBO Journal*, **4**, 2757–63.

Mirra, S. S., Heyman, A., McKeel, D., *et al* (1991). The consortium to establish a registry for Alzheimer's disease (CERAD). Part 2. Standardisation of the neuropathologic assessment of Alzheimer's disease. *Neurology*, **41**, 479–86.

Montaldi, D., Brooks, D., McColl, J., *et al.* (1990). Measurements of regional cerebral blood flow and cognitive performance in Alzheimer's disease. *Journal of Neurology, Neurosurgery and Psychiatry*, **53**, 33–8.

Morris, R. G. (1984). Dementia and the functioning of the Articulatory Loop System. *Cognitive Neuropsychology*, **1**, 77–97.

Morris, R. G. (1991). Neuropsychological studies of memory functioning in Alzheimer-type dementia. In *Memory: Neurochemical and abnormal perspectives*, (ed. J. Weinmann and J. Hunter), pp. 163–87. Harwood Academic Publishers, London.

Morris, R. G. (1992). Patterns of short-term memory impairment in Alzheimer's disease. In *Memory functioning in dementia*, (ed. L. Backman), pp. 3–25. Elsevier Science Publishers, Amsterdam.

Morris, R. G. (1994*a*). Recent developments in the neuropsychology of dementia. *International Journal of Psychiatry*, **4**, 85–107.

Morris, R. G. (1994*b*). Working memory in Alzheimer's disease. *Neuropsychology*, **8**, 544–54.

Morris, R. G. (1994*c*). Working memory in Alzheimer's disease: A dysconnection syndrome? *International Conference on Working Memory*, Magdalene College, Cambridge.

Morris, R. G. and Baddeley, A. D. (1988). Primary and working memory functioning in Alzheimer-type dementia. *Journal of Experimental and Clinical Psychology*, **51**, 757–66.

Morris, R. G. and Kopelman, M. D. (1986). The memory deficits in Alzheimer-type dementia: A review. *Quarterly Journal of Experimental Psychology*, **38**, 575–602.

Morrison, J., Scherr, S., Lewis, D., Campbell, M., Bloom F., Rogers, J., *et al.* (1986). The laminar and regional distribution of neocortical somatostatin and neuritic plaques: implications for Alzheimer's disease as a global neocortical disconnection syndrome. In (ed. A. Scheibel, A. Wechsler, and M. Brazier), pp. 115–31. *The biological substrates of Alzheimer's disease.* Academic Press, Orlando.

Moseley, I. (1993). Imaging the adult brain. *Journal of Neurology, Neurosurgery and Psychiatry*, **38**, 7–21.

Mountjoy, C. Q., Tomlinson, B. E., and Gibson, B. E. (1982). Amyloid senile plaques and cerebral blood vessels. A semi-quantitative investigation of a possible relationship. *Journal of Neurological Science*, **57**, 89–103.

Norman, D. and Bobrow, D. G. (1975). On data-limited and resource-limited processes. *Cognitive Psychology*, **7**, 44–67.

Norman, D. A. and Shallice, T. (1986). Attention to action: Willed and automatic control of behavior. In *Advances in research and theory:* Vol. 4. *Consciousness and self-regulation* (ed. R. J. Davidson, G. E. Schwartz, and D. Shapiro), pp. 1–18. Plenum Press, New York.

O'Connor, K. P., Shaw, J. C., and Ongley, C. O. (1979). The EEG and differential diagnosis in psychogeriatrics. *British Journal of Psychiatry*, **135**, 156–62.

Pandya, D.N. and Barnes, C.L. (1987). Architecture and connections of the frontal lobe. In *The frontal lobes revisited*, (ed. E. Perecman), pp. 41–72. IRBN Press, New York.

Parasuraman, R. and Haxby, J. V. (1993). Attention and brain function in Alzheimer's disease: A review. *Neuropsychology*, **7**, 242–72.

Parasuraman, R., Greenwood, P. M., Haxby, J. V., and Grady, C. L. (1992). Visuospatial attention in dementia of the Alzheimer's type. *Brain*, **115**, 711–33.

Parkin, A. J., Leng, N., and Hunkin, N. M. (1990). Differential sensitivity to context in diencephalic and temporal lobe amnesia. *Cortex*, **26**, 373–80.

Paulescu, E., Frith, C. D., and Frackowiak, R. S. J. (1993). The neural correlates of the verbal components of working memory. *Nature*, **362**, 342–45.

Pearson, R. C. A., Esiri, M. M., Hiorns, R. W., Wilcock, G. K., and Powell, T. P. S. (1985). Anatomical correlates of the distribution of the pathological changes in the neocortex in Alzheimer's disease. *Proceedings of the National Academy of Sciences USA*, **82**, 4531–4.

Penniello, M., Lambert, J., Eustache, F., Petit-Taboue, *et al.* (1995). A PET study of the functional neuroanatomy of writing impairment in Alzheimer's disease: The role of the left supramarginal and left angular gyrus. *Brain*, **118**, 697–706.

Petersen, S. E., Fox, P. T., Posner, M. I., Mintum, M., and Raichle, M. E. (1988). Positron emission tomographic studies of the cortical anatomy of single word processing. *Nature*, **331**, 585–9.

Philpot, M. (1994). The neurophysiology of dementia. In *Dementia.* (ed. A. Burns and R. Levy), pp. 371–85. Chapman & Hall, London.

Posner, M. I., Cohen, Y., Choate, L. S., Hockey, R., and Maylor, E. (1984*a*). Sustained concentration: passive filtering or active orienting? In *Preparatory states and processes* (ed. S. Kornblum and J. Requin), pp. 49–65. Erlbaum, Hillsdale, NJ.

Posner, M. I., Walker, J. A., Friedrich, F. J., and Rafal, R. D. (1984*b*). Effects of parietal injury on covert orienting of attention. *Journal of Neuroscience*, **4**, 1863–74.

Rogers, J. and Morrison, J. H. (1985). Quantitative morphology and regional and laminar distributions of senile plaques in Alzheimer's disease. *Journal of Neuroscience*, **5**, 2801–8.

Ruessman, K., Sondag, H. D., and Beneicke, U. (1990). P300 latency of the auditory evoked potential in dementia. *International Journal of Neuroscience*, **54**, 291–6.

Saper, C. (1986). *Is* Alzheimer's disease transmitted from neuron to neuron via normal neuronal connections? Paper presented at the meeting of the *British Association for Psychopharmacology*, Jesus College, Cambridge.

Seab, J. P., Jagust, W. J., Wong, S. T. S., *et al.* (1988). Quantitative NMR measurements of hippocampal atrophy in Alzheimer's disease. *Magnetic Resonance Imaging*, **8**, 200–8.

Shallice, T. (1981). Phonological agraphia and the lexical route in writing. *Brain*, **112**, 1549–61.

Shallice, T. (1988). *From neuropsychology to mental structure.* Cambridge University Press.

Shallice, T. and Vallar, G. (1990). The impairment of auditory-verbal short-term storage. In *Neuropsychological impairments of short-term memory*, (ed. G. Gillar and T. Shallice), pp. 11–53). Cambridge University Press.

Squire, L. R. (1992). Memory and the hippocampus: A synthesis from findings with rats, monkeys, and humans. *Psychological Review*, **9**, 195–231.

Stuss, D. T. and Benson, D. (1987). The frontal lobes and control of cogniti and memory. In *The frontal lobes revisited* (ed. E. Perecman), pp. 141–58. IRBN Press, New York.

Terry, R. D. (1990). Normal aging and Alzheimer's disease: growing problems. In *Neuropathology*, (ed. P. A. Cancilla, R. S. Vogel, and N. Kaufman), pp. 41–5. Williams & Wilkins, Baltimore.

Terry, R. D., and Katzman, R. (1983). Senile dementia of the Alzheimer's type. *Annals of Neurology*, **14**, 497–506.

Terry, R., Masliah, E., Salmon, D., Butters, N., De Teresa, L., Hansen, L., *et al.* (1990). Structure-function correlations in Alzheimer's disease [Abstract]. *Journal of Neuropathology and Experimental Neurology*, **49**, 318.

Tomlinson, B. E., Blessed, G., and Roth, M. (1970). Observations on the brains of non-demented old people. *Journal of Neurological Sciences*, **11**, 205–42.

Tucker, D. M., Roth, D. L., and Blair, T. B. (1986). Functional connections among cortical regions: topography of EEG coherence. *Electroencephalography and Clinical Neurophysiology*, **63**, 242–50.

Tulving, E. (1983). *Elements of episodic memory.* University Press, New York.

Van Hoesen, G. (1990). The dissection by Alzheimer's disease of cortical and limbic neural systems relevant to memory. In *Brain organization and memory* (ed. J. L. McGaugh, N. M. Weinberger, and G Lynch), pp. 234–61. Oxford Science Publications, Oxford.

Visser, S. L., (1985). EEG and evoked potentials in the diagnosis of dementias. In *Senile dementia of the Alzheimer's type* (ed. J. Traber and W. H. Gispen), pp. 102–16. Springer-Verlag, Berlin.

Weintraub, S. and Mesulam, M.-M. (1987). Right cerebral dominance in spatial attention: Further evidence based on ipsilateral neglect. *Archives of Neurology*, **44**, 621–5.

Whitehouse, P. J., Price, D. L., Clark, A. W., *et al.* (1981). Alzheimer's disease: evidence for selective loss of cholinergic neurons in the nucleus basalis. *Annals of Neurology*, **10**, 122–6.

Whittaker, S. C., and Siegfried, J. B. (1983). Origin of wavelets in the visual evoked potential. *Electroencephalography and Clinical Neurophysiology*, **55**, 91–101.

Wilcock, G. K., and Esiri, M. M. (1982). Plaques, tangles and dementia: A quantitative study. *Journal of Neurological Science*, **56**, 353–6.

Williams, P. A., Jones, G. H., Briscoe, M., *et al.* (1991). P300 and reaction time measures in senile dementia of the Alzheimer's type. *British Journal of Psychiatry*, **159**, 410–14.

Wright, C. E. and Furlong, P. L. (1988). Visual evoked potentials in elderly patients with primary or multi-infarct dementia. *British Journal of Psychiatry*, **152**, 679–672.

Wright, C. E., Harding, G. F. A., and Orwin, A. (1984). Presenile dementia—the use of the flash and pattern VEP in diagnosis. *Electroencephalography and Clinical Neurophysiology*, **57**, 405–15.

Yamamoto, T. and Hirano, A. (1985). Nucleus raphe dorsalis in Alzheimer's disease: neurofibrillary tangles and loss of large neurones. *Annals of Neurology*, **17**, 573–7.

Zola-Morgan, S. and Squire, L. R. (1990). The primate hippocampal formation: Evidence for a time-limited role in memory storage. *Science*, **250**, 288–90.

Zola-Morgan, S., Squire, L. R., and Amaral, D. G. (1986). Human amnesia and the medial temporal region: Enduring memory impairment following a bilateral lesion limited to field CA1 of the hippocampus. *Journal of Neuroscience*, **6**, 2950–67.

FOURTEEN

The cognitive psychopharmacology of Alzheimer's disease

H. Valerie Curran and Michael D. Kopelman

INTRODUCTION

Much of the current research on Alzheimer's disease is focused on molecular genetics, and one goal of such studies is to identify deficient enzymes and biochemical processes which require replacement or augmentation. It follows from this that increasing our knowledge first of which neurotransmitters are depleted in Alzheimer's disease and second what functional roles those transmitters play in cognitive function, remains an important research approach. These two topics are the focus of this chapter. The related topic of the efficacy of pharmacological agents in replacement therapy in Alzheimer dementia is considered in Chapter 18.

The first section overviews our current state of knowledge about which neurotransmitters are affected in Alzheimer's disease. Although several neurotransmitters have been implicated, cholinergic depletion is still the most clearly documented neurochemical loss. In turn, a good deal of research has focused on cholinergic blockade as a means of investigating the functional role of acetylcholine in memory, which is discussed in the second section. Psychopharmacological studies have shown that substances which have very different actions from cholinergic blockers can nevertheless produce similar impairments of cognitive function. These studies, in turn, raise questions about the specificity of the amnesic effects of cholinergic blockade and these are addressed in the final section.

NEUROTRANSMITTERS IN ALZHEIMER DEMENTIA

Acetylcholine

Several studies have reported a substantial loss of cholinergic neurones in the nucleus basalis, septal nucleus, and dorsal band of Broca of the basal forebrain, nuclei which project to the neocortex, hippocampus, and amygdala (Arendt *et al.* 1983; Mann *et al.* 1984, 1986; Whitehouse, 1982). There is widespread, cortical and subcortical reduction in choline acetyl transferase levels (Bowen *et al.* 1976; Perry *et al.* 1987; Rossor *et al.* 1984; Wilcock *et al.* 1982; 1984); and this abnormality is associated with a reduction in cholinergic synthesis in biopsy samples, (Francis *et al.* 1985; Sims *et al.* 1980). Post-synaptic muscarinic receptors appear to be intact, but nicotinic and presynaptic muscarinic receptors appear to be somewhat depleted (Flynn and Mash, 1986; Mash *et al.* 1985; Perry, E.K. *et al.* 1978; Perry, T.L. *et al.* 1987). The direction in which cholinergic changes proceed remains controversial (Arendt *et al.* 1985; Mann *et al.* 1986; Perry 1986; However, Esiri *et al.* (1990) have demonstrated that the topographical distribution of cholinergic depletion appears to correlate well with the density of neubofibrillary tangles, consistent with the notion that the disease spreads along corticocortical connections and between the neocortex and medial temporal structures (see Chapter 13).

Noradrenaline

There is a loss of neurones in the locus coeruleus from which ascending adrenergic pathways arise. This cell loss is greatest in patients under 80 at the time of their death (Bondareff *et al* 1982; Mann *et al.* 1984). There is a reduction in cortical noradrenaline, occurring mainly in younger subjects (Mann *et al.* 1980; Rossor *et al.* 1984). In addition, there is a reduction in the activity of phenylethanolamine-*N*-methyl transferase, which converts adrenaline to noradrenaline, the reduction in the hippocampus being correlated with measures of ante-mortem cognitive impairment (Burke *et al.* 1987).

Dopamine

Dopamine reduction occurs in the caudate nucleus (Palmer *et al.* 1986) and in other subcortical sites including the amygdala (Rossor and Iversen 1986). Concentrations in the cerebral cortex are generally preserved (Rossor and Iversen 1986), although there may be some depletion of frontal dopamine (Mann *et al.* 1987). The dopaminergic cells of the ventral tegmental area, projecting to the limbic and frontal areas of the cortex, are markedly depleted in Alzheimer's disease, and neurofibrillary tangles are commonly found in this region (Mann *et al* 1987). On the other hand, the cells of the substantia nigra, projecting to the basal ganglia, are relatively unaffected.

Vasopressin

Mazurek *et al* (1986) found reduced levels in the hippocampus, nucleus accumbens, and globus pallidus, although Rossor *et al.* (1980) found only a non-significant trend for a reduction in vasopressin levels in Alzheimer's disease.

Serotonin

A variable degree of loss of large neurones in the (serotinergic) raphe nucleus has been reported, in association with the presence of neurofibrillary tangles (Mann *et al.* 1984; Yamamoto and Hirano 1985). There is a reduction of serotonin levels in the temporal and frontal cortex (Benton *et al.* 1982; D'Amato *et al.* 1987), and there is also a reduction in serotoninergic binding sites in these regions (Cross *et al.* 1986; D'Amato *et al.* 1987). According to D'Amato *et al.* (1987), the reduction of serotoninergic markers in Alzheimer's disease is comparable in severity with the reduction in cholinergic markers. By contrast, Bowen and colleagues (1992*a*, *b*) reported that in half of the cortical areas they assayed, there was no evidence of reduced presynaptic activity.

Glutamate and glycine

Reductions in CSF concentrations of glutamate and glycine have been reported in Alzheimer patients, and glutamate content appeared to show some significant correlations with cognitive measures (Smith *et al.* 1985). In that study, other amino acids showed no significant correlations with cognitive scores. A substantial reduction in free glutamate in the terminal zone of the 'perforant pathway' in the entorhinal cortex has also been reported which can be attributed to a degeneration of a specific population of neurones in that region (Hyman *et al.* 1987). Ellison *et al.* (1986) found a significant reduction of glutamate in the inferior temporal gyrus, but not in other cortical regions; and Perry *et al.* (1987) failed to find any significant cortical reduction.

Glutamate appears to be the main excitatory neurotransmitter to the pyramidal neurones of the hippocampus (Shepherd 1988); and Bowen (1990) has reported that degeneration of columns of corticocortical glutamatergic pyramidal cells in circumscribed (parietotemporal) areas of the cerebral cortex occurs early in Alzheimer's disease. Moreover, Bowen and his colleagues (1992*a*, *b*) suggest that glutamatergic transmission may normally be the chief factor that sustains the activity of corticocortical neurones in the cortex. Thus the degeneration in the parietotemporal cortex probably reduces excitory input into neurones. Penney *et al.* (1990) have found a substantial loss of NMDA binding sites (widely thought to play a critical role in memory processes) and a moderate loss of glutamate binding, in autoradiographic studies of

Alzheimer brains, suggesting that the potential for facilitating activity at these receptors may be limited.

Gaba

GABA is the inhibitory neurotransmitter within the interneurones of the hippocampus, producing post-synaptic inhibition within the pyramidal neurones by feedback and feed-forward mechanisms (Shepherd 1988). GABA shows a reduction of approximately 20–30% in the temporal cortex of younger Alzheimer patients (Rossor *et al.* 1982, 1984). However, GABA may not be significantly diminished in other cortical or subcortical regions, nor in older Alzheimer patients (Ellison *et al.* 1986 Rossor *et al.* 1982, 1984). One study found a decreased GABA content in the frontal and occipital lobes (Perry *et al.* 1987), and another obtained a reduction at post-mortem in the frontal and temporal lobes (Lowe *et al.* 1988); there is evidence that GABA-A and GABA-B receptors are both reduced in the frontal cortex of Alzheimer patients (Chui *et al.* 1987). However, Lowe *et al.* (1988) failed to find reduced GABA levels ante-mortem in biopsy samples from Alzheimer patients, suggesting that this may be a late manifestation of the disorder.

Somatostatin

Many neuritic plaques and many neurones containing tangles are immunoreactive to somatostatin (Morrison *et al.* 1985; Roberts *et al.* 1985); and there is evidence of a widespread neocortical reduction in somatostatin levels, which is most profound in the temporal or parietal cortex, but is not found in the basal forebrain or other subcortical structures (Beal *et al.* 1986; Tamminga *et al.* 1987). There is also evidence that a reduction in CSF markers of somatostatin correlates with cognitive abnormalities (Soininen *et al.* 1984; Tamminga *et al.* 1987). On the other hand, Palmer *et al.* (1988) reported reduced somatostatin levels post-mortem, but not in ante-mortem biopsy samples. Tissue samples were taken from the temporal lobe in both cases, and the biopsy group had had Alzheimer symptoms for a mean duration of three years against eight years in the post-mortem group. This suggests that somatostatin depletion, like GABA depletion (Lowe *et al.* 1988; Palmer *et al.* 1988; may be a relatively late manifestation of the disorder.

Neuropeptides and amino acids

There is a report that substance P is significantly reduced in the cerebral cortex and hippocampus, especially the inferior temporal gyrus (Beal and Mazurek 1987). Neuropeptide Y was found to be reduced in one study in association with changes in somatostatin (Kowall and Beal 1988), but other studies have found normal neuropeptide Y levels (Rossor and Iversen 1986). A further study reported a reduction in corticotrophin-releasing factor in the frontal, temporal, and occipital lobes, which correlated with the reduction of choline acetyl transferase (Whitehouse *et al.* 1987). In general, levels of cholecystokinin, vasoactive intestinal polypeptide, neurotensin, thyrotropin-releasing hormone, aspartate, alanine, taurine, and glutathione have all been reported as normal (Ellison *et al.* 1986; Perry *et al.* 1987; Rossor and Iversen 1986).

PSYCHOPHARMACOLOGICAL STUDIES

Based on the considerable evidence that cholinergic neurones, enzymes, and synthesis are all depleted in Alzheimer patients, many studies have assessed the effects of cholinergic blockade in normal subjects using the anticholinergic drug scopolamine (SP). There is also evidence, particularly in younger patients, of substantial reductions in cortical levels of noradrenaline, serotonin, somatostatin, and glutamate. Findings with respect to dopamine, vasopressin, GABA, and the neuropeptides are more equivocal. Of the possible role of these substances in human memory, acetylcholine and the GABA/glutamate system have received the most research attention.

Acetylcholine and memory

One way of examining the effects of a putative neurotransmitter agent is to assess the cognitive effects of administering a substance which antagonizes or 'blocks' the actions of that agent. Scopolamine (hyoscine) selectively antagonizes the muscarinic actions of acetycholine (at very high doses, it can also antagonize nicotinic receptors) (Weiner 1980). Since the original work of Drachmann and Leavitt (1974), the amnesic effects of this drug have been studied extensively over the last 20 years. Most studies administer scopolamine to healthy young adults and then assess changes in performance on tests of attention and memory. Only a few studies have examined the effects of the drug in older adults and in Alzheimer's patients (e.g. Molchan *et al.* 1992; Sunderland *et al.* 1987).

A plethora of tasks have been used to assess the effects of SP on attention and memory, and even within each type of task, there has been considerable variation in specific task requirements. Different routes of administration of the drug (oral, intramuscular, intravenous) affect absorption rates and have to be taken into account when evaluating findings across different studies. However, whatever the route of administration, there is usually quite a clear dose–response effect (e.g. Nuotto 1983; Parrott 1986; Safer and Allen 1971; Wesnes and Warburton 1984).

In general, tasks which require remembering a few items for a period of seconds are not affected by scopolamine. These include, for example, digit or blockspan, where sequences of digits or spatial locations are repeated back immediately in serial order. The drug does impair performance on Sternberg's (1969) memory scanning task (Alford *et al.* 1991; Wesnes *et al.* 1988). However, this may well be due to the sedative effect of SP, slowing response speeds which reflect a quantitative effect on performance rather than a qualitative effect on memory (error rates are generally unaffected). Scopolamine impairs short-term recall in some versions of the Brown–Peterson task which requires three items to be remembered following short periods of distraction (Beatty *et al.* 1986; Caine *et al.* 1981), This may reflect the greater information-processing load that this task imposes (Kopelman and Corn 1988).

Results of some elegant studies by Rusted using dual-task paradigms imply that a main locus of SP's effects is on the 'central executive' component of working memory (Rusted 1988; Rusted and Warburton 1988; see Chapter 4). This may also underlie SP's impairment of performance on attentional tasks which is generally more marked the greater the complexity of the task and therefore the greater the demands on 'Central processing resources (Broks *et al.* 1988; Dunne and Hartley 1985; Warburton 1979, 1981). Indeed, Sahaki (1987) argues that attentional impairment may be the main locus of scopolamine's effect on cognition. In a thoughtful recent review of these issues, Rusted (1994) argues that impairment of a supposedly unitary or 'all-purpose' central executive mechanism cannot encompass the range of effects of SP on attention and memory. If a single executive mechanism allocated resources from a common pool, then one would expect attentional and memory impairments to co-occur with SP. However, studies which have systematically examined correspondence between the drug's attentional and memory effects have *not* shown a clear pattern of correspondence (Curran *et al.* 1991) (see also Kopelman and Corn 1988; Preston *et al.* 1989). These points are expanded on later.

The effects of cholinergic blockade on tests tapping episodic memory are consistent, and clearly dose-related. Scopolamine impairs performance on tasks requiring the supra-span recall or recognition of verbal or non-verbal materials (Collerton 1986; Kopelman 1986; Sahakian

1987). This deficit can be attenuated if not fully reversed by concurrent administration of a cholinergic agonist or anticholinesterase (Drachman 1977; Mohs and Davis 1985). Older healthy adults and Alzheimer patients show lower dose thresholds for the manifestation of scopolamine-induced learning impairments (Molchan *et al.* 1992; Sunderland *et al.* 1987). A variation on the free recall task is the selective reminding procedure (Buschke and Full 1974) where the subject is prompted on each trial with only those words which were not recalled successfully during the previous trial. This is also sensitive to disruption by SP (Broks *et al.* 1988 Caine *et al.* 1981; Molchan *et al.* 1990, 1992; Sunderland *et al.* 1987; Wesnes *et al.* 1990) as is the learning of paired associates (Beatty *et al.* 1986; Curran *et al.* 1991; Kopelman and Corn 1988; Nuotto 1983).

In general, it appears that the more effort-ful or resource-demanding a task is, the more marked the effect of cholinergic blockade on performance. Experimental manipulations which affect normal memory performance (for example recognition versus recall: levels of processing; delay/interference between acquisition and retrieval) produce a broadly parallel pattern of influences on the performance of SP-treated subjects. Only the more recent studies have examined the pattern of memory deficits in any clear detail (eg. Beatty *et al.* 1986; Bishop *et al.* 1996; Curran *et al.* 1991; Kopelman 1991; Knopman 1991; Kopelman and Corn 1988; Nissen *et al.* 1987; Rusted 1988; Rusted *et al.* 1991; Rusted and Warburton 1988; Schifano and Curran 1994; Tröster *et al.* 1989).

In contrast to the clear anterograde impairments induced by the drug, no study has found any evidence of *retrograde* impairments of memory with SP. Further, most studies find that the drug does not appear to impede people's ability to *retrieve* items of general knowledge or other well-established memories. For example the performance of healthy young subjects is generally intact on tasks like verbal fluency, in which subjects are required to retrieve as many words as possible beginning with a particular letter or belonging to a particular category (e.g. Beatty *et al.* 1986; Curran *et al.* 1991; Knopman 1991; Nissen *et al.* 1987). Several studies have, however, reported performance deficits on verbal fluency, but these have tended to use very high doses and/or intravenous administration (Caine *et al.* 1981; Drachman and Leavitt 1974), and so impairment may relate to motor sedation. Molchan *et al.* (1992) and Sunderland *et al.* (1987) showed that fluency impairments in older volunteers were evident only with the highest (0.5 mg IV) dose of SP used. Surprisingly, two studies report facilitated fluency following SP (Dunne *et al.* 1993; Lines *et al.* 1991). Bishop *et al.* (1996) used a sentence verification task which requires speeded retrieval from semantic memory, and found that a higher dose

(0.6 mg SC) increased both response times and errors compared with a lower dose (0.3 mg SC). No study to date has examined the effects of SP on the *acquisition* of new factual information into semantic memory.

Tasks tapping procedural memory are also largely resistant to SP-induced impairments. For example Nissen *et al.* (1987) showed clear impairments on verbal recall and recognition tests with intact ability on a perceptual-motor learning task (serial reaction time). Similar findings are reported by Knopman (1991). However, other types of procedural learning tasks are sometimes found to show scopolamine-induced impairments. For example Frith *et al.* (1989) have found that scopolamine did affect the rate of learning of a perceptual–motor tracking task.

Using a wide range of memory assessments, Kopelman and Corn (1988) compared findings for cholinergic blockade with the results obtained in similar studies of Alzheimer and Korsakoff patients. They showed that scopolamine did not affect the more passive aspects of 'primary' memory (for example span tests and a measure of verbal, short-term forgetting in which the 'distractor task' was kept constant throughout). In this, it resembled the Korsakoff syndrome and contrasted with the marked deficits seen in Alzheimer-type dementia. On the other hand, cholinergic blockade did produce impairment on a visuospatial, short-term forgetting test, and on a verbal test in which the distractor task was varied and made more difficult, thereby increasing the 'information-processing load' of the task. Cholinergic blockade produced a pattern of impairment on episodic memory similar to that seen in the anterograde amnesia of Korsakoff and many Alzheimer patients. There was a pronounced impairment in learning verbal and visuospatial material on both recall and recognition memory tests, a normal forgetting rate once learning had been accomplished, and preservation of the rate of learning a perceptual–motor skill. Further, cholinergic blockade did not affect priming (the general facilitation of a response from having recently seen a stimulus), but did impair cued recall. This pattern is commonly found in studies of amnesic patients (Graf *et al.* 1984) and in some studies of Alzheimer patients (Christensen *et al.* 1992; (Partridge *et al.* 1990). Knopman (1991) found that scopolamine produced impairment in the free recall of word lists, but did not affect a word-completion priming task, a motor serial reaction task, or repetition priming on a tachistoscopic word identification task. These findings would appear to confirm that scopolamine resembles organic amnesia in leaving called 'implicit memory' (Schacter 1987) unaffected, whereas 'explicit memory' is impaired. The sparing of priming as assessed by perceptual tasks, such as word-stem or fragment completion, appears to be a consistent finding following scopolamine administration (Bishop *et al.* 1996; Knopman 1991; Schifano and Curran 1994).

Kopelman and Corn (1988) concluded that cholinergic blockade produced a pattern of anterograde amnesia consistent with that seen in the Korsakoff syndrome and many Alzheimer patients, but that it did not mimic the extensive retrograde loss seen in both disorders, nor the full range of 'primary' or 'working' memory deficits which occur in Alzheimer-type dementia.

Acetylcholine, attention, and memory

Considerable debate centres on the issue of the relationship between the attentional and amnesic effects of scopolamine. Some studies have found fairly uniform impairments across different types of test (Parrott 1986; Wesnes *et al.* 1988). Other studies have reported that scopolamine can produce amnesic effects at doses which do not impair performance on tests of attention or vigilance (Caine *et al.* 1981; Crow and Grove-White 1973; Crow *et al.* 1975; Kopelman and Corn 1988; Sunderland *et al.* 1987). Dunne and Hartley (1985) and Broks *et al.* (1988) have argued that scopolamine can disrupt attentional processes without affecting overall memory performance. The most recent studies suggest that the amnesic properties of scopolamine cannot be accounted for by covarying effects on attention. Further, as discussed below, it is possible that effects of the drug on memory and attentional processes are *independent*.

Not only is there debate about the relationship between scopolamine's attentional and amnesic effects, but it is also clear that this drug has sedative effects, and so the question arises as to whether lowered arousal levels contribute to performance impairments on both attentional and memory tests. Kopelman and Corn (1988) found that cholinergic blockade produced a significant decrement on a subjective measure of arousal and on one of three 'attention' tests administered, but covarying for the latter had a negligible effect upon the significant impairments obtained for anterograde memory tests. Likewise, Curran *et al.* (1991) performed an analysis of covariance for subjectively rated sedation and three psychomotor measures against tests of memory, mental rotation, reasoning, vigilance, and perceptual-motor skills. They found that subjectively rated sedation was more closely related to performance on the psychomotor tasks than the memory tasks; and that covarying for sedation or psychomotor performance did not affect the significant effects of the drug on immediate recall of paired-associates or immediate and delayed recall of a prose passage. Wesnes *et al.* (1988) found impairments across a battery of memory and attention tests, and subsequent analysis (Wesnes 1992) using factor analytic techniques suggested the effects of the drug on attention were independent from those on memory. Potter *et al.* (1991) measured event-related potentials (ERPs) during a task requiring continuous recognition memory for visually presented words. They found that, in a placebo condition, correctly recognized words evoked more positive ERPs than did distractor words. Scopolamine caused a substantial impairment in task performance, but it did not reduce the size of these old-new word ERP differences. It was concluded that the old/new ERP effects were unlikely to reflect the level of functioning of cholinergically innovated brain regions contributing to recognition memory (which the authors suggest depends upon familiarity judgements), but may have been more closely associated with retrieval than acquisition processes. Finally, Rusted *et al.* (1991) examined the separate and combined effects of scopolamine and nicotine on verbal free recall, finding that a single dose of nicotine improved recall performance on lengthy but not short word lists, but had no effect on the scopolamine-induced recall deficits observed for both lists of words. These results were interpreted in terms of the independence of attention and memory processes, and the authors suggested that whereas nicotine improves attention, scopolamine has a specific effect upon memory processes.

With regard to this attentional deficit, Rusted (1988) argued that cholinergic blockade produces a selective effect on the 'central executive' component of working memory, consistent with the pattern of impairment in early Alzheimer patients (Baddeley *et al.* 1986; Morris 1986). However, she acknowledged that some other factor (perhaps related to the chronicity or severity of cholinergic depletion) needs to be postulated to account for the well-documented impairment of Alzheimer patients on simple span tests. Her argument was essentially that the pattern of deficit in 'working memory' following cholinergic blockade is *qualitatively* similar to that which occurs in Alzheimer's disease, and that *quantitative* differences in the extent of impairment account for discrepancies, for example, on span test performance.

More recently, Rusted (1994) has argued that impairment of a unitary, 'all purpose' central executive is not a sufficient explanation of the effects of cholinergic blockade. As mentioned previously, impairment of a single resource system would mean that memory and attentional impairments should occur together, and studies do not show this clear correspondence. Rusted (1994) takes up arguments by Frith (1992) who, in discussing psychological aspects of consciousness, associates attention not with a single resource pool but with two separate functions: (1) selectivity of information for processing and (2) capacity limitations. Frith argues that there may be separate mechanisms responsible for each and that these may be mediated by different neurobiological substrates. Differences in the pattern of impairments following cholinergic blockade as compared with Alzheimer's may reflect differential depletion in putative neurotransmitters subserving different executive mechanisms.

Catecholamines and memory

There have been a number of studies examining the effect of adrenergic agents upon memory and, in particular, investigating vasopressin which may modulate noradrenergic neurotransmission (De Wied and van Ree 1982). Much of this work derives from animal studies; and there is considerable controversy concerning whether vasopressin exerts a direct action on memory itself or has a secondary effect via a beneficial action on arousal and/or mood (De Wied 1984 Gash and Thomas 1983; Sahgal 1984;). Weingartner *et al.* (1981) and Millar *et al.* (1987) both suggested that vasopressin has a direct, beneficial effect on 'explicit' memory in healthy subjects, whereas Snel *et al.* (1987) postulated an action upon 'tonic attentional processes' rather than either the storage or retrieval of memories.

Frith *et al.* (1985) and Clark *et al.* (1986) studied the effect of low doses of clonidine on the grounds that it would inhibit noradrenaline release. Frith *et al.* (1985) found that healthy subjects were impaired by this drug on a paired-associate learning task, but that span tests and a measure of semantic memory were unaffected. On the other hand, Clark *et al.* (1986) found that the most striking effects were on subjective arousal, and that there was a significant impairment at both 'focused' and 'divided' attention tasks. In short, it seems likely that adrenergic agents have a direct effect upon processes mediating 'attention' and 'arousal', but it remains controversial whether they have direct mnemonic effects beyond this.

An elegant study by Cahill *et al.* (1994) assessed the effects of the beta-adrenergic receptor antagonist, propanolol, on memory for an emotionally arousing story compared with a carefully matched neutral story. As expected, subjects given placebo when told the stories recalled more of the emotional than the neutral story when tested one week later. Subjects given propanolol recalled the neutral story as well as placebo subjects, but were impaired on the emotional story, leading Cahill *et al.* (1984). to conclude that enhanced memory for emotional experience is mediated by the beta-adrenergic system. Again, however, one could argue that the enhanced memory is mediated by arousal and the effect of the drug was on arousal rather than memory.

GABA, benzodiazepines, and memory

Benzodiazepines (BZs) act on specific benzodiazepine receptors and *potentiate* the action of GABA, which is the major inhibitory neurotransmitter in the brain. BZ receptors are found throughout the brain, but highest concentrations are in the cerebral cortex, limbic system, and cerebellar cortex. GABA is depleted in late Alzheimer's disease (see above), but the severe depletion of glutamate, the excitatory neurotransmitter (Hyman *et al.* 1987) within the entorhinal cortex, may be more critical for the memory loss.

There have been literally hundreds of studies of the effects of benzodiazepines on memory. Unlike research with SP, this is not driven by a specific hypothesis about the role of GABA in cognition or cognitive dysfunction. Rather, the extensive research on BZs and memory has been driven by clinical issues since BZs are widely prescribed as tranquillizers and sleeping pills (for reviews see Curran 1986, 1991). Their use as premedicants before anaesthesia is also widespread, in part because anaesthetists value the anterograde amnesia for operative procedures that the drugs produce (see, for example Ghoneim and Mewaldt 1990).

Despite their differing pharmacological action, the effects of BZs on memory and attention are remarkably similar to those of SP. 'Primary' memory, as assessed by span tasks or the 'recency component' of free recall, is unaffected (e.g. Brown *et al.* 1982; Curran *et al.* 1986; Ghoneim and Mewaldt 1975; 1987). When subjects are given a larger quantity of information to learn or when recall or recognition is tested after a delay, benzodiazepines produce a marked anterograde impairment in 'explicit' or 'episodic' memory (e.g. Curran *et al.* 1987; 1988) Ghoneim and Mewaldt 1975, 1977; which is similar to scopolamine (Curran *et al.* 1991; Frith *et al.* 1984). Once learning has been accomplished, the rate of forgetting is normal (Brown *et al.* 1983), and like SP, BZs do not produce any retrograde deficits (Ghoneim and Mewaldt 1975, 1977).

The main locus of the episodic memory impairment produced by BZs appears to be acquisition and/or consolidation of new information. Retrieval of material learned shortly before drug administration is not impaired and indeed can sometimes be improved or facilitated by the drug (Brown *et al.*; 1991; Curran *et al.* 1987; Choneim *et al.* 1984; Weingartner *et al.* 1995). Whether this facilitation simply reflects reduced interference from poor post-drug learning, or some form of retrieval disinhibition is not yet known. Nor is it apparent whether SP produces a similar facilitation.

Although poor encoding of contextual information has been put forward as a mechanism for BZ-induced anterograde amnesia (Brown and Brown 1990), studies have not provided unanimous support. Increased prior list intrusions in free recall tasks are noted fairly often (e.g. Curran *et al* 1993). In a recent study modelled on that of Schacter *et al.* (1984) on 'source amnesia' in amnesic subjects, both memory for made-up facts and for the context in which those facts had been learned were severely impaired by the potent benzodiazepine, lorazepam, (Curran and Tulving, submitted). However, for subjects given lorazepam, over half of the facts which they did remember they claimed to have learnt from TV or magazines rather than during the actual experiment. Thus there was some evidence for disproportionate source amnesia induced by the drug.

Like research with scopolamine, studies of the effects of benzodiazepines on the retrieval of well-established (semantic) knowledge have used only one or two types of tasks. Verbal fluency is generally intact (Curran 1991), and one study reported facilitation of fluency to a 'difficult' category-cue following lorazepam (File *et al.* 1992). On sentence verification tasks, performance is slower, but errors are rare (Bishop *et al.* 1996). Procedural learning tasks show very similar effects of both benzodiazepines and scopolamine, with learning curves on the active drug generally paralleling those for placebo (Bishop *et al.* 1996; Curran 1991; Ghoneim and Mewaldt 1990; Knopman 1991).

Again, like scopolamine, studies have shown preserved perceptual priming following administration of several types of benzodiazepines (for example diazepam, oxazepam, alprazolam, triazolam), but, surprisingly, impairment following the benzodiazepine, lorazepam (Bishop and Curran 1995; Brown *et al.* 1989; Curran and Gorenstein 1993; Danion *et al.* 1992; Knopman 1991; Sellal *et al.* 1992; Vidailhet *et al.* 1994). The impairment of perceptual priming induced by lorazepam is attenuated by co-administration of the benzodiazepine antagonist, flumazenil (Bishop and Curran 1995). One study directly compared SP with lorazepam (Schifano and Curran 1994), but reported equivocal results: lorazepam's impairment of performance on a word-stem completion was not significant. However, that study used only one dose of lorazepam, and the sedative and attentional effects of the two drugs were not matched. A more recent study by Bishop *et al.* (1996) showed that when those effects were matched for two doses each of lorazepam and scopolamine, only the former impaired stem-completion. They concluded that the two drugs produce a similar profile of effects on explicit memory but differ in their effects on implicit memory. This provides further evidence of a dissociation of the neurochemical systems underlying these two kinds of remembering.

PHARMACOLOGICAL AND COGNITIVE SPECIFICITY OF EFFECTS

Although SP and BZs are pharmacologically very different from each other, it will be clear from the above accounts that the pattern of their effects on memory are remarkably similar. Indeed, the few attempts to distinguish their memory effects by directly comparing these drugs have had limited success (Curran *et al.* 1991; Frith *et al.* 1984; Ghoneim and Mewaldt 1975, 1977; Jones *et al.* 1979; Richardson *et al.* 1984). Both SP and BZs produce marked anterograde impairments of episodic memory whilst leaving semantic, procedural, and working memory relatively intact (see Tulving 1985).

This similarity may reflect a common neurochemical action, since it has been proposed that GABA-ergic mechanisms may act to inhibit cholinergic activity in the cortex via interaction at the level of the basal forebrain (Sarter *et al.* 1988*a*, *b*). In research with rats, it has been shown that injection of a benzodiazepine into the medial septum reduced acetycholine release in the hippocampus by 50%; injecting a benzodiazepine antagonist (flumazenil) increased acetylcholine release in the hippocampus by 95% (Imperato *et al.* 1994).

Relevant research with humans is seen in studies which have used cross-reversal designs, attempting to attenuate the effects of either a benzodiazepine with a cholinergic agonist or scopolamine with a benzodiazepine antagonist. On the whole, the few studies to date provide little evidence of cross-reversal of the drugs' memory effects, indicating separate neurochemical mediation (Dorow *et al.* 1987; Ghoneim and Mewaldt 1977; Preston *et al.* 1989). However, interpretation of these studies is not clear-cut as the relative doses of agonist/antagonist are crucial. This point is made especially clear by several studies attempting to reverse the effects of benzodiazepine agonists with benzodiazepine antagonists. Lower doses reverse sedative and psychomotor effects, but much higher doses appear necessary for reversing amnesic effects (Curran and Birch 1991; O'Boyle *et al.* 1983). The similarity in the effects of the two types of drugs may also reflect common mediation of memory impairments by the sedative or attentional effects of both scopolamine and BZs.

We have already discussed these points in the context of research on cholinergic blockade. There is a virtually parallel debate in research with the benzodiazepines, which is discussed elsewhere (Curran 1991). Evidence for specific amnestic effects stems from studies showing that doses of the benzodiazepine antagonist, flumazenil, which reverse sedative and attentional effects do not reverse amnestic effects (Curran and Birch 1991). Further, on repeated dosing, tolerance to sedative and attentional effects develops before tolerance to memory impairments (Curran *et al.* 1994; Ghoneim *et al.* 1984; Tata *et al.* 1994). Curran (1991) and Weingartner *et al.* (1993) concluded that sedation contributes to, but does not completely account for, the amnesic effects of benzodiazepines. A recent study matched the sedative effects of doses of scopolamine and lorazepam with those of an antihistamine (diphenhydramine) (Poovibunsuk *et al.* in preparation). All three drugs produced similar psychomotor impairments (and similar effects on early components of ERPs), but only scopolamine and lorazepam produced impairments of explicit memory (and effects on later components of ERPs). This would imply that sedation and amnesic effects can be largely independent of each other. Finally, drugs which act centrally can alter mood state, and this may also be a factor to consider when interpreting its cognitive effects, as well illustrated in the study by Cahill *et al.* (1994) described previously.

CONCLUSIONS

Depletions of acetylcholine, noradrenaline, serotonin, and glutamate seem important in the neurochemistry of Alzheimer's disease, and depletion of GABA may be a late development. Cholinergic depletion is the most consistent finding in Alzheimer dementia, and various studies of cholinergic blockade have shown that cholinergic depletion would be expected to produce a substantial anterograde amnesia, although retrograde amnesia has to be explained in different terms (Kopelman 1992*a*, *b*). The depletion of glutamate, an excitatory neurotransmitter within the NMDA hippocampal system, may also be important in producing the anterograde amnesia in Alzheimer dementia. Benzodiazepines which facilitate the transmission of GABA produce anterograde amnesia of a similar form to that produced by cholinergic blockade. To what extent this reflects an interaction between GABA-ergic and cholinergic systems is not yet established. Less is known about the specific cognitive effects of other neurotransmitters, but the catecholamines appear to act primarily upon attention, arousal, and mood. As psychopharmacological studies expand, we will come to understand better the link between particular neurotransmitter depletions and specific cognitive deficits, thereby allowing a more rational basis for the development of putative therapeutic agents.

REFERENCES

Alford, C., Bhatti, Z., Curran, S., McKay, G., and Hindmarch, I. (1991). Pharmacodynamic effects of buspirone and clobazam, *British Journal of Clinical Pharmacology*, **32**, 91–7.

Arendt, T., Bigl, V., Arendt, A., and Tennstedt, A. (1983). Loss of neurons in the nucleus basalis of Meynert in Alzheimer's disease, paralysis agitans and Korsakoff's disease. *Acta Neuropathologica*, Berlin, **61**, 101–8.

Arendt, T., Bigle, V., Tennstedt, A., and Arendt. A. (1985). Neuronal loss in different parts of the nucleus basalis is related to neuritic plaque formation in cortical target areas in Alzheimer's disease. *Neuroscience*, **14**, 1–14.

Baddeley, A. D., Logie, R., Bressi, S., Della Sala, S., and Spinnler, H. (1986). Dementia and working memory. *Quarterly Journal of Experimental Psychology*, **38A**, 603–18.

Beal, M. F. and Mazurek, M. F. (1987) Substance P-like immuno-reactivity is reduced in Alzheimer's disease cerebral cortex. *Neurology*, **37**, 1205–9.

Beal, M.F., Mazurek, M.F., Svendsen, C.N., Bird, E.D. and Martin, J.B. (1986). Widespread reduction of somatostatin-like immunoreactivity in the cerebral cortex in Alzheimer's disease. *Annals of Neurology*, **20**, 489–95.

Beatty, W.W., Butters, N., and Janowsky, D.S. (1986). Patterns of memory failure after scopolamine treatment: implications for cholinergic hypotheses of dementia. *Behavioural and Neurological Biology*, **45**, 196–211.

Benton, J.S., Bowen, D.M., Allen, S.J., Haan, E.A., Davison, A.N., Neary, D., *et al.* (1982). Alzheimer's disease as a disorder of the isodendritic core. *Lancet*, **1**, 456.

Bishop, K. I. and Curran, H. V. (1995). Psychopharmacological analysis of implicit and explicit memory: a study with lorazepam and the benzodiazepine antagonist, flumazenil, *Psychopharmacology*, 121, 267–78

Bishop, K. I., Curran, H. V., and Lader, M. (1997). Do scopolamine and lorazepam have dissociable effects upon human memory? A dose-response study with normal subjects *Experimental and Clinical Psychopharmacology*, in press.

Bondareff, W., Mountjoy, C.Q., and Roth, M. (1982). Loss of neurons of origin of the adrenergic projection to the cerebral cortex (nucleus locus ceruleus) in senile dementia. *Neurology*, **32**, 164–8.

Bowen, D.M. (1990). Treatment of Alzheimer's disease: molecular pathology versus neurotransmitter-based therapy. *British Journal of Psychiatry*, **157**, 327–30.

Bowen, D.M., Smith, C.B., White, P., and Davison, A.N. (1976). Neurotransmitter-related enzymes and indices of hypoxia in senile dementia and other abiotrophies. *Brain*, **99**, 459–96.

Bowen, D.M., Francis, P.T., Pangalos, M., Stephens, P.H., and Proctor, A.W. (1992). Treatment strategies for Alzheimer's disease. *Lancet*, **339**, 132–3.

Broks, P, Preston, G.C., Traub, M., Poppleton, P., Ward, C., and Stahl, S. (1988). Modelling dementia: effects of scopolamine on memory and attention. *Neuropsychologia*, **26**, 685–700.

Brown, J. and Brown, M.W. (1990) The effects of repeating a recognition test on lorazepam-induced amnesia: evidence for impaired contextual memory as a cause of amnesia. *The Quarterly Journal of Experimental Psychology*, **42** A, (2), 279–90.

Brown, J., Lewis, V., Brown, M., Horn, G., and Bowes, J. B. (1982). A comparison between transient amnesias induced by two drugs (Diazepam or Lorazepam) and amnesia of organic origin. *Neuropsychologia*, **20**, 55–70.

Brown, J., Brown, M.W., and Bowes, J. B. (1983). Effects of Lorazepam on rate of forgetting, on retrieval from semantic memory and on manual dexterity. *Neuropsychologia*, **21**, 501–12.

Brown, M.W., Brown, J., and Bowes, J. (1989). Absence of priming coupled with substantially preserved recognition in lorazepam induced amnesia. *Quarterly Journal of Experimental Psychology*, **41A**, 599–617.

Burke, W.J., Chung, H.D., Nakra, B.R.S., Grossberg, G.T., and Joh, T.H. (1987). Phenylethanolamine-*N*-methyltransferase activity is decreased in Alzheimer's disease brains. *Annals of Neurology*, **22**, 278–80.

Buschke,H. and Fuld, P.A. (1974). Evaluating storage, retention, and retrieval in disordered memory and learning. *Neurology*, **24**, 1019–25.

Cahill, L., Prins, B., Weber, M., and McGaugh, J.L. (1994). Beta-adrenergic activation and memory for emotional events *Nature*, **3H**, 702–4.

Caine, E.D., Weingartner, H., Ludlow, C.L., Cudahy, E.A., and Wehry, S. (1981). Qualitative analysis of scopolamine-induced amnesia. *Psychopharmacology*, **74**, 74–80.

Christensen, H., Maltby, N., Jorm, A.F., Creasy, H., and Broe, G.H. (1992). Cholinergic blockade as a model of the cognitive deficits in Alzheimer's disease. *Brain*, **115**, 168–99.

Chui, D.C.M., Penney, J.B., and Young, A.B. (1987). Cortical $GABA^B$ and $GABA^A$ receptors in Alzheimer's disease: a quantitative autoradiographic study. *Neurology*, **37**, 1454–9.

Clark, C.R., Geffen, G.M., and Geffen, L.B. (1986). Role of monoamine pathways in attention and effort. *Psychopharmacology*, **90**, 35–9.

Collerton, D. (1986). Cholinergic function and intellectual decline in Alzheimer's disease. *Neuroscience*, **19**, 1–28.

Cross, A.J., Crow, T.J., Ferrier, I.N., and Johnson, J.A. (1986). The selectivity of serotonin S2 receptors in Alzheimer-type dementia. *Neurobiology of Aging*, **7**, 3–7.

Crow, T.J. and Grove-White, I.G. (1973). An analysis of the learning deficit following hyoscine administration to man. *British Journal of Pharmacology*, **49**, 322–7.

Crow, T.J., Grove-White, I.G., and Ross, D.G. (1975) The specificity of the action of hyoscine on human learning. *British Journal of Clinical Pharmacology*, **2**, 367–8.

Curran, H.V. (1986) Tranquillising memories: a review of the effects of benzodazepines on human memory. *Biological Psychology*, **23**, 179–213.

Curran, H.V. (1991) Benzodiazpines, memory and mood: a review. *Psychopharmacology*, **105**, 1–8.

Curran, H.V. and Birch, B. (1991) Differentiating the sedative, psychomotor and amnesic effects of benzodiazepines: a study with midazolam and the benzodiazepine antagonist, flumazenil, *Psychopharmacology*, **103**, 519–23.

Curran, H. V. and Gorenstein, C. (1993) Differential effects of lorazepam and oxazepam on priming, *International Clinical Psychopharmacology*, **8**, 37–42.

Curran, H.V. and Tulving, E. Semantic learning and source forgetting in lorazepam-induced amnesia. Manuscript submitted for publication.

Curran, H.V., Schiwy, W., and Lader, M. (1987) Differential amnesic properties of benzodiazepines: a dose-response comparison of two drugs with similar elimination half-lives. *Psychopharmacology*, **92**, 358–64.

Curran, H.V., Schiwy, W., Eves, F., Shine, P., and Lader, M. (1988) A 'levels of processing' study of the effects of benzodiazepines on human memory, *Human Psychopharmacology*, **3**, 21–5.

Curran, H.V., Schifano, F., and Lader, M. (1991) Models of memory dysfunction? A comparison of the effects of scopolamine and lorazepam on memory, psychomotor performance and mood. *Psychopharmacology*, **103**, 83–90.

Curran, H.V., Gardiner, J. M., Java, R. I., and Allen D. (1993) Effects of lorazepam upon recollective experience in recognition memory. *Psychopharmacology*, **110**, 374–8.

Curran, H. V., Bond, A. J., O'Sullivan, G., Bruce, M., Marks, I., Lelliot, P., *et al.* (1994) Memory functions, alprazolam and exposure therapy: A controlled longitudinal study of agoraphobia with panic disorder, *Psychological Medicine*, **24**, 969–76.

D'Amato, R.J., Zweig, R.M., Whitehouse, P.J., Wenk, G.L., Singer, H.S., Mayeux, *et al.* (1987) Aminergic systems in Alzheimer's disease and Parkinson's disease. *Annals of Neurology*, **22**, 229–36.

Danion, J. M., Peretti, S., Grange, D., Bilik, M., Imbs, J. L., and Singer, L. (1992) Effects of chlorpromazine and lorazepam on explicit memory, repetition priming and cognitive skill learning in healthy volunteers, *Psychopharmacology*, **108**, 345–51.

De Wied, D. (1984) The importance of vasopressin in memory. *Trends in Neuroscience*, **7**, 62–4.

De Wied, D. and van Ree, J.M. (1982) Neuropeptides, mental performance and ageing. *Life Sciences*, **31**, 709–19.

Dorow, R., Berenberg, D., Duka, T., and Sauerbrey, N. (1987) Amnestic effects of lormetazepam and their reversal by the benzodiazepine antagonist Ro 15–17 88. *Psychopharmacology*, **93**, 507–14.

Drachman, D.A., (1977) Memory and cognitive function in man: does the cholinergic system have a specific role? *Neurology*, **27** 783–90.

Drachman, D.A., and Leavitt, J. (1974) Human memory and the cholinergic system. *Archives of Neurology*, **30** 113–21.

Dunne, M.P. and Hartley, L.R. (1985) The effects of scopolamine upon verbal memory: evidence for an attentional hypothesis. *Acta Psychologica*, **58**, 205–17.

Dunne, M. P., Statham, D., Raphael, B., Kemp, R., and Kelly, B. (1993) Further evidence that scopolamine can improve verbal fluency, *Journal of Psychopharmacology*, **7**, 159–63.

Ellison, D.W., Beal, M.F., Mazurek, M.F., Bird, E.D., and Martin, J.D. (1986) A post-mortem study of aminoacid neurotransmitters in Alzheimer's disease. *Annals of Neurology*, **20** 616–21.

Esiri, M.M., Pearson, R.C.A., Steele, J.E., Bowen, D.M., and Powell, T.P.S. (1990) A quantitative study of the neurofibrillary tangle and the choline acetyltransferase activity in the cerebral cortex and the amygadala in Alzheimer's disease. *Journal of Neurology, Neurosurgery and Psychiatry*, **53**, 161–5.

File, S.E., Sharma, R., and Shaffer, J. (1992) Is lorazepam-induced amnesia specific to the type of memory or to the task used to assess it? *Journal of Psychopharmacology*, **6**, 76–80.

Flynn, D.D. and Mash, D.C. (1986) Characterisation of L–H nicotine binding in human cortex: comparison between Alzheimer's disease and the normal. *Journal of Neurochemistry*, **47**, 1948–54.

Francis, P.T., Palmer, A.M., Sims, N.R., Bowen, D.M., Davison, A.N., Esiri, M., *et al.* (1985) Neurochemical studies of early-onset Alzheimer's disease. *New England Journal of Medicine*, **313**, 7–11.

Frith, C.D., (1992) Consciousness information processing and the brain. *Journal of Psychopharmacology*, **6** 436–40.

Frith, C.D., Richardson, J.T.E., Samuel, M., Crow, T.J., and McKenna, P.J. (1984) The effects of intravenous diazepam and hyoscine upon human memory. *Quarterly Journal of Experimental Psychology*, **36A**, 133–44.

Frith, C.D.J., Ferrier, I.N., and Crow,, T.J. (1985) Selective impairment of paired associate learning after administration of a centrally-acting adrenergic agonist (clonidine). *Psychopharmacology*, **87**, 490–3.

Frith, C.D., McGinty, M.A., Gergel, I., and Crow, T.J. (1989). The effects of scopolamine and clonidine upon the performance and learning of a motor skill. *Psychopharmacology*, **98**, 120–5.

Gash, D.M., and Thomas, G.J. (1983) What is the importance of vasopressin in memory processes? *Trends in Neurosciences*, **6**, 197–8.

Ghoneim, M.M. and Mewaldt, S.P. (1975) Effects of diazepam and scopolamine on storage, retrieval, and organisational processes in memory. *Psychopharmacologia* (Berlin), **44**, 257–62.

Ghoneim, M.M. and Mewaldt, S.P. (1977) Studies on human memory: the interactions of diazepam, scopolamine, and physostigmine. *Psychopharmacology*, **52**, 1–6.

Ghoneim, M.M., Mewaldt, S.P., and Henriches, J.R. (1984) Dose-response analysis of the behavioural effects of diazepam: 1. Learning and memory. *Psychopharmacology*, **82**, 291–5.

Ghoneim, M.M. and Mewaldt S.P. (1990). Benzodiazepines and human memory: a review *Anesthesiology*, **72**, 926–38.

Graf, P., Squire, L.R., and Mandler, G. (1984) The information that amnesic patients do not forget. *Journal of Experimental Psychology: Learning, Memory and Cognition*, **11**, 501–18.

Hyman, B.T., Van Hoesen, G.W., and Damasio, A.R. (1987) Alzheimer's disease: glutamate depletion in the hippocampal perforant pathway zone. *Annals of Neurology*, **22**, 37–40.

Imperato, A., Dazzi, L., Obinu, M. C., Gessa, G. L., and Biggio, G. (1994) The benzodiazepine receptor antagonist flumazenil increases acetylcholine release in rat hippocampus. *Brain Research*, **647**, 167–71.

Jones, D.M.M., Jones, M.E.L., Lewis, M.J. and Spriggs, T.L.B. (1979) Drugs and human memory: effects of low doses of nitrazepam and hyoscine on retention. *British Journal of Clinical Pharmacology*, **7**, 479–83.

Knopman, D. (1991) Unaware learning versus preserved learning in pharmacologic amnesia: similarities and differences. *Journal of Experimental Psychology, Learning, Memory and Cognition*, **17**, 1017–29.

Kopelman, M.D. (1986) The cholinergic neurotransmitter system in human memory and dementia: a review. *Quarterly Journal of Experimental Psychology*, **38A**, 535–73.

Kopelman, M.D. (1992*a*) The 'new' and the 'old': components of the anterograde and retrograde memory loss in Korsakoff and Alzheimer patients. In *The neuropsychology of memory* (2nd edn) (ed. L.R. Squire and N. Butters), pp. 130–46. Guilford, New York.

Kopelman, M.D. (1992*b*) Storage, forgetting, and retrieval in the anterograde and retrograde amnesia of Alzheimer dementia. In *Memory functioning in dementia* (ed. L. Backman), pp. 45–7. Elsevier Science Publishers, Amsterdam.

Kopelman, M.D. and Corn, T.H. (1988) Cholinergic 'blockade' as a model for cholinergic depletion: a comparison of the memory deficits with those of Alzheimer-type dementia and the alcoholic Korsakoff syndrome. *Brain*, **111**, 1079–110.

Kowall, N.W. and Beal, M.F. (1986) Cortical somatostatin, neuropeptide Y, and NADPH diaphorase neurons: normal anatomy and alterations in Alzheimer's disease. *Annals of Neurology*, **23**, 105–14.

Lines, C.R., Preston, G.C., Broks, P., and Dawson, C.E. (1991) The effects of scopolamine on retrieval from semantic memory. *Journal of Psychopharmacology*, **5**, 234–7.

Lowe, S.L., Francis, P.T., Procter, A.W., Palmer, A.M., Davison, A.N., and Bowen,

D.M. (1988) Gamma-aminobutyric acid concentration in brain tissue at two stages of Alzheimer's disease. *Brain*, **111**, 785–99.

Mann, D.M.A., Lincoln, J., Yates, P.O., Stamp, J.E., and Topper, S. (1980) Changes on monamine containing neurones of the human CNS in senile dementia. *British Journal of Psychiatry*, **136**, 533–41.

Mann, D.M.A., Yates, P.O., and Marcyniuk, B. (1984) Alzheimer's presenile dementia, senile dementia of Alzheimer type, and Down's syndrome in middle age form: an age related continuum of pathological changes. *Neuropathology and Applied Neurobiology*, **10**, 185–207.

Mann, D.M.A., Yates, P.O., and Marcyniuk, B. (1986) A comparison of nerve cell loss in cortical and subcortical structures in Alzheimer's disease. *Journal of Neurology, Neurosurgery, and Psychiatry*, **49**, 310–12.

Mann, D.M.A., Yates, P.O., and Marcyniuk, B. (1987) Dopaminergic neurotransmitter changes in Alzheimer's disease and Down's syndrome at middle age. *Journal of Neurology, Neurosurgery and Psychiatry*, **50** 341–4.

Mash, D.C., Flynn, D.D., and Potter, L.T. (1985) Loss of M2 muscarinic receptors in the cerebral cortex in Alzheimer's disease and exceptional cholinergic denervation. *Science*, **228**, 1115–17.

Mazurek, M.F., Beal, M.F., Bird, E.D., and Martin, J.B. (1986) Vasopressin in Alzheimer's disease: a study of post-mortem brain concentrations. *Annals of Neurology*, **20**, 665–70.

Millar, K., Jeffcoate, W.J., and Walden, C.P. (1987) Vasopressin and memory improvement in normal short-term recall and reduction of alcohol-induced amnesia. *Psychological Medicine*, **17**, 335–41.

Mohs, R.C. and Davis, K.L. (1985) Interaction of choline and scopolamine in human memory. *Life Sciences*, **37**, 193–7.

Molchan, S. E., Mellow, A. M., Lawlor, B. A., Weingartner, H. J., Cohan R. M., Cohan, M. R., and Sunderland, T. (1990). TRH attenuates scopolamine-induced memory impairment in humans, *Psychopharmacology*, **100**, 84–9.

Molchan, S. E., Martinez, R. A., Hill, J. L., Weingartner, H. J., Thompson, K., Vitiello, B., *et al.* (1992) Increased cognitive sensitivity to scopolamine with age and a perspective on the scopolamine model, *Brain Research Reviews*, **17**, 215–26.

Morris, R.G. (1986) Short-term forgetting in senile dementia of the Alzheimer's type. *Cognitive Neuropsychology*, **3**, 77–97.

Morrison, J.H., Rogers, J., Scherr, S., Benoit, R., and Bloom, F.E. (1985) Somatostatin immunoreactivity in neuritic plaques of Alzheimer patients. *Nature*, **314**, 90–2.

Nissen, M.J., Knopman, D.S., and Schacter, D.L. (1987) Neurochemical dissociation of memory systems. *Neurology*, **37**, 789–94.

Nuotto, E. (1983) Psychomotor, physiological and cognitive effects of scopolamine and ephedrine in healthy man. *European Journal of Clinical Pharmacology*, **24**, 603–9.

O'Boyle, C., Lambe, R., Darragh, A., Taffe, W., Brick, I., and Kenny, M. (1983) Ro 15–1788 antagonises the effects of diazepam in man without affecting its bioavailability, *British Journal of Anaesthesia*, **55**, 349–55.

Palmer, A.M., Proctor, A.W., Stratmann, G.L., and Bowen, D.M. (1986) Excitatory amino acid-releasing and cholinergic neurones in Alzheimer's disease. *Neuroscience Letters*, **66**, 199–204.

Palmer, A.M., Stratmann, G.C., Proctor, A.W., and Bowen, D.M. (1988) Possible neurotransmitter basis of behavioural changes in Alzheimer's disease. *Annals of Neurology*, **23**, 616–620.

Parrot, A.C. (1986) The effects of transdermal scopolamine and 4 dose levels of oral scopolamine (0.15, 0.3, 0.6, and 1.2 mg) upon psychological performance. *Psychopharmacology*, **89**, 347–54.

Partridge, F.M., Knight, R.G., and Feehan, M.J. (1990) Direct and indirect memory performance in patients with senile dementia. *Psychological Medicine*, **20**, 111–18.

Penny, J.B., Maragos, W.F., Greenamyre, J.T., Debowey, D.L., Hollingsworth, Z., and Young, A.B. (1990) Excitatory amino acid binding sites in the hippocampal region of Alzheimer's disease and other dementias. *Journal of Neurology, Neurosurgery and Psychiatry*, **53**, 314–20.

Perry, E.K., (1986) The cholinergic hypothesis—ten years on. *British Medical Bulletin*, **42**, 63–9.

Perry, E.K., Tomlinson, B.E., Blessed, G., Bergmann, K., Gibson, P.H., and Perry, R.H. (1978) Correlation of cholinergic abnormalities with senile plaques and mental test scores in senile dementia. *British Medical Journal*, **2**, 1457–9.

Perry, T.L., Yong, V.W., Bergeron, C., Hansen, S., and Jones, K. (1987) Amino acids, glutathione, and glutathione transferase activity in the brains of patients with Alzheimer's disease. *Annals of Neurology*, **21**, 331–6.

Potter, D.B., Pickles, C.D., Roberts, R.C., and Rugg, M.D. (1991) The effects of scopolamine on event-related potentials in a continuous recognition memory task. *Psychophysiology*, **29**, 29–37.

Preston, G.C., Ward, C., Lines, C.R., Poppleton, P., Haigh, J.R.M., and Traub, M. (1989) Scopolamine and benzodiazepine models of dementia: cross-reversals by Ro 15–1788 and physostigmine. *Psychopharmacology*, **98**, 487–94.

Poovibunsuk, P., Curran, H. V., and Lader, M.H. Parallel dissociation of the amnestic and sedative effects, and the event-related potential effects, of scopolamine, lorazepam and an antihistamine. Manuscript in preparation.

Richardson, J.T.E., Frith, C.D., Scott, E., Crow, T.J., and Cunningham-Owens, D. (1984). The effects of intravenous diazepam and hyoscine upon recognition memory. *Behavioural Brain Research*, **14**, 193–9.

Roberts, G.W., Crow, T.J., and Polak, J.M. (1985) Location of neuronal tangles in somatostatin neurones in Alzheimer's disease. *Nature*, **314**, 92–4.

Rossor, M. and Iversen, L.L. (1986) Non-cholinergic neurotransmitter abnormalities in Alzheimer's disease. *British Medical Bulletin*, **42**, 70–4.

Rossor, M.N., Iversen, L.L., Mountjoy, C.Q., *et al* (1980) Arginine vasopressin and choline acetyl transferase and choline acetyl transferase in brains of patients with Alzheimer-type dementia. *Lancet*, **ii**, 1369–70.

Rossor, M.N., Garrett, N.J., Johnson, A.L., Mountjoy, C.Q., Roth, M., and Iversen, L.L. (1982) A post-mortem study of the cholinergic and GABA systems in senile dementia. *Brain*, **105**, 313–30.

Rossor, M.N., Iversen, L.L., Reynolds, G.P., Mountjoy, C.Q., and Roth. M. (1984) Neurochemical characteristics of early and late onset types of Alzheimer's disease. *British Medical Journal*, **288**, 961–4.

Rusted, J.M. (1988) Dissociative effects of scopolomine on working memory in healthy young volunteers. *Psychopharmacology*, **96**, 487–92.

Rusted, J. (1994) Cholinergic blockade and human information processing: are we asking the right questions, *Journal of Psychopharmacology*, **8**, 54–9.

Rusted, J.M. and Warburton, D.M. (1988) The effects of scopolamine on working memory in healthy young volunteers. *Psychopharmacology*, **96**, 145–52.

Rusted, J. Eaton-Williams, P., and Warburton, D. (1991) Distinguishing between attentional and amnestic effects in information processing: the separate and combined effects of scopolamine and nicotine on verbal free recall. *Psychopharmacology*, **104**, 363–6.

Safer, D.J. and Allen, R.P. (1971) The central effects of scopolamine in man. *Biological Psychiatry*, **3**, 347–55.

Sahakian, B. J. (1987) Cholinergic drugs and human cognitive performance, In *Handbook of psychopharmacology*, (ed. L. L. Iverson, S. D. Iverson, and S. H. Snyder), pp. 393–424. Plenum Press, New York.

Sahgal, A. (1984) A critique of the vasopressin-memory hypothesis. *Psychopharmacology*, **83**, 215–28.

Sarter, M., Shneider, H. H., and Stephens, D. N. (1988*a*). Treatment strategies for senile dementia: antagonist beta-carbolines. *Trends in Neuroscience*, **11**, 13–17.

Sarter, M., Bodewitz, G., and Stephens, D. N. (1988*b*) Attenuation of scopolamine-induced impairment of spontaneous alternation by antagonist but not inverse agonist and agonist Beta-carbolines. *Psychopharmacology*, **94**, 491–5.

Schacter, D.L. (1987) Implicit memory: history and current status. *Journal of Experimental Psychology: Learning, Memory and Cognition*, **13**, 501–18.

Schacter, D.L., Harbluk, J.L., and McLachlan, D.R. (1984). Retrieval without recollection: an experimental analysis of source amnesia. *Journal of Verbal Learning and Verbal Behavior*, **23**, 593–611.

Schifano, F. and Curran, H. V. (1994) Pharmacological models of memory dysfunction? I A comparison of the effects of scopolamine and lorazepam on word valence ratings, priming and recall, *Psychopharmacology*, **115**, 430–4.

Sellal, F., Danion, J. M., Kauffmann-Mueller, F., Grange, D., Imbs, J. L., Van Der Linden, M., *et al.* (1992) Differential effects of diazepam and lorazepam on repetition priming in healthy volunteers, *Psychopharmacology*, **108**, 371–9.

Shepherd, G.M. (1988) A basic circuit of cortical organization. In *Perspectives in memory research* (ed. M.S. Gazzaniga). MIT Press, Cambridge, MA.

Sims, N., Bowen, D., Smith, C., Flack, R., Davison, A., Snowden, J., *et al.* D. (1980) Glucose metabolism and acetylcholine synthesis in relation to neuronal activity in Alzheimer's disease. *Lancet*, **1**, 333–4.

Smith, C.C.T., Bowen, D.M., Francis, P.T., Snowden, J.S., and Neary, D. (1985) Putative amino acid transmitters in lumbar CSF and patients with histologically-verified Alzheimer's dementia. *Journal of Neurology, Neurosurgery and Psychiatry*, **48**, 469–71.

Snel, J., Taylor, J., and Wegman, M. (1987) Does DGAVP influence memory, attention and mood in young healthy men? *Psychopharmacology*, **92**, 224–8.

Sternberg, S,(1969) Memory scanning: mental processes revealed by reaction time experiments *American Scientist*, **57**, 421–57.

Sunderland, T., Tariot, P.N., Cohen, R.M., Weingartner, H., Mueller, E.A., and Murphy, D.L. (1987) Anticholinergic sensitivity in patients with dementia of the Alzheimer-type and age-matched controls: a dose-response curve. *Archives of General Psychiatry*, **44**, 418–25.

Tamminga, C.A., Foster, N.L., Fedio, P., Bird, E.D., and Chase, T.N. (1987) Alzheimer's disease: low cerebral somatostatin levels correlate with impaired cognitive function and cortical metabolism. *Neurology*, **37**, 161–5.

Tata P., Rollings, J., Collins M., Pickering, A., and Jacobson R. (1994). Lack of cognitive recovery following withdrawal from long-term benzodiazepine use *Psychological Medicine*, **24**, 203–13.

Tröster, A.I., Beatty, W.W., Staton, R.D., and Rorabaugh, A.G. (1989) Effects of scopolamine on anterograde and remote memory in humans. *Psychobiology*, **17**, 12–18.

Tulving, E. (1985) How many memory systems are there? *American Psychologist*, **40**, 385–98.

Vidailhet, P., Danion, J. M., Kauffmann-Muller, F., Grange, D., Giersch, A., Van Der Linden, M., *et al.* (1994) Lorazepam and diazepam effects on memory acquisition in priming tests. *Psychopharmacology*, **115**, 397–406.

Warburton, D. M. (1979) Neurochemical basis of consciousness, In *Chemical influences on behaviour*, (ed. K. Brown and S. J. Cooper). Academic Press, London.

Warburton, D. M. (1981) Neurochemical bases of behaviour, *British Medical Bulletin*, **37**, 121–5.

Weiner, N. (1980) Atropine, scopolamine, and related antimuscarinic drugs. In *Goodman and Gilman's the pharmacological basis of therapeutics* (6th edn), (ed. A.G. Gilman, L.S. Goodman, and A. Gilman), pp. 120–37. Macmillan, New York; Ballière Tindall, London.

Weingartner, H., Gold, P., Ballenger, J.C., Smallberg, S.A., Summers, R., Rubinow, D.R., *et al.* (1981) Effects of vasopressin on human memory functions. *Science*, **211**, 601–3.

Weingartner, H. J., Joyce, E. M., Sirocco, K. Y., Adams, C. M., Eckhardt, M. J., George, T., *et al.* (1993) Specific memory and sedative effects of the benzodiazepine triazolam. *Journal of Psychopharmacology*. **7**, 305–15.

Weingartner, H. J., Sirocco, K., Curran, H.V., and Wolkowitz, O. (1995) Memory facilitation following the administration of the benzodiazepine triazolam. *Journal of Clinical and Experimental Psychopharmacology*, **3**, 298–303

Wesnes, K. (1992) The design, validity and applications of scopolamine model of dementia. Paper presented at *British Psychological Society Annual Conference, (Abstracts)* p. 13.

Wesnes, K. and Warburton, D.M. (1984) Effects of Scopolamine and nicotine on human rapid information processing performance. *Psychopharmacology*, **82** 147–50.

Wesnes, K., Simpson, P., and Kidd, A. (1988) An investigation of the range of cognitive impairments induced by scopolamine 0.6 mg sc. *Human Psychopharmacology*, **82**, 27–41.

Wesnes, K., Anand, R., Simpson, P., and Christmas, L. (1990). The use of a scopolamine model to study the potential nootropic effects of aniracetam and piracetam in healthy volunteers, *Journal of Psychopharmacology*, **4**(4), 219–32.

Whitehouse, P.J., Price, D.L., Struble, R.G., Clark, A.W., Coyle, J.T., and Delong, M.R. (1982) Alzheimer's disease and senile dementia: loss of neurons in the basal forebrain. *Science*, **215**, 1237–9.

Wilcock, G.K., Esiri, M.M., Bowen, D.J., and Smith, C.C.T. (1982) Alzheimer's disease: correlation of cortical choline acetyltransferase activity with the severity of dementia and histological abnormalities. *Journal of Neurological Sciences*, **57**, 407–17.

Yamamoto, T. and Hirano, A. (1985) Nucleus raphe dorsalis in Alzheimer's disease: neurofibrillary tangles and loss of large neurons. *Annals of Neurology*, **17**, 573–7.

FIFTEEN

Genetic subtypes of Alzheimer's disease and cognitive functioning

Sarah K. Agnew

EPIDEMIOLOGICAL STUDIES

An hereditary basis for Alzheimer-type dementia (AD) was proposed in 1925 by Meggendorfer and later, in 1932, by Schottky, but it was not until the descriptions of large pedigrees that an autosomal dominant mode of inheritance, with full penetrance, was recognized (Bird *et al.* 1988; Cook *et al.* 1979; Feldman *et al.* 1963; Frommelt *et al.* 1991; Heston *et al.* 1966; Lowenberg and Waggoner 1934; Martin *et al.* 1991; McMenemey *et al.* 1939; Nee *et al.* 1983). Estimates of the prevalence of a family history vary. Detailed epidemiological studies have suggested that a family history may be found in 5–50% of cases (Farrer *et al.* 1989; Fitch *et al.* 1988; Heston *et al.* 1981; Heyman *et al.* 1983). The variation may, in part, be attributable to differences in age at onset. Certainly, age at onset appears to be a moderating variable as far as family history is concerned.

Heston *et al.* (1981) found a lifetime risk of AD in siblings of young-onset affected cases of 45% versus the 10% found in the siblings of older-onset cases. The genetic influence in young-onset cases was confirmed by Heyman *et al.* (1983). The relationship of age at onset and family history however, may reflect a bias in incidence rather than genetic variables playing a bigger part in early-onset disease. The mode of inheritance may not be apparent in the older-onset cases where potential carriers fail to live to express the illness. Fitch *et al.* (1988) found that 43% of AD cases had a family history, determined by the presence of more than one case in the family. In one third of these cases the disease was expressed after 70 years of age. More recent epidemiological studies have further confirmed this influence to be greater in the younger population, as Heston *et al.* (1981) originally suggested (La Rue *et al.* 1992; Van Duijn *et al.* 1991*b*).

It must be appreciated that the majority of cases, regardless of age of onset, do not have a family history of dementia (Van Duijn *et al.* 1991*b*). This is confirmed by studies showing discordance in monozygotic twins (Kumar *et al.* 1991; Nee *et al.* 1987). Nee *et al.* (1987) found a similar proportion of concordance between monozygotic and dizygotic twins and argued for the presence of environmental factors in the development of the disease. Twin studies, however, are plagued with ascertainment bias by the fact that dizygotic twins are far more prevalent than monozygotic twins in the general population (Breitner *et al.* 1990).

Epidemiological studies have highlighted the unique qualities of young-onset, autosomal dominant, familial Alzheimers disease (adFAD), for multidisciplinary studies of the disease process. The clarity of inheritance has resulted in studies of adFAD dominating the familial literature. The preceding discussion addresses the key issues in this population relating to the focus of the present study; they concern the clinical issues associated with age at onset irrespective of family history, the major molecular genetic advances in adFAD and corresponding phenotypic expression, and finally the neuropsychological investigations of adFAD cases.

GENETIC HETEROGENEITY

Chromosome 21 linkage and the *APP* gene

The molecular genetic studies of adFAD, and more specifically those that resulted in the identification of specific mutations on Chromosome 21 co-segregating with the disease, were largely directed by three fundamental discoveries. The first, and perhaps most established, pointer for genetic investigations was the finding of AD pathology (characteristic senile plaques and neurofibrillary tangles) in trisomy 21 Down's syndrome cases (e.g. Ropper and Williams 1980). The second and third relate to a component protein of senile plaques, found to be beta-amyloid protein (Glenner and Wong 1984); by determining the amino acid sequence of this protein, the gene was cloned and found to code for a larger molecule—the amyloid precursor protein (APP). The gene was located on the long arm of Chromosome 21 (Tanzi *et al.* 1987).

Linkage studies in adFAD focused on Chromosome 21. These were fruitful in that linkage of the disease was demonstrated, in four families, to markers on the long arm of Chromosome 21 [St George-Hyslop *et al.* 1987]. Since these markers were in the region of the *APP* gene, further work concentrated on the sequencing of the *APP* gene and particularly the exons which encode for the beta-amyloid protein. This resulted in the identification of a point mutation in the *APP* gene, at codon 717, which co-segregated with the affected members of a particular British family (Goate *et al.* 1991). This was predicted to result in a valine to isoleucine amino acid substitution. Following this discovery, two further mutations resulting in different substitutions were found at the same site (valine to phenylalanine (Murrell *et al.* 1991) and valine to glycine (Chartier-Harlin *et al.* 1991). More recent work has identified a double mutation at a different locus (*APP* 670/671) in a Swedish adFAD pedigree (Mullan *et al.* 1992*a*). To date, these remain the only identified mutations co-segregating with adFAD. The demonstration of at least four mutations of the *APP* gene provide evidence for allelic, as well as genetic heterogeneity.

Linkage to markers on other chromosomes

The initial finding of genetic linkage to Chromosome 21 resulted in a surge of studies attempting to replicate this important advance. Despite some support (Goate *et al.* 1989), other studies failed to confirm the initial findings (e.g. Schellenberg *et al.* 1988). A pooling of resources from different centres resulted in the conclusion that genetic heterogeneity existed in adFAD (St George-Hyslop *et al.* 1990). Furthermore, the screening of other young-onset families for mutations in the *APP* gene proved relatively unfruitful (Crawford *et al.* 1991; Schellenberg *et al.* 1991).

Recently, linkage to markers on Chromosome 14 has been demonstrated (Mullan *et al.* 1992*b*; Schellenberg *et al.* 1992; Van Broeckhaven *et al.* 1992). Speculations regarding potential candidate genes continues with the emphasis on those which may play a role in the metabolism of beta-amyloid protein.

Continued linkage studies in late-onset families confirmed linkage to markers on Chromosome 19 (Pericak-Vance *et al.* 1991). This has been attributed to the inheritance of different polymorphisms for apolipoprotein E, which exists in three common forms: E2, E3, and E4. Inheritance of the E4 allele, particularly homozygosity, confers considerable increased risk of developing AD, probably due to its increased binding affinity to beta amyloid (Strittmatter *et al.* 1993).

PHENOTYPIC EXPRESSION

Only limited reports of the phenotypes of genetically different families have been published and have been overshadowed by the continuing genetic advances. As yet, it appears that mean age at disease onset within families is the only feature consistent with phenotypic heterogeneity. Chromosome 14-linked families show a mean age at onset in the early 40s, whereas those demonstrating linkage to Chromosome 19 show a mean onset after the age of 65. Variation is also observed within the *APP* gene mutation families; the mutation resulting in the valine to isoleucine substitution shows a mean disease onset in the

50, whereas those resulting in the valine to glycine and valine to phenylalanine substitutions, show a mean disease onset in the 40s. Moreover, it is known from epidemiology studies that age at onset is genetically determined (Huff *et al.* 1988), and that the majority of variance in age at onset in adFAD is accounted for between rather than within families (Van Diujn *et al.* 1991*a*). Two clinical studies support these findings, with phenotypic heterogeneity in terms of age at onset being observed in affected cases from different German families, with Russian ancestry (Bird *et al.* 1989, 1992). These families have autopsy confirmation of AD. Bird *et al.* (1989), also, found evidence for phenotypic heterogeneity in their finding of psychiatric, schizophrenic-like initial symptoms in the affected cases from one of the families studied.

The extent to which the behavioural presentation reflects genetic differences remains to be seen. For the meantime, reports of direct clinical and neuropsychological comparisons are restricted to those of adFAD cases, with unknown genetic status, and sporadic Alzheiner's disease (SAD) cases. Future, more detailed comparative studies of cases with specific mutations will lend information to support evidence, from age at onset differences, of phenotypic heterogeneity.

Distinguishing clinical features in adFAD have been observed, although these are apparently specific to the nature of inheritance of the condition, rather than the reported genetic heterogeneity. Myoclonus, seizures, and extrapryamidal signs show a higher incidence in adFAD than SAD (Feldman *et al.* 1963; Frommelt *et al.* 1991; Goudsmit *et al.* 1981; Karlinsky *et al.* 1992; Kennedy *et al.* 1993; Lowenberg and Waggoner 1934). Other clinical group studies have failed to use strict criteria for 'familial' AD which render the results non-comparable with reports from specific autosomal dominant pedigrees. One clinical comparison of familial (categorized by just one other affected family member) and sporadic cases failed to identify differences between the two patient groups (Haupt *et al.* 1992). These results might be those expected from findings of similar neuropathology in adFAD and SAD patient groups (Lantos *et al.* 1992; Martin *et al.* 1991). The importance of investigating adFAD as a specific subgroup, hence, becomes apparent. Further studies, comparing genetically heterogeneous families, will identify these clinical features as potential phenotypic differences.

NEUROPSYCHOLOGICAL INVESTIGATIONS

Many neuropsychological findings have derived from cases in which the family history is somewhat dubious. Breitner and Folstein (1984) observed that AD patients with aphasia and apraxia were more likely to have a family history (greater than one affected family member). They further estimated that the first degree relatives of those aphasic and apraxic patients showed a 50% cumulative lifetime risk of becoming affected with the disease. These findings, however, were based on the initial diagnosis of aphasia from the ability to write a sentence in the Mini-Mental State Examination (MMSE). The limited testing, the lack of a control measure for overall severity of the disease and the criteria for being termed 'familial' renders the validity of these results questionable. Indeed, contradictory findings are observed when disease severity is taken into account (Duara *et al.* 1993. Knesevich *et al.* 1985). Duara and colleagues, recently found significantly higher confrontation naming scores (Boston Naming Test) in their familial group (defined by a 90% probability that multiple affected members had not aggregated by chance), as compared to a sporadic cohort. These results not only contradict those of Breitner and Folstein, but also challenge those early studies suggesting greater language impairment in young-onset cases. Furthermore, they are not directly applicable to adFAD due to the criteria used for the definition of 'family history'.

More detailed neuropsychological studies of adFAD have largely failed to show differences from SAD (Duara *et al.* 1993, Karlinsky *et al.* 1992; McGeer *et al.* 1990; Nee *et al.* 1983; Reisberg *et al.* 1989; Swearer *et al.* 1992), and these studies are supported by functional imaging studies showing similar patterns of metabolic dysfunction (Guze *et al.* 1992; McGeer *et al.* 1990). Reports of very early neuropsychological dysfunction in an adFAD case (Karlinsky *et al.* 1992) and a SAD case (Kurz *et al.* 1990) both with a one-year history of dementia, show a similar pattern of deficits. Studies of more demented adFAD cases show wide-ranging deficits, also consistent with those observed in SAD (Nee *et al.* 1983; Reisberg *et al.* 1989). Direct comparisons using the same tests and procedures have, until recently, not been made, due to the logistics of compiling rare adFAD subjects for a group study.

Three studies exist in the literature to date. The first comprises seven adFAD cases and reports a similar pattern of neuropsychological deficits to SAD cases, when matched for disease severity (Swearer *et al.* 1992). This study has been referred to briefly in discussion of mildly affected adFAD cases and age at disease onset. These authors compared the neuropsychological features of seven affected individuals from just two families with those of 23 severity matched SAD cases. Assessment of severity was made using a six-point functional ability scale in which degree of difficulty in the home and work environments was rated. The study, essentially investigates potential group differences in performance on the neuropsychological tests administered. These comprised tests of verbal and visuospatial abilities and included the verbally and visuospatially mediated sub-tests of the Wechsler Adult Intelligence Scale—revised (WAIS-R) along with three further tests in each case. Memory functions were assessed using sub-tests of the Wechsler Memory Scale (WMS) and the word list learning from Rey's Auditory Verbal Learning Test. Average cognitive profiles were developed for the two patient groups by comparing the patients' scores with the mean normal score on each test. The results were analysed using a two-way analysis of variance, in which age and patient group acted as independent variables. A similar neuropsychological profile was observed in each of the two groups. This was of a mild to moderately impaired verbal performance and concentration, slowed psychomotor speed and severely impaired delayed recall of verbal material. They found that age, and not group membership, was the most significant variable in terms of test performances. Both the young controls and the young-onset adFAD cases showed better performances than their older counterparts on tests of abstract reasoning, psychomotor speed, and tracking. They concluded that it was age and not diagnostic category that was the determinant of any observed differences in level of performance on neuropsychological tests.

The second direct comparison of adFAD and SAD cases reports the group results of 113 loosely termed familial cases on a variety of neuropsychological measures (Duara *et al.* 1993). These results have been briefly discussed earlier. Of this group of 'familial' patients, adFAD cases represent 17% (20 cases). An analysis of variance of the neuropsychological test results of this adFAD subgroup and the SAD group yielded no significant difference on any one measure. Further comment is not possible due to their failure to present the data from this subgroup, independent of the other 93 classified 'familial' cases. It should be noted that the adFAD cases in this study have a mean age at onset of 73 years and are consequently not comparable with the young-onset adFAD cases in the present investigations.

The most recent comparison demonstrates clear differences in the cognitive functioning of 17 adFAD and 26 SAD cases, matched in terms of severity of overall dementia. Agnew (1993) examined the differential relationships of tests within each patient group and found a significantly higher proportion of adFAD cases with preserved naming skills. Indeed confrontation naming was the only skill on which adFAD patients performed at a higher level than their SAD counterparts. The result was not attributable to differences in ages at disease onset within the two groups or to genetic heterogeneity within the familial group. This finding suggests that adFAD cases show a pathological pathway that is distinct from SAD cases.

Further, recently detailed neuropsychological profiles from individual adFAD cases have substantiated this suggestion. Kennedy *et al.*

(1993) documented the neuropsychological profiles of two affected cases carrying the reported *APP* gene mutation at codon 717 (valine to glycine) and showed a relative preservation of confrontation picture naming. Kennedy *et al.* (1995) demonstrated neuropsychological homogeneity in three affected members of a family showing linkage to Chromosome 14. The profiles were characterized by an initial memory deficit with early dyscalculia and an impairment in speech production with relative absence of anomia. An interesting feature, previously undocumented in AD, was that of a speech production deficit. Farlow *et al.* (1994) detailed the neuropsychological investigations of three asymptomatic gene carriers from a pedigree with the *APP* gene mutation at codon 717 (valine to phenylalanine). One of these patients showed deficits in recent memory, information processing speed, simple sequential tracking, and concept reasoning. Spared functions included confrontation naming, verbal fluency, and visuoperceptual ability. This study highlights the unique opportunity in this condition to document early cognitive changes not only in the affected individuals (because diagnosis can be made comparatively early in the disease process), but also in those individuals 'at risk' from contracting the disease. One longitudinal investigation of an 'at risk' individual from a Chromosome 14-linked pedigree further demonstrates the importance of comprehensive neuropsychological investigation in these cases. Newman *et al.* (1994) showed cognitive anomalies in an 'at-risk' case 26 months prior to clinical diagnosis. These were a moderately selective verbal memory deficit, in the context of mild general intellectual impairment. Subsequent testing showed the progressive deterioration of visual memory and a relatively mild decline of perceptual and spatial skills; language and literacy skills remained comparatively intact. These recent studies provide the clearest indication that cognitive change precedes clinical change and they demonstrate the importance of early neuropsychological investigation. Furthermore, mounting evidence of preserved naming skills in adFAD cases directly contradicts the anomia widely reported in SAD cases (Appell *et al.* 1982; Bayles and Tomoeda 1983; Cummings *et al.* 1985) and is central in distinguishing adFAD from SAD.

To conclude, adFAD represents a particular aetiological subtype of AD showing similar neuropathological changes. There is increasing evidence, however, that this subtype can be distinguished in both neuropsychological and clinical terms. Recent genetic studies show adFAD to be a genetically and allelically heterogeneous condition (Rossor 1993; Schellenberg *et al.* 1991; St George-Hyslop *et al.* 1987). Phenotypes, as yet, have only been distinguished in terms of age at disease onset. It remains to be seen whether the suggestion of neuropsychological heterogeneity (Kennedy *et al.* 1995) is substantiated. What is clear is that investigations of the clinical and neuropsychological features of adFAD must use genetically homogeneous subject groups.

REFERENCES

Agnew, S. (1993). The neuropsychology of Autosomal dominant familial Alzheimer's disease. Ph.D. thesis, University of London.

Appell, J., Kertesz, A., and Fisman, M. (1982). A study of language functioning in Alzheimer's disease. *Brain and Language*, **17**, 73–91.

Bayles, K. and Tomoeda, C. (1983). Confrontation naming impairment in dementia. *Brain and Language*, **19**, 98–114.

Bird, T., Lampe, T., Nemens, E., *et al.* (1988). Familial Alzheimer's disease in American descendants of the Volga Germans: probable genetic founder effect. *Annals of Neurology*, **23**, 25–31.

Bird, T., Sumi, S., Nemens, E., *et al.* (1989). Phenotypic heterogeneity in familial Alzheimer's disease: a study of 24 kindreds. *Annals of Neurology*, **25**, 12–25.

Bird, T., Nemens, E., Nochlin, D., (1992). Familial Alzheimer's disease in Germans from Russia: A model of genetic heterogeneity in Alzheimer's disease. In *Heterogeneity of Alzheimer's disease*, (ed. F. Boller, F. Forette, and Z. Khachaturian), pp. 118–29. Springer-Verlag, Berlin.

Breitner, J. and Folstein, M. (1984). Familial Alzheimer dementia: A prevelant disorder with specific clinical features. *Psychological Medicine*, **14**, 63–80.

Breitner, J., Murphy, E., Folstein, M., and Magruder-Habib, K. (1990). Twin studies of Alzheimer's disease: an approach to aetiology and prevention. *Neurobiology of Aging*, **11**, 207–12.

Chartier-Harlin, M-C., Crawford, F., Houlden, H., *et al.* (1991). Early onset Alzheimers disease caused by mutations at codon 717 of the Bamyloid precursor protein gene. *Nature*, **353**, 844–6.

Cook, R., Ward, B., and Austin, J. (1979). Studies in aging of the brain: IV. Familial Alzheimer disease: relation to transmissible dementia, aneuploidy and microtubular defects. *Neurology*, **29**, 1402–12.

Crawford, F., Hardy, J., Mullan, M., *et al.* (1991). Sequencing of exons 16 and 17 of the beta-amyloid precursor protein gene in 14 families with early onset Alzheimer's disease fails to reveal mutations in the betamyloid sequence. *Neuroscience Letters*, **133**, 1–2.

Cummings, J., Benson, F., Hill, M., and Read, S. (1985). Aphasia in dementia of the Alzheimer type. *Neurology*, **35**, 394–97.

Duara, R., Lopez-Alberola, B., Barker, W., *et al.* (1993). A comparison of familial and sporadic Alzheimer's disease. *Neurology*, **43**, 1377–84.

Farlow, M., Murrell, J., Ghetti, B., *et al.* (1994). Clinical characteristics in a kindred with early onset Alzheimer's disease and their linkage to a G-T change at position 2149 of the amyloid precursor protein gene. *Neurology*, **44**, 105–11.

Farrer, L., O'Sullivan, D., Cupples, A., *et al.* (1989). Assessment of genetic risk for Alzheimer's disease among 1st-degree relatives. *Annals of Neurology*, **25**, 485–93.

Feldman, R., Chandler, K., Levy, L., and Glaser, G. (1963). Familial Alzheimer's disease. *Neurology*, **13**, 811–24.

Fitch, N., Becker, R., and Heller, A. (1988). The inheritance of Alzheimer's disease: a new interpretation. *Annals of Neurology*, **23**, 14–19.

Frommelt, P., Schnabel, R., Kuhne, W., *et al.* (1991). Familial Alzheimer's disease: a large, multigeneration German kindred. *Alzheimer's disease and Associated Disorders*, **5**, 36–43.

Glenner, G. and Wong, C. (1984). Alzheimer's disease: Initial report of the purification and characterisation of a novel cardiovascular amyloid protein. *Biochemical and Biophysical Research Communications*, **120**, 885–90.

Goate, A., Haynes, A., Owen, M., *et al.* (1989). Predisposing locus for Alzheimer's disease on Chromosome 21. *Lancet*, **89**, Feb. 18, 1(8634); 352–55.

Goate, A., Chartier-Harlin, M-C., Mullan, M., *et al.* (1991). Segregation of a missense mutation in the amyloid precursor protein gene with familial Alzheimer's disease. *Nature*, **349**, 704–6.

Goudsmit, J., White, B., and Weitkamp, L., *et al.* (1981). Familial Alzheimer's disease in two kindreds of the same geographic and ethnic origin. *Journal of the Neurological Sciences*, **49**, 79–89.

Guze, B., Hoffman, J., Mazziota, J., *et al.* (1992). PET and FAD: a pilot study. *Journal of the American Geriatric Society*, **40**, 120–23.

Haupt, M., Kurz, A., Pollmann, S., and Romero, B. (1992). Alzheimer's disease: identical phenotype of familial and non-familial cases. *Journal of Neurology*, **239**, 248–50.

Heston, L., Lowther, D., and Levanthal, C. (1966). Alzheimer's disease: a family study. *Archives of Neurology*, **15**, 225–33.

Heston, L., Mastri, A., Anderson, E., and White, J. (1981). Dementia of the Alzheimer type: clinical genetics, natural history, and associated conditions. *Archives of General Psychiatry*, **38**, 1085–90.

Heyman, A., Wilkinson, W., Hurwitz, B., *et al.* (1983). Alzheimer's disease: genetic aspects and associated clinical disorders. *Annals of Neurology*, **14**, 507–15.

Huff, F., Auerbach, J., Chakravarti, A., and Boller, F. (1988). Risk of dementia in relatives of patients with Alzheimer's disease. *Neurology*, **38**, 786–90.

Karlinsky, H., Vaula, G., Haines, J., *et al.* (1992). Molecular and prospective phenotypic characterisation of a pedigree with familial Alzheimer's disease and a missence mutation in codon 717 of the B-amyloid precursor protein. *Neurology*, **42**, 1445–53.

Kennedy, A., Newman, S., McCaddon, A., *et al.* (1993). Familial Alzheimer's disease: A pedigree with a mis-sense mutation in the amyloid precursor protein gene (amyloid precursor protein 717 valine-glycine). *Brain*, **116**, 309–24.

Kennedy, A., Newman, S., Frackowiak, R., *et al.* (1995). Chromosome 14 linked familial Alzheimer's disease: A clinico-pathological study of a single pedigree. *Brain*, **118**, 185–205.

Knesevich, J., Toro, F., Morris, J., and La Barge, E. (1985). Aphasia, family history and the long course of senile dementia of the Alzheimer-type. *Psychiatry Research*, **14**, 255–63.

Kumar, A., Shapiro, M., Grady, C., *et al.* (1991). Anatomic, metabolic, neuropsychological and molecular genetic studies of three pairs of identical twins discordant for dementia of the Alzheimer type. *Archives of Neurology*, **48**, 160–9.

Kurz, A., Romero, B., and Lauter, H. (1990). The onset of Alzheimer's disease. A longitudinal case study and a trial of a new diagnostic criteria. *Psychiatry*, **53**, 53–61.

Lantos, P., Luthert, P., Hanger, D., *et al.* (1992). Familial Alzheimer's disease with the amyloid precursor protein position 717 mutation and sporadic Alzheimer's disease have the same cytoskeletal pathology. *Neuroscience Letters*, **137**, 221–4.

La Rue, A., Matsuyamas, S., McPherson, S., *et al.* (1992). Cognitive performance in relatives of patients with probable Alzheimer's disease: an age at onset effect. *Journal Clinical and Experimental Neuropsychology*, **14**, 533–8.

Lowenberg, K. and Waggoner, R. (1934). Familial organic psychosis (Alzheimer's type). *Archives of Neurology and Psychiatry*, **31**, 737–54.

McGeer, E., Peppard, R., McGeer, H., *et al.* (1990). 18-Fluorodeoxyglucose PET studies in presumed Alzheimer cases, including 13 serial scans. *Canadian Journal of Neurological Sciences*, **17**, 1–11.

McMenemey, W., Worster-Drought, C., Flind, J., and Williams, H. (1939). Familial presenile dementia: report of case with clinical and pathological features of Alzheimer's disease. *Journal of Neurology and Psychiatry*, **2**, 293–302.

Martin, J., Gheuens, J., Bruylan, M., *et al.* (1991). Early-onset Alzheimer's disease in 2 large Belgian families. *Neurology*, **41**, 62–8.

Meggendorfer, F. (1925). Uber familiengeschichtliche Untersuchungen bei arteriosklerotischer und seniler Demenz. *Zentralblatt für Neurologie und Psychiatrie*, **40**, 359.

Mullan, M., Crawford, F., Axelman, K., *et al.* (1992*a*). A pathogenic mutation for probable Alzheimer's disease in the APP gene at the N-terminus of B-amyloid. *Nature Genetics*, **1**, 345–7.

Mullan, M., Houlden, H., Windelspecht, M. *et al.* (1992*b*) A locus for familial early onset Alzheimer's disease on the long arm of chromosome 14, proximal to the one-antichymotrypsin gene. *Nature Genetics*, **2**, 340–2.

Murrell, J., Farlow, M., Ghetti, B., and Benson, M. (1991). A mutation in the amyloid precursor protein associated with hereditary Alzheimer's disease. *Science*, **254**, 97–9.

Nee, L., Polinsky, R., Eldridge, R., *et al.* (1983). A family with histologically confirmed Alzheimer's disease. *Archives of Neurology*, **40**, 203–8.

Nee, L., Eldridge, R., Sunderland, T., *et al.* (1987). Dementia of the Alzheimer type: clinical and family study of 22 twin pairs. *Neurology*, **37**, 359–63.

Newman, S., Warrington, E., Kennedy, A., and Rossor, M. (1994). The earliest cognitive change in an individual with familial Alzheimer's disease: Presymptomatic neuropsychological features in a pedigree with autopsy confirmed familial Alzheimer's disease. *Journal of Neurology, Neurosurgery and Neuropsychiatry*, **57**, 967–72.

Pericak-Vance, M., Bebout, J., Gaskell, P., *et al.* (1991). Linkage studies in familial Alzheimer's disease: evidence for chromosome 19 linkage. *American Journal of Human Genetics*, **48**, 1034–50.

Reisberg, B., Ferris, S., Franssen, E. (1989). Clinical features of a neuropathologically verified familial Alzheimer's cohort with onset in the fourth decade: comparison with senile onset Alzheimer's disease and etiopathogenic implications. *Alzheimer's Disease and Related Disorders*, **3**, 43–54.

Ropper, A. and Williams, R. (1980). Relationship between plaques, tangles and dementia in Down's syndrome. *Neurology*, **30**, 639–44.

Rossor, M. (1993). Alzheimer's disease. *British Medical Journal*, **307**, 779–82.

St George-Hyslop, P., Haimes, J., Farrer, L. *et al.* (1987). Genetic linkage studies suggest that Alzheimer's disease is not a single homogeneous disorder. *Nature*, **325**, 733–6.

St George-Hyslop, P., Haines, J., Farrer, L., *et al.* (1990). Genetic studies suggest that Alzheimer's disease is not a single homogeneous disorder. *Nature*, **347**, 184–90.

Schellenberg, G., Bird, T., Wijsman, E., *et al.* (1988). Absence of linkage of chromosome 21q21 markers to familial Alzheimer's disease. *Science*, **241**, 1507–10.

Schellenberg, G., Anderson, L., O'Dahl, S., *et al.* (1991). APP 717, APP693 and PRIP gene mutations are rare in Alzheimer's disease. *American Journal of Human Genetics*, **49**, 511–17.

Schellenberg, G., Bird, T., Wijsman., E., *et al.* (1992). Genetic linkage evidence for a familial Alzheimer's disease locus on chromosome 14. *Science*, **258**, 668–71.

Schottky, J. (1932). Über Prasenile Verblodungen. *Neurological Psychology*, **140**, 333–97.

Strittmatter, W., Saunders, A., Schmechel, D., *et al.* (1993). Apolipoprotein E: High avidity binding to beta amyloid and increased frequency of type 4 allele in late onset familial Alzheimer's disease. *Journal of Neuropathology and Experimental Neurology*, **50**, 82–94.

Swearer, J., O'Donnell, B., Drachman, D., and Woodward, B. (1992). Neuropsychological features of familial Alzheimer's disease. *Annals of Neurology*, **32**, 687–94.

Tanzi, R., Gusella, J., Watkins, P., *et al.* (1987). Amyloid beta protein gene: cDNA, mRNA distribution and genetic linkage near the Alzheimer locus. *Science*, **235**, 880–4.

Van Broeckhaven, C., Backhovens, H., Cruts, M., *et al.* (1992). Mapping of gene predisposing to early onset Alzheimer's disease to chromosome 14q24.3. *Nature Genetics*, **2**, 334–339.

Van Duijn, C., Broeckhoven, C., Hardy, J. *et al.* (1991*a*). Evidence for allelic heterogeneity in familial early-onset Alzheimer's disease. *British Journal of Psychiatry*, **158**, 471–4.

Van Duijn, C., Clayton, D., Chandra, V., *et al.* (1991*b*). Familial aggregation of Alzheimer's disease and related disorders: a collaborative re-analysis of case control studies. *International Journal of Epidemiology*, **20**, S13–S20.

IV. Implications for treatment and rehabilitation

SIXTEEN

The assessment of dementia

Edgar Miller

INTRODUCTION

This chapter is concerned with the psychological assessment of people with dementia or suspected dementia. Potentially this is an extremely wide field. A vast number of different techniques and instruments might be legitimately be employed in examining such patients (see, for example, Morris and McKiernan 1994). In order to keep this chapter to a manageable size, some restriction has to be placed on the material to be covered.

In the first place, concern will be restricted to standard forms of assessment that might be used in an ordinary clinical practice rather than procedures that might be employed on a more individual basis as in the carrying out of research studies. It will also be limited to forms of assessment directed at answering basic questions. These are such questions as whether the individual being examined might have a dementing disorder and, if so, its possible nature.

A further limitation to the present chapter is that it will be largely, if not entirely, concerned with the sorts of measures and procedures that would be used by psychologists which have been developed systematically and validated. The use of more *ad hoc* or 'bedside' types of clinical examination that might be used by psychiatrists and neurologists as part of routine clinical practise will not be covered. Descriptions of the latter can be found in a number of other sources (e.g. Cummings and Benson 1992; Strub and Black 1977).

Even restricting the scope in this way still leaves a considerable amount of material that could be included, much of which has been reviewed in other contexts Morris and McKiernan (1994). This chapter will therefore concentrate on the basic issues and principles, and will eschew any attempt to provide anything like a comprehensive account of all the possible instruments described in the literature. The particular instruments mentioned will be chosen because they are of especial importance or because they illustrate particular points.

It might be useful for some readers to have a more general introduction to neuropsychological assessment, for instance suitable sources include Crawford *et al.* (1992) and Lezak (1983).

BACKGROUND ISSUES

Before getting into the details of assessment it is useful to be aware of a number of background issues. These relate to two main areas. First, it is necessary to consider the nature of the people who are being assessed and, second, the nature of the techniques or instruments available for their assessment.

Factors relating to the individual

People being assessed in relation to dementia or possible dementia tend to be older and typically of above retirement age. Dementia is, of course, a disorder mostly associated with old age although it may become manifest in middle age. However, younger cases are relatively rare.

A major problem is that older people are much more liable to suffer from other disorders and handicaps and many of these may have consequences for psychological assessment. For example, the prevalence of sensory impairment is much greater among the elderly. Poor vision and impaired hearing are common and can affect test performance (O'Neill and Calhoun 1975). Especially if some degree of mental impairment is also involved, people being investigated may not possess up-to-date and properly adapted prostheses to correct for sensory loss. It is therefore sensible in any psychological assessment of older people to check that vision and hearing, with appropriate correction or enhancement, are adequate for the task. Where uncorrected sensory impairments exist, it can sometimes be extremely difficult to judge to what extent poor test performance is due to a true mental impairment as opposed to a failure to appreciate what is required due to poor sensory functioning.

There is also a greater risk for a number of physical problems which may also interact with psychological functioning. Cardiovascular problems are again far from uncommon and have been associated with some impairment of cognitive functioning (Abrahams and Birren 1973; Hale 1992). It has similarly been suggested that diabetes can be associated with mild cognitive deficits (Worrall *et al.* 1993).

Another health factor that can cause difficulty in the assessment of older people is the occurrence of infections. Infections, like urinary tract and chest infections, can occur relatively commonly in older people. They are not as obvious as in those who are younger since they do not always result in a raised temperature, which tends to be the most usual and obvious sign of illness. It is also the case that older people are much more prone to become mentally confused when suffering from an infection. What this means is that an older person can present with an apparent dementia with poor performance on cognitive tests, and yet this may be solely the consequence of a readily treatable medical condition such as a urinary tract or chest infection.

Finally, older people are also much more prone to suffer the toxic side effects of drugs, especially mental confusion. The fact that they are more liable to have general health problems means that older people are more likely to be on medication. On top of this, multiple health problems are far from unknown and this can mean that a cocktail of drugs is involved. Whilst each drug may be appropriate in itself, the combined toxic effect of several drugs, with their complex interactions, can have a marked impact on mental functioning.

The tendency to produce mental confusion and a picture like dementia as a result of infection or polypharmacy can complicate assessment and needs to be kept in mind. It is not always easy to eliminate these possibilities in a case of suspected dementia. A careful history of the onset of symptoms may be helpful, but this depends upon being able to question someone who knows the individual well, since mentally confused patients are often unable to provide an adequate history on their own. In the traditional medical literature, mental confusion due to these causes is linked to a clouded sensorium with impaired attention, whereas these are not features of dementia. This may well be true, but the presence of these allegedly key features is not always clear cut thus making their assessment difficult and not wholly reliable. This is especially so since levels of consciousness may fluctuate over time making the timing of the examination quite crucial.

It should also be noted that these possible complicating factors all act in one direction. This is to produce a deterioration in cognitive performance which may result in the erroneous decision that the individual suffers from a dementing disorder.

Factors relating to psychological measures

Turning to problems associated with the assessment instruments, a major difficulty is that many potentially useful tests do not have norms that extend into the older age ranges. Among the few tests with norms for older subjects are the Wechsler Adult Intelligence Scale—Revised (WAIS-R) and the revised Wechsler Memory Scale (WMS-R) where the age range extends to 74 years in both instances. Even so it is not uncommon to have to deal with people who are appreciably over 74 years of age. If norms for older people are available they tend to be less carefully and extensively developed. This would not matter so much if a good range of instruments was developed specifically for use with the elderly. With the exception of many screening tests for dementia, this has not been the case.

An important characteristic of dementia is the trend towards a steady deterioration in mental functioning. This means that a major problem in some contexts can be to find instruments that can still detect differences in cognitive functioning in severely impaired patient typically require some basic level of competence for adequate performance and this basic level is above that exhibited by many subjects with moderate dementia or worse. From the point of view of identifying dementia this is not an appreciable problem since subjects are typically quite clearly suffering from dementia by the time that they fail to score on the usual cognitive tests. Where it does become a problem is in relation to such issues as trying to plot change or deterioration over time.

IDENTIFICATION OF DEMENTIA

A central issue is whether a patient is suffering from a dementia and, if so, which type. In practice, psychological approaches to answering this question are not used in a vacuum. They typically arise in a clinical context in which other means of attempting to answer the same question will also be employed. These other means involve a general (medical) clinical examination and history taking as well as the use of radiological procedures, mainly CT and NMR scanning. No single approach to the diagnostic exercise in this area comes close to giving entirely reliable results. This means that best practice involves the judicious evaluation of information from a number of assessment modalities. Where this information is consistent decision making is easy. However, there are no simple and straightforward rules for dealing with conflicting evidence.

Screening tests

A large number of what might be best described as screening tests for dementia have been devised. This is the one area referred to in an early section where a considerable number of instruments have been devised primarily and validated for populations in the age ranges associated with dementia. Typically these screening tests consist of a set of questions, often around 20 or 30 in number, which cover basic information and cognitive functions. They may require the subject to give basic personal information (name, home address, etc.), answer simple questions based on common knowledge (for instance who is the present Prime Minister or President of the USA), and remember simple items of information, such as a fictitious name and address, to recall a few minutes later.

Probably the best known and used most extensively of these screening tests is the Mini-Mental State Examination (MMSE) of Folstein *et al.* (1975). Other examples of similar scales are the Blessed Scale (Blessed *et al.* 1968), the ADAS of Rosen *et al.* (1984) and the Mattis Dementia Rating Scale (Mattis 1976). However, a large number of similar instruments could also be mentioned (see Nelson *et al.* 1986) and new scales are constantly being added to the literature (e.g. Brazzelli *et al.* 1994).

Screening tests of this type can be useful especially since they are quick and easy to administer. They do have decidedly less than perfect validity in discriminating those with dementia from non-demented subjects. Inaccuracies tend most commonly to be in the direction of producing false-positives. Whilst they have too much error to be reliably used on their own to diagnose dementia in individual cases, they can be of practical value in identifying individuals for whom further and much more extensive assessment would be warranted.

With a large number of similar instruments readily available, choosing a particular screening test is not easy. The published validity studies will obviously be important but it should be noted that there is a tendency for further validity studies on a particular instrument to reveal an attenuation in the level of diagnostic discrimination. All other things being equal, it is possible to argue a case for choosing a scale like the MMSE that has been shown repeatedly to have worthwhile levels of validity rather than a recently published instrument with an unreplicated claim for a slightly higher level of validity. In addition, there may well be cultural differences in the ability to answer questions requiring the giving of general information (for example, asking a British person who is the current President of the USA). It may therefore be safer, given the choice, to stick with a scale developed and validated in the same cultural context as that in which it is being used.

Test batteries and diagnostic systems

Attempts have been made to develop reliable diagnostic criteria for dementia such as the NINCDS–ADRDA criteria (Blacker *et al.* 1994; McKhann *et al.* 1984). These include neuropsychological features considered important in diagnosis. Specific neuropsychological test batteries have also been put forward by a number of other groups, including that of the Consortium to Establish a Registry for Alzheimer's Disease (CERAD) and the University of California Alzheimer's Disease Research Center (UCSD–ADRC) test battery (see Morris *et al.* 1989; Salmon and Butters 1992).

As well as screening instruments such as the MMSE, these batteries contain a range of measures covering different aspects of cognition including, for example, memory, constructional praxis, different verbal functions, and visuospatial abilities. Such batteries can take a considerable length of time to administer (4 hours in the case of the UCSD–ADRC battery). It is not always clear that some of the tests included contribute very much to diagnosis, although some of them may be of value for other purposes. For example within the CERAD battery, which has good overall levels of reliability and validity, only a limited number of measures actually contribute appreciably to the discrimination of cases of early dementia from non-dementing controls (Welsh *et al.* 1991, 1992). The tests of delayed recall and confrontational naming were the most effective in this role.

Worth noting in this context are certain more elaborate psychiatric diagnostic systems for the detection of dementia. These include the CAMDEX system (Roth *et al.* 1986) and AGECAT (Copeland *et al.* 1986). These take very much longer to administer than screening tests and rely on medical/psychiatric factors as well as psychological measures. In return they offer rather better levels of diagnostic discrimination.

Tests of individual functions

Intelligence

Given that the very term 'dementia' implies a deterioration in general intellectual functioning, it is tempting to see tests of general intelligence, such as the revised Wechsler Adult Intelligence Scale (WAIS-R), as having a potentially useful diagnostic role In practice, tests like the WAIS-R contribute very little to early detection, largely because of two factors. First, the development of intelligence tests is typically associated with a search to develop high levels of test–retest reliability. This in turn is associated with high stability and an insensitivity to change or deterioration in cognitive functioning, especially if this is far from extensive. Second, and linked to the first point, is the fact that performance on intelligence tests like the WAIS-R involve the use of long-established and well-practised skills. Such skills are particularly resistant to decline due to cerebral pathology (Miller 1984*a*).

One refinement to the use of intelligence tests in this context has been to try to develop indices of premorbid intellectual functioning against which present IQ levels can be judged. One way has been to use different subtest patterns of the Wechsler intelligence scales as indicators of present and premorbid ability (the so-called deterioration indices and subtest profiles). But these have proved to be rather unreliable and their use is subject to a number of criticisms which have been described in detail elsewhere (e.g. Miller 1977).

The difficulty that arises in using any form of analysis of the profile of subtest scores is well illustrated by Ryan and Bohac (1994). Relying on work that had established allegedly normal subtest profiles for the WAIS-R, they then examined a large number of cases with various forms of brain pathology in terms of their subtest profiles. Considering just the subset of the overall sample with Alzheimer-type dementia, only about 21% had what could be described as an abnormal or unusual profile. On this basis, subtest profiles hardly offer a high level of detection of Alzheimer-type dementia even without allowing for the fact that some normal subjects would be likely to produce unusual profiles.

By far the best validated of the methods for obtaining an indication of premorbid IQ has been the use of the National Adult Reading Test or NART (Nelson and O'Connell 1978). This makes use of the fact that the ability to read words appears to be highly resistant to deterioration due to brain pathology, at least if this is not extreme or the subject is in the early stages of a progressive disorder like dementia. The NART makes use of words in English whose spelling is irregular (for instance *naive* and *aeon*), so that the subject cannot make use of the usual rules of spelling to pronounce the words and so can only pronounce them correctly if there is previous familiarity with the words. Such reading performance correlates with IQ and can be used as an index of premorbid IQ against which present intelligence test performance can be compared. A more extensive description of work on the use of the NART as an index of premorbid intelligence is provided by Crawford (1992) and Morris and Kopelman (1992).

Memory

Of the tests relating to specific functions, it is tests of memory that have proved to be the most useful in discriminating between subjects with dementia and those without, at least in the early stages of dementia. In part, this may be because memory tests have possibly been the most extensively researched in this context. Nevertheless, it is also relevant that in AD, with its slow and insidious onset, it is usually failures in memory that first draw attention to the fact that the sufferer is undergoing some adverse changes (e.g. Miller 1977).

As a preliminary point, it must be admitted that the clinical assessment of memory is often unsatisfactory. Erickson and Scott (1977), in a major review, pointed out that advances in knowledge about memory processes were generally ignored in the design of clinical tests of memory. As Kapur (1988) has indicated, a decade later the situation had improved to some degree, but it is undoubtedly and almost inevitably the case that memory tests specifically designed for clinical usage lag a long way behind advances in more fundamental research into memory. From the present point of view it is more important that the memory tests which are used have good diagnostic discrimination, and whether they match easily on to current models of memory is more of a refinement. Nevertheless, to have tests which give both good discrimination and independently examine the various facets of memory, as indicated by more recent research into memory processes, would be highly desirable.

One of the most commonly used memory tests is the Wechsler Memory Scale, now available in a revised version (Wechsler 1987). This includes a number of subscales covering such aspects as both verbal and non-verbal memory, with retention over both short-and long-term intervals being tested. The age-related norms go up to 74 years, making it of potential relevance for use with at least some cases of suspected dementia. As Mayes and Warburg (1992) point out, it is highly likely that a large amount of data relating to the use of this test in various contexts will appear. A disadvantage with the WMS-R is that it does take an appreciable length of time to administer which might limit its ready acceptable by elderly subjects.

A range of other generally used tests of memory, or even batteries of memory tests, can be identified. A number of those with some standardization for elderly populations are listed by Morris and Kopelman (1992) and more recently by Morris and McKiernan (1994) Two significant tests are the Recognition Memory Test (Warrington 1984) and the Rivermead Behavioural Memory Test (Wilson *et al.* 1985). The former presents the subject with sets of verbal (words) on non-verbal (faces) stimuli and then requires the recognition of the presented stimulus from pairs which contain one distracter item. The Rivermead Behavioural Memory Test represents an attempt to offer a more 'ecologically valid' test of memory in that it aims to mimic the memory requirements of everyday life. For example one subtest requires the subject to remember to carry out a particular action when cued to do so by a bell.

A memory test specifically designed to discriminate people with dementia and with norms that go well into the older age ranges, is the Object Learning Test of Kendrick *et al.* (1979). This is a relatively simple test in that it requires subjects to examine four cards containing sets of pictures of objects and then to try to recall as many names of the objects as possible after the presentation of each card. It has been found to be highly acceptable to elderly subjects. It is designed to be used in tandem with a simple and quick test of psychomotor speed, the Digit Copying Test. Kendrick's group has been rather overconcerned with the differential diagnosis between dementia and depression, based on what is now known to be the dubious assumption that almost all subjects incorrectly regarded as possibly suffering from dementia will be depressed. Initial validation data suggested extremely high levels of diagnostic accuracy, although further work did not reveal such outstanding results (Gibson *et al.* 1980). The best diagnostic results are obtained when subjects are retested after a 6-week interval.

The work on the Object Learning Test offers the additional sophistication that Kendrick *et al.* (1979) tried to take base rates into account in their normative data, they assumed that the a priori diagnosis was likely to be depression in 68% of cases being investigated for possible dementia and true dementia in the other 33%. Whilst base rates are of great potential importance in making decisions about the likely cause of a person's problems, it is unlikely that the 67/33% split used by Kendrick and his colleagues will be true of all settings in which the tests are likely to be used.

Whilst discussing memory and memory testing it is appropriate to sound a note of caution. Whilst failures in memory may be the thing which most commonly alerts others to the fact that some form of adverse change is taking place in the individual, this does not mean that those who present to health-related services complaining of memory difficulties are necessarily in the early stages of a dementing illness. As a number of studies have shown, the vast majority of those in middle age and early old age who present with such complaints do not appear subsequently to have a dementing illness (Bolla *et al.* 1991; Feehan *et al.* 1991; O'Brien *et al.* 1992). Most of those who present with memory complaints probably have a functional cause and this is most typically, but by no means invariably, depression. The indication is that if it is the patient's relatives rather than the patient him/herself who make the complaint of memory loss then this is rather more likely to be indicative of a dementing illness.

Language

Impairment of language also occurs in dementia and is often clinically apparent in the early stages (Miller 1989; Miller and Morris 1993). Tests of language can therefore also contribute to diagnosis. The most commonly encountered language impairment in dementia is in naming (e.g. Miller 1989; Welsh *et al.* 1992). Two tests of naming with at least some normative data, although not across the whole of the age range of interest, are the Boston Naming Test (Kaplan *et al.* 1983) and the Graded Naming Test (McKenna and Warrington 1983).

Another potentially useful simple language-related test that appears to show some decline in the early stages of Alzheimer type dementia is verbal fluency (e.g. Hart *et al.* 1988; Miller 1984*b*). In some contexts, tests of verbal fluency have been regarded as tests of semantic memory rather than language (see Miller 1989), but the distinction between semantic memory and language in this context is rather arbitrary.

Other cognitive functions

The, by now, extensive literature on dementia indicates that more or less any psychological function is likely to deteriorate in dementia (e.g. Miller and Morris 1993; Parks *et al.* 1993). This means that, in principle at least, tests of almost any psychological function could be used in the detection of dementia. In practice, continually adding more and more different types of test to those already described is unlikely to give much of an increase in accuracy in detecting dementia. This is so even if measures with suitable age-related norms can be found.

A possible exception to this statement are tests of visuospatial ability. Design copying tests whereby subjects are shown abstract designs and then have to copy these from memory, such as Benton's (1974) Visual Retention Test, are sometimes useful. These are sometimes regarded as memory tests since they do require memory for adequate performance, yet they are arguably just as dependent upon the subject's ability to analyse spatial relationships.

DISTINGUISHING BETWEEN DIFFERENT FORMS OF DEMENTIA

Since dementia is not a unitary condition, the further question arises as to the type of dementia that might be involved. It is certainly true that dementias of different types do tend to have different psychological characteristics (Miller and Morris 1993; Parks *et al.* 1993). To what extent can neuropsychological examinations differentiate between the different forms of dementia?

Two of the most common forms of dementia are Alzheimer-type dementia and cerebrovascular dementia, and some effort has gone into devising means to discriminate between these two types. Two clinically significant features are the history of the disorder and the general medical status of the patient. Not surprisingly, cerebrovascular dementia is more common in those who have other evidence of cardiovascular disease. It is also the case that those with cerebrovascular dementia caused by a series of small brain haemorrhages may exhibit a clear history of sudden exacerbations in mental disturbance followed by periods in which the level of disturbance fails to progress or may even partially recover. A problem here is that the person being examined may not be able to give an adequate history on which to judge reliably the presence of a stepwise progression. It may also be impossible to talk to someone who has continuous knowledge of the patient and is able to provide the necessary information.

From a psychological point of view, it would be expected that an Alzheimer-type dementia would be associated with a more even spread of disturbance across different psychological functions, whilst cerebrovascular dementia would have a more patchy pattern of impairment linked to the specific loci of vascular events. In practice this is not a reliable means of discrimination because cerebral atrophy, as it occurs in Alzheimer-type dementia, is not necessary evenly spread, especially in the early stages (Neary *et al.* 1986, 1988). It is also the case that series of small, dispersed vascular events can disrupt a wide range of functions. One particular suggestion is that dementia due to vascular causes will exhibit a greater preponderance of frontal deficits (Kertesz and Clydesdale 1994). It should be borne in mind, however, that predominantly frontal atrophy can occur in dementia linked primarily to atrophic changes in the brain. Neary *et al.* (1986, 1988)

It is certainly possible to develop batteries of tests that will discriminate groups of patient with Alzheimer-type dementia from those with dementia due to vascular causes (Mendez and Ashla-Mendez 1991; Perez *et al.* 1975*a, b*), and to determine particular test profiles that may more commonly arise in one type of dementia rather than another. Whilst highly statistically significant mean differences may arise, this is always in the context of considerable areas of overlap between the groups. This makes the resulting cut-off scores or test profiles less reliable when used with individual cases.

The problem of distinguishing between the allegedly 'cortical' dementias (for instance Alzheimer-type dementia) and the so-called 'subcortical' dementias as found in such conditions as Parkinson's disease, progressive supranuclear palsy, Huntington's chorea, and the like, on the basis of psychological findings does not really arise. This is because the disorders associated with the subcortical dementias have characteristic motor disorders, other physical symptoms, and even genetic links. This is in no way to deny that differences in the nature of the psychological impairments encountered in these different conditions do arise (see Miller and Morris 1993; Parks *et al.* 1993),

In practice, the differential assignment of patients into different types of dementia should not be made on the basis of neuropsychological examination alone. Neuropsychological data can sometimes give an indication that the type of dementia involved is more likely to be of one particular type than another, but such indications should not be accepted with great confidence.

Computerized testing

The use of automated testing has been discussed for some considerable time (e.g. Miller 1968), but it is the advent of microcomputers that has really made this form of assessment practicable. Automated or computer-based assessment has a number of advantages, of which the most important are that it allows test materials to be presented in a rigorously standardized manner and also the accurate recording of response times. Although it is difficult, if not impossible, to present certain forms of test material commonly used in conventional assessment new forms of assessment are made possible, particularly in the realm of interactive assessment.

Two sets of computerized test materials have been developed specifically for use with subjects who may be elderly and who may be suffering from dementia. Carr *et al.* (1986*a*, *b*) have developed a battery with five subtests which include verbal and non-verbal memory tests, a lexical decision test, and a matching-to-sample test. The battery is specifically designed to be suitable for use with elderly patients by means of such things as having a large display to make it easier for those with poor vision and using brief instructions to minimize memory problems.

Morris *et al.* (1987) have developed the Cambridge Automated Neuropsychological Test Automated Battery (CANTAB) which incorporates such things as a delayed matching-to-sample test and a visual recognition test specifically based on test paradigms used with experimental animals. Other tests in the battery include a computerized version of the Tower and Hanoi Test and a version of the Corsi Block Span Test. As yet this battery has largely been used in experimental studies (e.g. Sahakian *et al.* 1988). Again the presentation of tests in the battery is designed to make them easy for cognitively impaired subjects to use.

Confirmatory reports of the validity of these batteries in routine clinical use are still awaited. Nevertheless, the work reported so far indicates that computer-based testing of this kind can be used quite effectively with elderly patients and those with marked cognitive impairment. It is likely that the role of computer-based assessment will be extended in the future.

NON-COGNITIVE FACTORS

In attempting to identify possible cases of dementia it is important to consider other explanations of apparent poor functioning. For example older people with depression may present in a state which mimics dementia; the patient is withdrawn and inactive, says very little, appears unable to provide everyday pieces of information, has not been looking after him/herself properly, and so on. There may also be complaints from the patient or those close to him/her of memory loss.

It is therefore necessary on occasions to take the possibility of depression seriously. Clinical criteria for determining the presence of depression and related disorders are provided in a number of sources, such as the 4th edition of the *Diagnostic and statistical manual* (DSM IV) of the American Psychiatric Association (APA 1994). In addition, a number of scales exist to assess the severity of depression. One such of particular value in older people is the Geriatric Depression Scale of Yesavage *et al.* (1983). Depression is often accompanied by physical features (for instance motor retardation and bowel disturbances), yet these same, or very similar, physical disturbances are common in older people and can arise for a number of reasons other than being depressed. In examining depression in older people it is therefore appropriate to use a scale which minimizes the significance of these physical manifestations. The Geriatric Depression Scale was constructed with just this point in mind.

It should be noted, however, that some patients in the early stages of a dementing illness can also be depressed. In other words, depression and dementia are not mutually exclusive states. Later on in the course of dementia, depression is much less likely since emotional responses tend to get flattened.

FURTHER ISSUES RELATING TO DIAGNOSTIC INSTRUMENTS

In identifying people with dementia a major concern for any test, or battery of tests, that is to be used is that of diagnostic validity—in the sense of the test's ability to discriminate between subjects with and without dementia or to distinguish between those with different forms of dementia. Validity is usually established by demonstrating that the test or battery as a whole can discriminate between subjects known to have the relevant characteristics (for example Alzheimer-type dementia and normal subjects of similar age).

A number of issues can arise in such validation exercises. The first of these is that it is not sufficient for instruments to discriminate between groups. Given the appropriate circumstances a group with, say, Alzheimer-type dementia may have a mean score that is very highly significantly different in statistical terms from that of normal controls and yet there can still be considerable overlaps between the two distributions. In diagnostic exercises it is the ability of the diagnostic instrument to make valid distinctions on the basis of individual subjects that matters, and this typically requires a level of validity that is much harder to achieve than that of discriminating between group means. It would be useful if validity studies of all neuropsychological diagnostic tests reported sensitivity and specificity data as a matter of routine. (For an account of sensitivity and specificity and the means of determining these characteristics see Hennekens and Buring 1987.)

A second issue in validity studies is that tests are often validated against groups of subjects whose diagnostic status is well established. In the case of dementia obtaining cases where the diagnosis is relatively certain involves using those that are well established. Well-established cases will have clearer levels of impairment and thus be easier to detect. The outcome will be that the validity study is likely to overestimate the instruments' ability to discriminate newer cases. Yet it is these possible newer cases in whom the diagnostic issue most commonly arises and with whom the diagnostic instrument will most commonly be used.

A possible way round this dilemma is to validate the test by applying it to samples of subjects exactly like those with whom the test is designed to be used (for example possible new cases where firm diagnosis is most difficult). The sample is then followed up for, say, 12 months and then reassessed fully. The test is then validated against its ability to predict the diagnosis at a future stage, where the passage of time will reveal much more reliably which subjects were truly demented. This, of course, makes validation studies rather longer and more tedious, but is likely to lead to much more accurate information on validity.

The third and last significant issue is that of base rates. This problem has already been mentioned above and is discussed in greater detail elsewhere (e.g. Meehl and Rosen 1955). The basic point is that the decisions which can legitimately be based on the outcome of a diagnostic test are influenced by the 'antecedent probabilities' of the different possible outcomes (where the antecedent probability refers to the proportion within the population to which the test is being applied who actually exhibit the condition that needs to be identified). If the aim is to identify cases of dementia from those without dementia, then a subject who scores below the cut-off point for dementia on the test may be suffering from dementia. However, allowing for the fact that no diagnostic test ever gives perfect discrimination, then this same subject could be a 'false-positive', namely someone without dementia who just happens to do very poorly on the test. The smaller the proportion of people within the sample being tested who really do suffer from dementia, the bigger the chance that a test score in the dementia range is a false-positive. Indeed, in the extreme case, the situation may arise where a score in the range allegedly indicating dementia is more likely to reflect a false-positive than a true case of dementia.

FINAL COMMENT

The neuropsychological assessment of the patient with suspected dementia is quite complex, in that it is possible to employ a variety of different tests relating to a wide range of psychological domains. It is, however, generally the case that if careful assessment of memory, language, and possibly one other function fails to show any sign of impairment of the kind indicative of dementia, then further and more extensive testing becomes less likely to yield anything of interest, at least from the point of view of identifying possible cases of dementia.

In general, it is also the case that, where error occurs, it is more likely to be in the direction of falsely identifying a patient as suffering from a dementing illness than the reverse. The reverse kind of error (a false-negative) certainly can occur, but tends to be rather less frequent. This is because a large number of factors (affective disorder, sensory impairment, infection, etc.) other than dementia can be responsible for a poor test performance. The number of causes that can push test performance in the reverse direction is much more limited.

Whilst the identification of dementia by psychological means is far from wholly accurate, useful levels of diagnostic validity can be obtained which compare favourably in the detection of early dementia with other forms of assessment, especially the general clinical examination and radiological methods. The fact that the key defining characteristic of dementia is a deterioration of cognitive functioning also means that neuropsychological assessment must be regarded as a major form of investigation for people with a suspected dementing disorder.

REFERENCES

Abrahams, J. T. and Birren, J. E. (1973). Reaction time as a function of age and behavioral predisposition to coronary heart disease. *Journal of Gerontology*, **28**, 471–8.

APA (1994). *Diagnostic and statistical manual of mental disorders* (4th ed). American Psychiatric Association, Washington, DC.

Benton, A. L. (1974). *The Revised Benton Visual Retention Test* (4th edn). Psychological Corporation, New York.

Blacker, D., Albert, M.S., Bassett, S.S., Go, R.C.P., Harrell, L.E., and Folstein, M.F. (1994). Reliability and validity of NINCDS–ADRDA criteria for Alzheimer's disease. *Archives of Neurology*, **51**, 1198–204.

Blessed, G., Tomlinson, B.E., and Roth, M. (1968). The association between quantitative measures of dementia and senile change in the cerebral grey matter of elderly subjects. *British Journal of Psychiatry*, **114**, 797–811.

Bolla, K.I., Lindgren, K.N., Bonaccorsy, C., and Bleaker, M.I. (1991). Memory complaints in older adults: fact or fiction? *Archives of Neurology*, **48**, 61–4.

Brazzelli, M., Capitani, E., Della Salla, S., and Zuffi, M. (1994). A neuropsychological instrument adding to the description of patients with suspected cortical dementia: the Milan overall dementia assessment. *Journal of Neurology, Neurosurgery and Psychiatry*, **57**, 1510–17.

Carr, A.T., Woods, R.T., and Moore, B.J. (1986*a*). Automated cognitive assessment of elderly patients: a comparison of two types of response device. *British Journal of Clinical Psychology*, **25**, 305–6.

Carr, A.T., Woods, R.T., and Moore, B.J. (1986*b*). Developing a micro-computer based automated testing system for use with psychogeriatric patients. *Bulletin of the Royal College of Psychiatrists*, **10**, 309–12.

Copeland, J.R.M., Dewey, M.E., and Griffith-Jones, H.M. (1986). A computerised diagnostic system and case nomenclature for elderly subjects: GMS and AGECAT. *Psychological Medicine*, **16**, 89–99.

Crawford, J.R. (1992). Current and premorbid intelligence measures in neuropsychological assessment. In *A handbook of neuropsychological assessment* (ed. J.R. Crawford, D.M. Parker, and W.W. McKinlay), pp. 21–49. Lawrence Erlbaum, Hove.

Crawford, J.R., Parker, D.M., and McKinley, W.W. (ed) (1992). *A handbook of neuropsychological assessment*. Lawrence Erlbaum, Hove.

Cummings, J.L. and Benson, D.F. (1992). *Dementia: a clinical* approach (2nd edn). Butterworth-Heinemann, Boston.

Erickson, R.C. and Scott, M.L. (1977). Clinical memory testing: a review. *Psychological Bulletin*, **84**, 1130–49.

Feehan, M., Knight, R.G., and Partridge, F.M. (1991). Cognitive complaint and test performance of elderly patients suffering from depression or dementia. *International Journal of Geriatric Psychiatry*, **6**, 287–93.

Folstein, M.F., Folstein, S.E., and McHugh, P.R. (1975). Mini-Mental State: a practical method for grading the cognitive state of the patient for the clinician. *Journal of Psychiatric Research*, **12**, 189–98.

Gibson, A.J., Moyes, I.C.A., and Kendrick, D.C. (1980). Cognitive assessment of the elderly long-stay patient. *British Journal of Psychiatry*, **137**, 537–55.

Hale, W.E., Stewart, R.E., Moore, M.T., and Marks, R.G. (1992). Electrocardiographic changes and cognitive impairment in the elderly. *Journal of Experimental and Clinical Gerontology*, **14**, 91–102.

Hart, S., Smith, C.M., and Swash, M. (1988). Word fluency in patients with early dementia of the Alzheimer's type. *British Journal of Clinical Psychology*, **27**, 115–24.

Hennekens, C.H. and Buring, J.E. (1987). *Epidemiology in medicine*. Little, Brown and Company, Boston.

Kaplan, E., goodglass, H., and Weintrout, S. (1983). *Boston Naming Test manual*. Lea & Febiger, Philadelphia.

Kapur, N. (1988). *Memory disorders in clinical practice*. Butterworths, London.

Kendrick, D.C., Gibson, A.J., and Moyes, I.C.A. (1979). The revised Kendrick battery: clinical studies. *British Journal of Clinical Psychology*, **18**, 329–40.

Kertesz, A. and Clydesdale, S. (1994). Neuropsychological deficits in vascular dementia vs Alzheimer's disease: frontal lobe deficits prominent in vascular dementia. *Archives of Neurology*, **51**, 1226–31.

Lezak, M. (1983). *Neuropsychological assessment* (2nd edn). Oxford University Press, New York.

McKenna, P. and Warrington E.K. (1983). *Graded Naming Test*. NFER-Nelson, Windsor.

McKhann, G., Drachman, D., Folstein, M., Katzman, R., Price, D., and Stadlin, E.M. (1984). Clinical diagnosis of Alzheimer's disease: report of the NINCDS—ADRDA work group under the auspices of the Department of Health and Human Services Task Force on Alzheimer's disease. *Neurology*, 34, 939–44.

Mattis, S. (1976). Mental status examination of organic mental syndrome in the elderly patient. In *Geriatric psychiatry*, (ed. L. Bellack and T.B. Karasu), pp. 71–121. Grune & Stratton, New York.

Mayes, A. and Warburg, R. (1992). Memory assessment in clinical practice and research. In *A handbook of neuropsychological assessment*, (ed. J.R. Crawford, D.M. Parker, and W. W. McKinley), pp. 73–101. Lawrence Erlbaum, Hove.

Meehl, P.E. and Rosen, A. (1955). Antecedent probabilities and the efficiency of psychometric signs, patterns or cutting scores. *Psychological Bulletin*, **52**, 194–216.

Mendez, M.F. and Ashla-Mendez, M. (1991). Difference between multi-infarct dementia and Alzheimer's disease on unstructured neuropsychological tests. *Journal of Clinical and Experimental Neuropsychology*, **13**, 923–32.

Complex visual disturbance in Alzheimer's disease. *Neurology*, **40**, 439–43.

Miller, E. (1968). A case for automated clinical testing. *Bulletin of the British Psychological Society*, **21**, 75–8.

Miller, E. (1977). *Abnmormal ageing*. Wiley, Chichester.

Miller, E. (1984*a*). *Recovery and management of neuropsychological impairments*. Wiley, Chichester.

Miller, E. (1984*b*). Word fluency as a function of a measure of verbal intelligence and in relation to different types of cerebral pathology. *British Journal of Clinical Psychology*, **23**, 53–7.

Miller, E. (1989). Language impairment in Alzheimer type dementia. *Clinical Psychology Review*, **9**, 181–95.

Miller, E. and Morris, R. (1993). *The psychology of dementia*. Wiley, Chichester.

Morris, J.C., Heyman, A., Mohs, R.C., Hughes, J.P., van Belle, G., Fillenbaum, G., *et al.*, and the CERAD investigators (1989). The Consortium to Establish a Register for Alzheimer's Disease (CERAD), I clinical and neuropsychological assessment for Alzheimer's disease. *Neurology*, **39**, 1159–65.

Morris, R.G. and Kopelman, M.D. (1992). The neuropsychological assessment of dementia. In *A handbook of neuropsychological assessment* (ed. J.R. Crawford, D.M. Parker, and W.W. McKinley), pp. 295–321. Lawrence Erlbaum, Hove.

Morris, R.G. and McKiernan, F. (1994). Neuropsychological investigations of dementia. In *Dementia* (ed. A. Burns and R. Levy), pp. 327–54. Chapman & Hall, London.

Morris, R.G., Evenden, J.L., Sahakian, B.J., and Robbins, T.W. (1987). Computer assisted assessment of dementia: comparative studies of neuropsychological deficits in Alzheimer-type dementia and Parkinson's disease. In *Cognitive neurochemistry* (ed. S. Stahl, S. Iverson, and E. Goodman), pp. 21–36. Oxford University Press.

Neary, D., Snowden, J.S., Bowen, D.H., Sims, N.R., Mann, D.M.A., Benton, J.S., *et al.* (1986). Neuropsychological syndromes in presenile dementia due to cerebral atrophy. *Journal of Neurology, Neurosurgery and Psychiatry*, **49**, 163–74.

Neary, D., Snowden, J.S., Northern, R., and Goulding, P. (1988). Dementia of the frontal lobe type. *Journal of Neurology, Neurosurgery and Psychiatry*, **51**, 353–61.

Nelson, A., Fogel, B.S., and Faust, D. (1986). Bedside cognitive screening instruments. A critical assessment. *Journal of Nervous and Mental Diseases*, **174**, 73–83.

Nelson, H. and O'Connell, A. (1978). Dementia: the estimation of premorbid intelligence using the new adult reading test. *Cortex*, **14**, 234–44.

O'Brien, J.T., Beats, B., Hill, K., Howard, R., Sahakien, B., and Levy, R. (1992). Do subjective memory complaints precede dementia? A three-year follow-up of patients with supposed 'benign senescent forgetfulness'. *International Journal of Geriatric Psychiatry*, **7**, 481–6.

O'Neill, P.M. and Calhoun, K.S. (1975). Sensory deficits and behavioral deterioration in senescense. *Journal of Abnormal Psychology*, **84**, 579–82.

Parks, R.W., Zec, R.F. and Wilson, R.S. (1993). *Neuropsychology of Alzheimer's disease and other dementias.* Oxford University Press, New York.

Perez, F.I., Gay, J.R.A., Taylor, R.L., and Rivera, V.M. (1975*a*). Patterns of memory performance in the neurologically impaired aged. *Canadian Journal of Neurological Science*, **2**, 347–55.

Perez, F.I., Rivera, V.M., Myer, J.S., Gay, J.R.A., Taylor, R.L., and Mathew, N.T. (1975*b*). Analysis of intellectual and cognitive performance in patients with multi-infarct dementia, vertebrobasilar deficiency with dementia and Alzheimer's disease. *Journal of Neurology, Neurosurgery and Psychiatry*, **38**, 533–40.

Rosen, W.G., Mohs, R.C. and Davis, K.L. (1984). A new rating scale for Alzheimer disease. *American Journal of Psychiatry*, **141**, 1356–64.

Roth, M., Tym, E., Mountjoy, Q.C., Huppert, F.A., Hendrie, H. Verma, S., and Goddard, R. (1986). CAMDEX: a standardized instrument for the diagnosis of mental disorder in the elderly with special reference to the early detection of dementia. *British Journal of Psychiatry*, **149**, 698–709.

Ryan, J.J. and Bohac, D.L. (1994). Neurodiagnostic implications of unique profiles of the Wechsler Adult Intelligence Scale—Revised. *Psychological Assessment*, **6**, 360–3.

Sahakian, B.J., Morris, R.G., Evenden, J.L., Heald, A., Levy, R., Philpot, M., *et al.* (1988). A comparative study of visuospatial memory and learning in Alzheimer-type dementia and Parkinson's disease. *Brain*, **111**, 695–718.

Salmon, D.P. and Butters, N.M. (1992). Neuropsychological assessment of dementia in the elderly. In *Principles of geriatric neurology* (ed. R. Katzman and J.W.Rowe), pp. 144–93. F.A. Davies, Philadelphia.

Strub, R.L. and Black, F.W. (1977). *The Mental Status Examination in neurology.* F.A. Davis, Philadelphia.

Warrington, E.K. (1984). *Recognition Memory Test.* NFER-Nelson, Windsor.

Wechsler, D. (1987). *Wechsler Memory Scale—revised.* The Psychological Corporation, San Antonio.

Welsh, K., Butters, N., Hughes, J., Mohs, R., and Heyman, A. (1991). Detection of abnormal memory decline in mild cases of Alzheimer's disease using CERAD neuropsychological measures. *Archives of Neurology*, **48**, 278–81.

Welsh, K., Butters, N., Hughes, J.P., Mohs, R.C., and Heyman, A. (1992). Detection and staging of dementia of Alzheimer's disease: use of the neuropsychological measures developed for the Consortium to Establish a Register for Alzheimer's Disease. *Archives of Neurology*, **49**, 448–52.

Wilson, B., Cockburn, J., and Baddeley, A. (1985). *The Rivermead Behavioural Memory Test.* Thames Valley Test Co., Reading, Berkshire, UK.

Worrall, G., Moulton, N., and Briffett, E. (1993). Effect of type II diabetes mellitus on cognitive function. *Journal of Family Practice*, **36**, 639–43.

Yesavage, J.A., Brink, T.L., Rose, T.L., Lum, D., Huang, V., Adey, M., *et al.* (1983). Development and validation of a Geriatric Depression Screening Scale: a preliminary report. *Gerontologist*, **20**, 260–6.

SEVENTEEN

Cognitive approaches to the management of dementia

Bob Woods

INTRODUCTION

Psychological approaches to the management of dementia have an extensive history (see early reviews by Miller 1977; Woods and Britton 1977). The word 'management' may be preferable to 'treatment' or 'therapy' in view of the connotations of lasting improvement and of change in the underlying disorder implicit in the other terms. Management may be taken to suggest the aims of ameliorating certain aspects of the disorder, reducing disability in certain circumstances, or lowering the frequency of behavioural problems associated with the disorder, without a particular expectation of the maintenance or the generalization of the effects of the intervention. Management also implies a continuing, rather than a time-limited, intervention.

The emphasis of this chapter will be on interventions with a cognitive focus; however, it must be borne in mind that cognitive impairments form only part of the characteristic symptoms of the dementias, and that other aspects, specifically the affective and behavioural, will also be important and are often interwoven with the cognitive features. The relationship of changes on measures of cognitive function to those in 'real-life' have been of particular concern. Out of these, memory dysfunction is often described as an early and virtually universal cognitive feature of the dementias and most of the studies to date have tended to focus on this topic almost to the exclusion of other domains. However, in this chapter an attempt will be made to highlight other areas of cognitive function that might usefully be targeted.

Several general management approaches to dementia with a strong cognitive flavour have been developed; the evidence for their efficacy will first be reviewed, before examining in more detail the specific cognitive strategies which might be utilized in management programmes. Finally, such strategies will be placed in the context of the broader picture of working with the individual person with dementia.

MANAGEMENT APPROACHES WITH A COGNITIVE FOCUS

Reality orientation

This long-established psychosocial approach has been used with older people with dementia for over 30 years, and an extensive literature, both evaluative and descriptive, is available (see Holden and Woods 1995; Miller and Morris 1993; Woods 1992 for full reviews).

Two major components of Reality Orientation (RO) are described. The 24-hour RO (or informal RO) involves a number of changes to the environment, with clear signposting of locations around the ward or home, extensive use of notices and other memory aids, and a consistent approach by all staff in interacting with the person with dementia. In its original form, it was intended that staff undertaking 24-hour RO would offer orientating information in each and every interaction; more recently, a modification has been described where staff are trained to take a more reactive stance, orientating the person only in response to his/her requests (Reeve and Ivison 1985; Williams *et al.* 1987). RO sessions (or RO classes) are structured group sessions, involving a small number of patients and staff, meeting regularly, often several times a week for half an hour or so. A wide variety of activities and materials are used to engage the patients with their surroundings, to maintain contact with the wider world, and to provide cognitive stimulation. A typical session would go over basic information (such as names of those in the group, day, date, time, and place), discuss a current relevant theme of interest, perhaps play a number or naming game, and finish with refreshments. Throughout there would be a tangible focus: a white-board for the current information; pictures or objects appropriate to the theme; personal diaries and notebooks for those able to record information for later use.

Holden and Woods (1995) have identified 21 studies meeting the criterion of reporting an evaluation of the effects of RO in comparison with either no-treatment or an alternative intervention. The studies vary in many ways:

1. *In the type of RO evaluated*: only one-third of studies included 24-hour RO; just two of these evaluated the extent to which this intensive approach was actually being implemented.

2. *In setting*: hospital wards, residential and nursing homes, day centres, and out-patients have all been used, with some variability in the specificity of the diagnosis of dementia.

3. *In measures used*: a wide variety of brief cognitive scales (mainly orientation tests) and behaviour rating scales have been adopted.

4. *In the length of the intervention period*: the briefest period was three weeks, the longest a year; frequency of RO sessions varied from twice daily to once a week; most studies had sessions five times a week.

5. *In design and methodological adequacy*: whilst some studies have randomly allocated patients to groups, others have had comparison groups in different wards/homes/units. Each approach has its problems, the former especially where 24-hour RO is included. Few studies have employed raters 'blind' to group membership; few have followed-up patients after the end of the intervention.

6. *In comparison groups included*: no-treatment has been most commonly used, but about a third of studies have offered an alternative group activity, sometimes as a 'placebo' to control for the effects of attention, at times as a viable alternative to RO sessions.

Despite these variations in methodology the conclusions are remarkably consistent. First, there is strong support for RO sessions being associated with increased scores on measures of verbal orientation, as compared with no-treatment control groups. One study to date (Williams *et al.* 1987) has reported cognitive changes that could be attributed specifically to 24-hour RO, but, as mentioned above, few studies have actually demonstrated its implementation. With the emphasis in RO on verbal orientation, these findings are perhaps not so surprising (although may require some explanation). More controversial are suggestions that more general cognitive improvements may occur. Some studies suggest that only those orientation items specifically taught are learned; others that from a battery of cognitive tests, only the orientation items show improvement. More recent reports have tended to support the notion that more wide-ranging improvements in new learning ability may follow cognitive stimulation of this type (e.g. Breuil *et al.* 1994; Zanetti *et al.* 1993).

The second main conclusion is that changes in function and behaviour are much more elusive than cognitive changes; in general, they have been the exception rather than the rule. There are many possible factors in this difference between the change in cognitive test performance and real-life function. Behavioural rating scales used have often been less sensitive to the small changes envisaged; an environment encouraging dependence (as many have been shown to do) may counteract any benefits from group sessions; questions may also be raised as to the extent to which verbal orientation underlies many of the areas of function, such as feeding and dressing, which comprise much of the content of the behaviour rating scales typically used. It may be argued that direct training of a particular skill will be required for behavioural change; several workers have shown this in relation to ward orientation—the person finding his/her way around the ward/home. Improvements in this domain have been shown in relation to specific training by Hanley *et al.* (1981) and associated with 24-hour RO by Reeve and Ivison (1985) and Williams *et al.* (1987). All these studies have in common a demonstrable intervention in the person's living environment; the former through direct training, the other two through the monitored evaluation of 24-hour RO; these studies have, in fact, shown the greatest range of behavioural improvement of all the studies reviewed.

The RO literature raises many questions, but does indicate that scope for cognitive management in dementia does exist. Some of the more detailed findings will be mentioned in later sections.

Reminiscence therapy

The use of past memories to establish a point of interest and contact has often been used in RO sessions, and has attracted interest as an approach in its own right (Gibson 1994; Woods and McKiernan 1995). Reminiscence work with older people more generally developed from psychotherapeutic considerations, emphasizing the place of life review in adaptation. Haight and Burnside (1993) draw attention to the way in which this psychotherapeutic use of life review has been confused with other reminiscence work, such as that with people with dementia. Here the cognitive roots of using this approach arise from the apparent preservation of remote memory in dementia; the person appears to remember events from their childhood, whilst unable to recall what he/she had for lunch. Of course, when this area has been systematically tested, recall for specific events from many years ago is not relatively preserved (Morris 1994); performance across the lifespan is depressed compared with age-matched controls. People with dementia—like normal older people—recall more memories from early life; such memories are often over-learned or well rehearsed, or have particular personal and/or emotional significance for the person concerned. Morris points out that studies of autobiographical memory indicate there is typically virtually no recall from the person's middle years; this disconnection must add greatly to the difficulty of regaining orientation to the present time.

Reminiscence therapy has been used with individuals and in small groups (Gibson 1994; Norris 1986; Thornton and Brotchie 1987; Woods *et al.* 1992). Photographs, music, and archive recordings and items from the past are used to stimulate a variety of personal memories. Evaluative studies with people with dementia are few, and a clear picture has yet to emerge. For example Baines *et al.* (1987) report results from two groups, with only one (which had first undergone RO sessions) showing improvements in orientation and function outside the group. There are reports of it being an enjoyable activity for many older people with dementia, with evident increases in interaction (Woods and McKiernan 1995), but there is little evidence of any effect on cognitive function or function outside the group setting. However, studies have tended to focus on non-cognitive aspects or on current orientation; it would be of interest to evaluate the impact of this approach on autobiographical memory in the first instance, perhaps using a measure such as the Autobiographical Memory Interview (Kopelman *et al.* 1990).

SPECIFIC COGNITIVE STRATEGIES

A number of more specific approaches to the improvement/maintenance of cognitive performance in people with dementia have been suggested; some have been applied, often in single-case studies; others are implications arising from the empirical literature on cognitive dysfunctions in the dementias, and await evaluation in practice. Essentially, the rationale underlying this area is to identify areas of function and processes that are relatively unimpaired, and to maximize their use, whilst placing less reliance on areas and processes where the impairment is greater. Similarly, the conditions under which performance is known to be enhanced are replicated wherever possible.

Reduce cognitive load

Studies on attention in AD suggest that whilst focused attention is relatively unimpaired, divided attention is less efficient (Nebes and Brady 1989). There is ample evidence that performance is impaired when two tasks are undertaken in parallel, even if the subsidiary task appears likely to require minimal processing capacity because of its automatic nature (Morris 1994; see also Chapter 4). These difficulties, reflecting reduced capacity of the central executive system in the working memory model, imply that the cognitive demands on people with dementia should be simplified as far as possible, and that efforts should be made to avoid competing demands on attention. For example 'background' noise during an activity session, or several people talking at once, or a lot of movement and noise during a meal might, for some patients, split attention sufficiently to impair performance at the primary activity.

Real life is, of course, full of complexity. Alberoni *et al.* (1992) have examined some of the processes involved in group conversations. People with dementia had difficulty in remembering who said what in a group conversation, particularly as the group size increased.

Patients tended to use spatial location as a cue, and performance was particularly disrupted when group members changed places. These difficulties were elicited in relation to patients watching a video-tape of a group conversation, rather than participating themselves, and in an actual conversation, with familiar people, the problems might not be so marked. Alberoni *et al.* suggest that one-to-one interactions might accordingly be the preferable focus for rehabilitation efforts, rather than group-work which has often been the norm in both RO and Reminiscence Therapy. Morris (1994) argues that these deficits mean group therapies 'can degenerate into a monologue between individual staff members and patients'. For example in reminiscence sessions Woods *et al.* (1992) showed that the majority of interactions taking place were between staff and patients; as would be predicted, they occurred more often between patients in a smaller group. The advantages of working in a group—peer support, a social atmosphere, shared experiences—need to be weighed against their undoubted cognitive demands, in repeatedly shifting and refocusing attention, as well as in keeping track of who says what in the group (Hart and Semple 1990). Where groups are used, they should be as small as possible, with members retaining the same seating position from session to session; background noise and distractions should be kept to a minimum, and care taken to ensure that only one person speaks at a time.

Other practical means of reducing the cognitive load for the person with dementia in communication may be identified (e.g. Hart and Semple 1990, p. 241 therein). The aim is to reduce the memory and/or information processing load. This can be achieved by using short, simple sentences. Where the sentence is more complex, the initial clauses should contain the crux of the communication, with later ones elaborating ('right-branching'). If later clauses arc needed to understand previous ones ('left-branching'), the person with dementia is likely to miss the point. The frequent use of pronouns places a load on immediate memory, which may simply be reduced by repeating the referents. Closed questions, which limit the number of response alternatives may assist the person who has difficulty in generating a sequence of ideas, even when this has been part of the person's knowledge base (a schema or 'script', Grafman *et al.* 1991). As a general principle, communication that has a high degree of redundancy, with salient points restated and a focus on the directly familiar and observable, is more likely to be effective. Supplementing the spoken word with pictorial information or objects, allows more efficient access to semantic memory. Non-verbal communication, which may show less decline in dementia, may also add to the redundancy of the verbal material, with eye-contact an important way of gaining and holding the person's attention.

In the area of memory ability, the aim is for memory and learning to become a less critical component of daily life. Examples would include labelling doors, signposting directions, placing required items in prominent positions, and so on. This approach, which has ready applicability to people with dementia, has links with the concept of a 'prosthetic environment' (Holden and Woods 1995); the environment is designed as far as possible to require the minimum of memory function to operate within it. Care must be taken not to overload the person with such a plethora of information boards and signs creating the irony that the person is unable to find the information they required in the first place. Providing accurate information is essential, if the person is to rely on these sources; this is not always achieved in practice.

External memory aids

External memory aids reduce the level of demand on effortful, self-initiated cognitive processes and provide support for the person in cueing and prompting retrieval of information—a key feature of effective cognitive training approaches (Backman 1992). Retrieval cues in dementia generally require a high degree of specificity in order to be effective. External aids which are rather non-specific, such as an alarm clock or a kitchen timer, reminding the person to do *something* are of relatively little use; the person may be prompted by the aid to remember something had to be done, but requires further assistance in recalling what it is they were meant to do! The effects of more specific aids have mainly been demonstrated through single-case studies. For example a 68-year-old patient with a severe memory impairment successfully used a diary to prompt continuing awareness of personal information taught to her in daily individual sessions (Woods 1983). Hanley and Lusty (1984) report a single-case study where an 84-year-old patient with dementia was able to achieve a higher level of orientation, using a watch and diary as retrieval cues. Specific training was required in the use of the cues; without this, the patient did not make use of them spontaneously. During the training phase, the patient kept a far greater proportion of her 'appointments' than previously, demonstrating a behavioural orientation, as well as being better able to answer the items of a personalized orientation measure.

In a series of studies Bourgeois (1990, 1992) evaluated the effects of a prosthetic memory aid on conversational skills in people with dementia. The aid consisted of photographs and pictures of past and more recent events, important people in the person's life, and so on, in a convenient robust wallet or book format. The person's spouse and other visitors were encouraged to use the aid when talking with the person. The results suggest that its use was associated with less ambiguous utterances and more statements of fact. The quality of conversation was assessed by independent raters as being significantly improved with the use of the aid as a focus for conversation. The aid is also reported to have proved useful in improving the quality of interaction between pairs of people with dementia. Although the aid is described as a prosthesis, its effects appear to be as much in prompting a number of memories related to each item, rather than simply acting as a replacement memory store for the specific information contained therein.

External memory aids have been explicitly used to reduce the load on the person's own memory and support retrieval in daily living tasks (Josephsson *et al.* 1993). In this study, four patients with dementia were evaluated on tasks such as preparing and consuming a drink or snack. Signs on drawers and cupboards indicated the location of required items. Physical demonstrations of task components were provided, for the patient to repeat. Verbal prompts and cues were also given. Improvements in task performance were shown by three patients; for two of these, continued environmental support and guidance was needed to maintain these gains. The remaining patient's lack of improvement was attributed to a high level of anxiety interfering with the learning process.

The need for staff input, at least initially, in reinforcing the use of the external aids is seen in the RO literature on signposting. Signs are usually more effective when combined with staff involvement, pointing out the signs and using them to orientate the person in training sessions (Gilleard *et al.* 1981; Hanley 1981). Such signposts may be viewed as retrieval cues; certainly some people with dementia are capable of benefiting from them, if prompted or trained in their use.

Internal memory strategies

Although widely used, generally, in memory re-training, internal memory strategies have had less impact in relation to dementia. Such strategies include the clustering of items to be recalled, or recalling the most recent items first, as well as more artificial strategies making use of various mnemonics. These might include the method of loci, where the person learns to visualize a route around their home or familiar place, and then commits a list of items to memory by visualizing each in turn at a different location on the route. Alternatively, the patient may be instructed to make a visual association between some aspect of another person's name and his/her appearance and facial features, to assist later recall. Verbal strategies might include working through the alphabet in an attempt to cue with the initial letter the retrieval of a word to be recalled. The problem in dementia is that usually the patient will have difficulty in learning and remembering to use the strategy; generally internal strategies have proved more difficult to implement and been associated with less clinically relevant gains than external memory aids (Bäckman 1992). An exception is a single-case reported by Hill *et al.* (1987); here a 66-year-old patient with dementia was taught to use visual imagery to remember the names associated with particular photographs of faces. The average interval over which the associations were retained increased from less than 3 minutes to over 6 minutes. The patient learned to identify a prominent facial feature and to make a visual image associated with the name; however, he rarely remembered to associate the feature with the image. Hill *et al.* point out that the effects were relatively modest, although the gains had not disappeared at one-month follow-up. At present, approaches such as this and the method of loci seem to demand a great deal of effort for relatively little return: as Twining (1991) advises, 'If you have to remember a list, just make sure it is written down, and then spend the time doing something you enjoy'.

New learning

There is compelling evidence of some limited potential for new learning in dementia (see Miller and Morris 1993). In particular, it is thought that once information is adequately encoded, the rate of forgetting after the first 10 minutes or so may be virtually normal. Several techniques to achieve initial learning have been described.

In spaced retrieval or expanded rehearsal (see, for example, Camp and Schaller 1989; Moffat 1989) only one item at a time is learned; on each trial the retrieval period is adjusted according to whether the item was successfully recalled during the preceding trial; if it was, it is doubled, if not, it is halved. In this way, the item becomes fully registered, and subject to a relatively normal rate of forgetting, rather than the immediate decay of the memory trace usually associated with dementia. The next item is only taught when the first is fully established. Although this seems (and is) a laborious process, there is some evidence that learning may generalize to items not specifically taught in some situations. For example Moffat (1989) indicated some generalization in retrieving the names of pictures of objects in a younger patient with Alzheimer's disease.

Bäckman (1992) suggests that learning potential is greatest where increased support is given both during learning and at the time of retrieval. More learning trials, with fewer items at a time, will be needed; more guidance in coding the material is required, in addition to more cues to aid retrieval. Studies conducted by Bäckman and his colleagues suggest that encoding information in the form of a motor act (such as acting out a movement associated with the word to be learned) is helpful, even where the degree of dementia is severe (see also Martin *et al.* 1985). An example of support at encoding and retrieval is provided by Sandman (1993). He showed that people with dementia improved their recall of a TV programme when they worked with their relatives on creating their own test questions on it (that is to say they established their own retrieval cues at the time of learning). Self-generated cues are likely to be the most effective.

From the same study comes a further example of how support at the time of encoding might be given, by making the event more distinctive and memorable. Care-givers of dementia sufferers planned a significant event with them, chosen to stand out from the usual routine. This might be a picnic, trips out, or a meal at a special restaurant. Patients were subsequently asked about details of the day, not directly related to the event, such as what they were wearing, who they met that day, and so on. Patients showed normal recall for items from these special days, whilst being significantly impaired on items from ordinary days. Care-givers are often encouraged to develop a routine, as this may reduce memory load; this should not, however, be at the cost of having nothing worth remembering.

These findings have some immediate practical implications. One is to 'de-emphasize memorization as a goal' (Sandman 1993). By making the experience as rich and meaningful as possible, memories associated with it will be enhanced. Helping the person to work on the material (but *not* asking them to remember it) and using retrieval cues are probably the best ways of enhancing performance.

Implicit and procedural memory

Implicit memory refers to performance of a task being enhanced without conscious or explicit recall of material. It is an aspect of memory generally viewed as relatively spared in dementia. An example is learning on a motor skills task (also described as procedural memory), where learning rates have been shown to be preserved in people with dementia (Miller and Morris 1993). Zanetti *et al.* (1994), in a brief report outline a rehabilitation programme for people with dementia based on procedural memory, requiring no explicit memory effort. Employing the time taken to perform various basic and instrumental acts of daily living tasks as the outcome measure, four patients are reported to have shown improvements after 3 weeks of daily one-hour training sessions. Improvements were noted on both the specific activities trained and control tasks not included in the programme.

A second example of implicit memory is 'priming', where exposure to an item enhances the processing of that, or a related item. As indicated in Chapter 7, under certain circumstances, AD patients can exhibit normal performance on priming tasks.

Making use of preserved implicit memory, by reducing reliance on effortful processing, and building on more automatic, well-preserved skills is an approach with much to commend it. These processes could be seen as underlying several approaches described previously, for example spaced retrieval (Bäckman 1992), retrieval cues (Josephsson *et al.* 1993), ward orientation training (e.g. Lam and Woods 1986). However, two caveats should be noted. First, the various forms of implicit memory may not all be affected in the same way by the person's dementia. Thus, Heindel *et al.* (1989) indicate that people with Huntington's disease show an impairment on procedural memory, but not on lexical priming, whereas people with Alzheimer-type dementia show the opposite pattern. Parkinson's disease patients with dementia were impaired on both types of implicit memory. Second, it should not be assumed that such techniques help the person achieve 'normal' memory. The person in fact may have little or no conscious memory of the event (as is suggested by the definition); what is being accessed are more automatic processes, achieving the goal by a different pathway. Indeed the person may feel they are guessing the answer (Downes 1987). However, to achieve a goal by a different route is a perfectly reasonable rehabilitation goal, and this approach is worth pursuing on this basis.

AN INDIVIDUALIZED APPROACH TO COGNITIVE MANAGEMENT IN DEMENTIA

Individual differences in the pattern and severity of cognitive deficits in people with dementia arise from the variety of conditions underlying the dementias, their progressive course, with a changing pattern over time, and the apparently almost haphazard localization of certain types of pathology. In applying cognitive strategies to management of the individual case, several factors must be considered.

Assess and build on strengths

It is essential that an individualized plan is developed, based on an understanding of the individual's pattern of abilities and deficits. Are there particular processes, modalities, or materials which are relatively well preserved, and that can be used extensively to compensate for the more impaired areas? For example, one patient may have relatively intact visual memory, but poor verbal learning ability; another might be able to benefit from written presentation of verbal material, having preserved word-reading ability, whereas the same items presented only in the auditory modality would be less well recalled. Studies such as those of Grafman *et al.* (1991), on script generation, and Heindel *et al.* (1989) on implicit memory, reflect differences in the pattern of functioning between patients with dementia. Unfortunately, the emphasis in the development of assessment measures has been so much on diagnosis (and impaired function) that the assessment and description of preserved abilities remains a complex task.

Work with care-givers

Most people with dementia are supported by family members, who often experience considerable strain (Morris *et al.* 1988). The care-giver's perspective is vital. What difficulties are seen as most significant? Is participation in a cognitive management programme simply an additional burden? Is there a danger of making a difficult relationship more fraught, perhaps where considerable criticism and tension already exists?

Notes of caution may be identified in the literature; negative effects on care-givers when the person with dementia attended a memory training group (Zarit *et al.* 1982); family carers reporting no improvement in conversation, despite independent raters noting significant improvements (Bourgeois 1990). The extent of the loss experienced by the care-giver must not be underestimated; interventions, even if effective, may be perceived as being peripheral to such loss.

Quayhagen and Quayhagen (1989) provide a relatively rare example of successfully involving family care-givers, who carried out daily sessions of cognitive stimulation, memory provoking exercises, and problem-solving techniques with their relative. The patients showed cognitive and emotional improvement; care-givers did not report greater burden or symptoms of depression, unlike a control group, who had in fact refused to take part in the training programme (and so may not be the best comparison group). Involving care-givers is a complex matter. Often others who are less involved, under less strain, and experiencing less loss may be better placed to take on direct involvement in interventions. Perhaps as early ascertainment of dementia becomes more common, greater family involvement may be feasible, before strain has begun to escalate.

Cognition and emotion

Dementia does not, of course, simply have a direct impact on cognitive functions such as memory, language and attention. Behavioural disturbance and the person's reaction to the disorder are also of great importance. For example anxiety or depression in a person with dementia will further reduce performance levels. Kitwood (1990) argues that under-functioning is commonplace in dementia, in that the person functions at a level below the limits set by the actual neurological impairment. The disparity is attributed to the person withdrawing, in reaction to devaluing, invalidating, dehumanizing aspects of the social environment. As well as having far-reaching implications for the care environment (Kitwood and Bredin 1992), this work does point to the need to consider the interaction of cognitive, emotional, and behavioural aspects. There are increasing reports of the use of psychotherapeutic techniques with people with dementia, including relaxation therapy (Welden and Yesavage 1982), cognitive behavioural therapy (Thompson *et al.* 1990), and psychodynamic approaches (Hausman 1992; Sinason 1992), assisting adjustment to the changes occurring. There is also a growing literature on interventions for behavioural problems in dementia (see Holden and Woods 1995).

The growth of interest in Validation therapy (Feil 1992) similarly indicates a movement to recognize affective aspects of dementia. In Validation therapy (Feil 1993) attempts are made to discern and respond to the emotional content of what the person says, rather than focusing on the factual, cognitive content. It has developed partly as a reaction to the over-cognitive application of RO, which applied insensitively can become confrontational, constantly 'correcting' the person rather than seeking to understand the attempted communication (Dietch *et al.* 1989). Evaluative studies are rather inconclusive to date (e.g. Bleathman and Morton 1992; Morton and Bleathman 1991), but clinicians are clearly finding the techniques a valuable aid to communication (Woods 1992).

At a theoretical level, Williams (1994) suggests that the Interacting Cognitive Subsystems model, developed by Teasdale and Barnard (1993), may be helpful. It proposes two meaning subsystems: Propositional and Implicational, reflecting cognitive and emotional representations, respectively. If the Implicational subsystem is intact, the Propositional subsystem will not be able to make sense of its output in relation to recent events, as propositional event memory is clearly impaired in dementia. Instead, it will use material relating to events perhaps many years previously to complete the fragmented description emerging from the Implicational subsystem. For example, the person's emotion of feeling lonely and abandoned, generated in the Implicational subsystem may only be interpretable propositionally, as, 'Where is my mother?' The task for the care-giver is to respond at a level that connects with the Implicational content. Reframing Validation in this way may assist in developing the approach from a theoretical foundation.

CONCLUSIONS

The extent and severity of cognitive changes in the dementias represent a real challenge to cognitive management approaches. Some approaches are available, and there are some promising indications of directions worth exploring. Clearly problems are more likely where episodic memory or even semantic memory are relied upon. Positive results are possible where the cognitive load is kept to a minimum, where procedural memory and certain aspect of implicit memory can be utilized, where strong support is provided for encoding *and* retrieval, with the use of retrieval cues where appropriate (see also Chapter 5). Programmes need to be fairly extensive, and to address how any improvements will be maintained. Finally, cognitive aspects in practice cannot be addressed in isolation from emotional and behavioural features.

REFERENCES

Alberoni, M., Baddeley, A., Della-Sala, S., Logie, R., and Spinnler, H. (1992). Keeping track of a conversation: impairments in Alzheimer's disease. *International Journal of Geriatric Psychiatry*, **7**, 639–46.

Bäckman, L. (1992). Memory training and memory improvement in Alzheimer's disease: rules and exceptions. *Acta Neurologia Scandinavica* (Suppl. 139), 84–9.

Baines, S., Saxby, P., and Ehlert, K. (1987). Reality orientation and reminiscence therapy: a controlled cross-over study of elderly confused people. *British Journal of Psychiatry*, **151**, 222–31.

Bleathman, C. and Morton, I. (1992). Validation therapy: extracts from 20 groups with dementia sufferers. *Journal of Advanced Nursing*, **17**, 658–66.

Bourgeois, M. S. (1990). Enhancing conversation skills in patients with Alzheimer's disease using a prosthetic memory aid. *Journal of Applied Behavior Analysis*, **23**, 29–42.

Bourgeois, M. S. (1992). *Conversing with memory impaired individuals using memory aids: a memory aid workbook.* Winslow Press, Bicester.

Breuil, V., Rotrou, J. D., Forette, F., Tortrat, D., Ganansia-Ganem, A., Frambourt, A., *et al.* (1994). Cognitive stimulation of patients with dementia: preliminary results. *International Journal of Geriatric Psychiatry*, **9**, 211–17.

Camp, C. J. and Schaller, J. R. (1989). Epilogue: spaced-retrieval memory training in an adult day-care center. *Educational Gerontology*, **15**, 641–8.

Dietch, J. T., Hewett, L. J., and Jones, S. (1989). Adverse effects of reality orientation. *Journal of American Geriatrics Society*, **37**, 974–6.

Downes, J. (1987). Classroom RO and the enhancement of orientation—a critical note. *British Journal of Clinical Psychology*, **26**, 147–8.

Feil, N. (1992). Validation therapy with late-onset dementia populations. In *Care-giving in dementia: research and applications* (ed. G. Jones and B. Miesen), pp. 199–218. Routledge, London.

Feil, N. (1993). *The Validation breakthrough: simple techniques for communicating with people with 'Alzheimer's type dementia'*. Health Professions Press, Baltimore.

Gibson, F. (1994). What can reminiscence contribute to people with dementia? In *Reminiscence reviewed: evaluations, achievements* (ed. J. Bornat), pp. 46–60. Open University Press, Buckingham.

Gilleard, C., Mitchell, R. G., and Riordan, J. (1981). Ward orientation training with psychogeriatric patients. *Journal of Advanced Nursing*, **6**, 95–8.

Grafman, J., Thompson, K., Weingartner, H., Martinez, R., Lawlor, B. A., and Sunderland, T. (1991). Script generation as an indicator of knowledge representation in patients with Alzheimer's disease. *Brain and Language*, **40**, 344–58.

Haight, B. K. and Burnside, I. (1993). Reminiscence and life review: explaining the differences. *Archives of Psychiatric Nursing*, **7**, 91–8.

Hanley, I. G. (1981). The use of signposts and active training to modify ward disorientation in elderly patients. *Journal of Behaviour Therapy and Experimental Psychiatry*, **12**, 241–7.

Hanley, I. G., McGuire, R. J., and Boyd, W. D. (1981). Reality orientation and dementia: a controlled trial of two approaches. *British Journal of Psychiatry*, **138**, 10–14.

Hanley, I.G. and Lusty, K. (1984). Memory aids in reality orientation: a single-case study. *Behaviour Research and Therapy*, **22**, 709–12.

Hart, S. and Semple, J. M. (1990). *Neuropsychology and the dementias*. Taylor & Francis, London.

Hausman, C. (1992). Dynamic psychotherapy with elderly demented patients. In *Care-giving in dementia: research and applications*, (ed. G. Jones and B. M. L. Miesen), pp. 181–98. Routledge, London.

Heindel, W. C., Salmon, D. P., Shults, C. W., Walicke, P. A., and Butters, N. (1989). Neuropsychological evidence for multiple implicit memory systems: a comparison of Alzheimer's, Huntington's and Parkinson's disease patients. *Journal of Neuroscience*, **9**, 582–7.

Hill, R. D., Evankovich, K. D., Sheikh, J. I., and Yesavage, J. A. (1987). Imagery mnemonic training in a patient with primary degenerative dementia. *Psychology and Aging*, **2**, 204–5.

Holden, U. P. and Woods, R. T. (1995). *Positive approaches to dementia care* (3rd edn). Churchill Livingstone, Edinburgh.

Josephsson, S., Backman, L., Borell, L., Bernspang, B., Nygard, L., and Ronnberg, L. (1993). Supporting everyday activities in dementia: an intervention study. *International Journal of Geriatric Psychiatry*, **8**, 395–400.

Kitwood, T. (1990). The dialectics of dementia: with particular reference to Alzheimer's disease. *Ageing and Society*, **10**, 177–96.

Kitwood, T. and Bredin, K. (1992). Towards a theory of dementia care: personhood and well-being. *Ageing and Society*, **12**, 269–87.

Kopelman, M., Wilson, B., and Baddeley, A. (1990). *The autobiographical memory interview*. Thames Valley Test Company, Titchfield, Hants.

Lam, D. H. and Woods, R. T. (1986). Ward orientation training in dementia: a single-case study. *International Journal of Geriatric Psychiatry*, **1**, 145–7.

Martin, A., Browers, P., Cox, C., and Fedio, P. (1985). On the nature of the verbal memory deficits in Alzheimer's disease. *Brain and Language*, **25**, 323–41.

Miller, E. (1977). The management of dementia: a review of some possibilities. *British Journal of Social and Clinical Psychology*, **16**, 77–83.

Miller, E. and Morris, R. (1993). *The psychology of dementia.* Wiley, Chichester.

Moffat, N. J. (1989). Home-based cognitive rehabilitation with the elderly. In *Everyday cognition in adulthood and late life,* (ed. L. W. Poon, D. C. Rubin, and B. A. Wilson), pp. 659–80. Cambridge University Press, Cambridge.

Morris, R. G. (1994). Recent developments in the neuropsychology of dementia. *International Review of Psychiatry,* **6**, 85–107.

Morris, R. G., Morris, L. W., and Britton, P. G. (1988). Factors affecting the emotional well-being of the caregivers of dementia sufferers. *British Journal of Psychiatry,* **153**, 147–56.

Morton, I. and Bleathman, C. (1991). The effectiveness of validation therapy in dementia: a pilot study. *International Journal of Geriatric Psychiatry,* **6**, 327–30.

Nebes, R. D. and Brady, C. B. (1989). Focused and divided attention in Alzheimer's disease. *Cortex,* **25**, 305–15.

Norris, A. (1986). *Reminiscence.* Winslow Press, London.

Quayhagen, M.P. and Quayhagen, M. (1989). Differential effects of family-based strategies on Alzheimer's disease. *Gerontologist,* **29**, 150–5.

Reeve, W. and Ivison, D. (1985). Use of environmental manipulation and classroom and modified informal reality orientation with institutionalized, confused elderly patients. *Age and Ageing,* **14**, 119–21.

Sandman, C. A. (1993). Memory rehabilitation in Alzheimer's disease: preliminary findings. *Clinical Gerontologist,* **13**, 19–33.

Sinason, V. (1992). The man who was losing his brain. In *Mental handicap and the human condition: new approaches from the Tavistock* (ed. V. Sinason), pp. 87–110. Free Association Books, London.

Teasdale, J.D. and Barnard, P.J. (1993). *Affect, cognition and change.* Erlbaum, Hove.

Thompson, L. W., Wagner, B., Zeiss, A., and Gallagher, D. (1990). Cognitive/behavioural therapy with early stage Alzheimer's patients: an exploratory view of the utility of this approach. In *Alzheimer's disease: treatment and family stress,* (ed. E. Light and B. D. Lebowitz), pp. 383–97. Hemisphere, New York.

Thornton. S. and Brotchie, J. (1987). Reminiscence: a critical review of the empirical literature. *British Journal of Clinical Psychology,* **26**, 93–111.

Twining, C. (1991). *The memory handbook.* Winslow Press, Bicester.

Welden, S. and Yesavage, J. A. (1982). Behavioral improvement with relaxation training in senile dementia. *Clinical Gerontologist,* **1**, 45–9.

Williams, J.M.G. (1994). Interacting cognitive subsystems and unvoiced murmurs: a review of *Affect cognition and change* by John Teasdale and Philip Barnard. *Cognition and Emotion,* **8**, 571–4.

Williams, R., Reeve, W., Ivison, D., and Kavanagh, D. (1987). Use of environmental manipulation and modified informal reality orientation with institutionalized confused elderly subjects: a replication. *Age and Ageing,* **16**, 315–18.

Woods, R. T. (1983). Specificity of learning in reality orientation sessions: a single-case study, *Behaviour Research and Therapy,* **21**, 173–5.

Woods, R. T. (1992). What can be learned from studies on reality orientation? In *Care-giving in dementia,* (ed. G. Jones and B. Miesen), pp. 121–36. Routledge, London.

Woods, R. T. and Britton, P. G. (1977). Psychological approaches to the treatment of the elderly. *Age and Ageing,* **6**, 104–12.

Woods, R. T. and McKiernan, F. (1995). Evaluating the impact of reminiscence on older people with dementia. In *The art and science of reminiscing: theory, research, methods and applications* (ed. B. K. Haight and J. Taylor), pp. 233–42. Taylor & Francis, Washington DC.

Woods, R. T., Portnoy, S., Head, D., and Jones, G. (1992). Reminiscence and life-review with persons with dementia: which way forward? In *Care-giving in dementia.* (ed. G. Jones and B. Miesen), pp. 137–61. Routledge, London.

Zanetti, O., Bianchetti, A., Montini, M., and Trabucchi, M. (1993). Reality orientation therapy in demented patients: useful or not? (Abstract). Presented at the *International Congress of Gerontology*, Budapest, Hungary.

Zanetti, O., Magni, E., Binetti, G., Bianchetti, A., and Trabucchi, M. (1994). Is procedural memory stimulation effective in Alzheimer's disease? *International Journal of Geriatric Psychiatry*, **9**, 1006–7.

Zarit, S. H., Zarit, J. M., and Reever, K. E. (1982). Memory training for severe memory loss: effects on senile dementia patients and their families. *Gerontologist*, **22**, 373–77.

EIGHTEEN

Neurobiological treatment of Alzheimer's disease

Marcus Richards

INTRODUCTION

Alzheimer-type dementia (AD) is the major neurodegenerative disorder of old age with substantial personal, social, and economic consequence. A large and serious international effort is therefore underway to develop effective and feasible treatments. AD can neither be prevented nor cured, yet accumulating evidence suggests that certain neurobiological interventions can retard the progression of disease features. Pharmacological strategies, particularly cholinergic therapy, are under intensive investigation. Other techniques, such as neural transplantation, have also been proposed, although, as yet, these remain untried within a clinical setting.

Pharmacological interventions have resulted in clinical global impressions of change in AD patients, but the most intriguing effects of these interventions have occurred in cognitive function. This chapter will therefore review available and proposed neurobiological therapies for AD, their effects on cognitive function, and problems encountered in interpreting these effects. Before embarking upon this, it is worth noting some basic issues in the design and interpretation of clinical trials.

Those include, for example, how to specify the goals of treatment, the design and interpretation of clinical trials, and dealing with the heterogeneity of AD, factors that are considered below.

What is treatment in AD?

The ultimate therapeutic goal for AD is to develop agents that will prevent or abolish the signs and symptoms of this disease. No such agent appears in prospect. An interim goal therefore is to improve the quality of sufferers' lives and those around them through agents that can mitigate these signs and symptoms, even if only for a limited period of time. As Wilcock and Dawbarn (1994) note, this improvement entails an increased ability of the patient to undertake activities of daily living (ADL) and a reduced level of stress in the carer. As AD progresses, improvements in ADL become more difficult to attain and the priority shifts to the amelioration of behavioural disturbances. In mild AD, however, pharmacological intervention can produce discernable improvements in cognitive function. A central question therefore concerns the definition of improvement. Wilcock (1993) proposed that the minimum acceptable benefit from an intervention should constitute a change in the score of a global cognitive test that represents a saving of six months of deterioration. This would amount to a change of two or three points on the total Mini-Mental Status Examination score (MMSE; Folstein *et al.* 1975). There are several difficulties with such a formula and the reader is referred to Wilcock (1993) for a full discussion of this issue.

The interpretation of clinical trial results

There are several stages through which testing of a novel pharmacological compound must undergo before it can be assessed in human patients. In addition, formal guidelines for the administration of controlled clinical trials for these compounds have been set forth. Thorough reviews of these procedures are provided by Canal *et al.* (1993). Claims for the clinical efficacy of a compound should be based on evidence of improvement in function under active treatment, in contrast to placebo. Trials should also be conducted under double-blind conditions, in which the identity of patients receiving active treatment and those receiving placebo is unknown to the patients and the investigators for the duration of the trial. When reading the report of such a trial, the reader should be aware of potential sources of bias. These include:

1. *Patient recruitment*: most clinical trials are conducted at medical centres with access to patients who have undergone a full clinical diagnostic assessment. In addition, most trials employ strict exclusion criteria concerning co-morbid conditions and confounding medication. This is not always the case, however, and the patient description section of a report should always be reviewed carefully.

2. *Statistical power*: as with all biomedical research, sample size, the variability and signal-to-noise ratio of the outcome measures, and their sensitivity to change will all govern the ability of investigators to detect significant effects.

3. *Drop-out rate*: the higher the drop-out rate, the less likely it is that patients who have successfully completed a trial will be representative of AD patients as a whole. Comparisons of baseline characteristics and outcome performance between patients continuing in a trial and patients withdrawn from a trial should therefore be reported.

Heterogeneity in AD

It is well known that patients who satisfy NINCDS–ADRDA criteria for AD (McKhann *et al.* 1984) constitute a clinically heterogeneous population. Several authors have described 'subtypes' of AD based on the presence or absence of neurological or psychotic features (Chui *et al.* 1985; Mayeux *et al.* 1985; Richards *et al.* 1993). Attempts have also been made to distinguish subtypes of AD based on cognitive performance (Siegfried 1991). For example some patients may be characterized by a dominant memory impairment, others by a prominent attentional deficit, and others by focal language or visuospatial dysfunction.

This variance in the clinical expression of AD is capable of reducing the sensitivity of any measure to detect change in response to an intervention. In the case of pharmacotherapy, this would be especially true if these clinical and neuropsychological subgroups correspond to pharmacological subgroups, since the latter will differentially respond to a particular agent (Siegfried 1991). Since it is impossible to identify responders and non-responders in advance, investigators are faced with three alternatives. One is to increase sample size, which is not always practical; another is to introduce a crossover design. Because of the progressive nature of AD, this is only feasible for trials of short duration, where care must be taken to avoid carry-over effects. A third is to use the so-called 'enrichment' procedure, where responders are preselected on the basis of an off-baseline pharmacological challenge, then entered into a randomized, double-blind, placebo-controlled study. This procedure is controversial and the proportion of responders selected from the total denominator for randomization should always be specified (Siegfried 1991).

With the above strictures in mind, which neurobiological interventions have been explored in AD and what are their effects on cognitive function?

These can be split broadly into approaches that concern cholinergic neurochemical transmission, since this is the dominant approach, and a more miscellaneous selection of other agents, as described below.

CHOLINERGIC THERAPY

The cholinergic hypothesis of AD is discussed in Chapter 14. Suffice it to say that a major strategic effort has been made to correct the putative cholinergic deficit in this disease. This effort can be divided into several distinct approaches and these are summarized in Table 17.1.

TABLE 17.1 Cholinergic therapy in AD

Method	Action	Agents
ACh precursor loading	ChAT acetylates choline to produce ACh	Choline Lecithin
AChE inhibition	Prevents the hydrolysis of synaptically released ACh	Physostigmine Tacrine (THA)
Cholinergic agonism	Increases the effect of ACh at the receptor site	Nicotine RS-86 Pilocarpine Arecoline Oxotremorine Bethanecol
ACh release enhancement	Increases ACh release	Phosphatidylserine (BC-PS) 4-aminopyridine
Neural transplantation	To regenerate ACh	Embryonic basal forebrain cells

ACh, acetylcholine; ChAT, choline acetyltransferase; AChE, acetylcholinesterase.

Acetylcholine precursor loading

Choline is acetylated rapidly by the enzyme choline acetyltransferase (ChAT) to give acetylcholine (ACh). An early strategy for increasing available CNS ACh therefore consisted of precursor loading through the direct administration of choline to patients. Unfortunately, intestinal bacteria break down this compound to trimethylamine, which smells of rotting fish (Levy 1994). However, phosphatidylcholine (lecithin) provides a more acceptable choline source. Little *et al.* (1985) administered a purified form of this compound to AD patients within a double-blind study. Factor analysis of their cognitive measures yielded two factors: (1) verbal learning and memory, consisting of paired associate learning, verbal fluency and orientation, and (2) visuospatial and constructional, which included tests of visual pattern recognition, visual matching, copying, and non-verbal reasoning. Little *et al.* found evidence of a moderate and temporary improvement in verbal learning and memory following active lecithin administration. However, this was observed in patients whose plasma choline levels were twice those of controls but not in those whose choline levels were greater than this. Heyman *et al.* (1987) found no beneficial effects of lecithin. In general, this compound has been regarded as relatively unsuccessful in the improvement of cognitive function in AD. One possible reason is provided by Marek *et al.* (1982), who calculated that extracellular choline levels would have to be increased more than 50-fold to enable the AD brain to synthesize ACh at a normal rate.

Although it has several modes of action, acetyl-L-carnitine has also been classified as an ACh precursor (Levy 1994). This compound has been shown to stimulate ACh release (Imperato *et al.* 1989) and is, in fact, structurally similar to ACh. Improvements in cognitive function have been reported in several double-blind studies. Livingston *et al.* (1991) administered tests of visual and verbal memory, verbal fluency, and visual construction to 71 demented patients, 50 of whom were diagnosed with probable AD. Although acetyl carnitine produced a trend towards better performance than controls in most of these tests, this effect only reached significance for a test of word recognition.

Spagnoli *et al.* (1991) administered a range of cognitive tests to assess verbal and non-verbal memory, non-verbal reasoning, selective attention, verbal judgement and comprehension, visual construction, and praxis. Patients taking acetyl carnitine showed slower deterioration in abstract reasoning (Raven's Progressive Matrices), verbal critical abilities, selective attention (target searching), and long-term verbal memory (Buschke Selective Reminding Test).

Improved selective attention was confirmed in a smaller study by Sano *et al.* (1992), also using a target searching task. In addition, these authors demonstrated improved performance in forward digit span, which is also sensitive to attention.

Cholinesterase inhibition

The development of acetylcholinesterase (AChE) inhibition constitutes the most widely discussed strategy in experimental AD therapy. AChE inhibitors prevent the hydrolysis of synaptically released ACh, thereby increasing the efficiency of cholinergic transmission.

Physostigmine

Physostigmine was the first such agent to be investigated, although its action is limited by a short half-life (Whitehouse 1993). Action of the oral form is also hindered by poor gastrointestinal absorption (Levy 1994). Nevertheless, several studies have demonstrated a significant improvement in word list learning, using the Buschke Selective Reminding Test in patients taking this compound in contrast to placebo (Beller *et al.* 1985; Sano *et al.* 1993; Stern *et al.* 1988; Thal *et al.* 1983). Similar results were found for non-verbal memory (Christie *et al.* 1981). A dose-related response was also reported in these studies. In most cases, the relationship occurred between physostigmine dose and cognitive test performance, although one study (Thal *et al.* 1983) reported a direct correlation between the latter and inhibition of cholinesterase in cerebrospinal fluid.

It should be noted that memory was the only cognitive domain assessed in these studies, so they cannot confirm that physostigmine specifically improves memory performance. Of interest therefore is an earlier study by Stern *et al.* (1987). These authors failed to demonstrate an effect of physostigmine on the Selective Reminding Test, but they reported significant improvements in WAIS-R Digit Symbol substitution and in a cancellation task, where patients were required to cross out diamond shapes from an array of distractors. Both these tasks require visuospatial analysis, speeded performance, and sustained attention. However, the relative contributions of these domains are unclear; on the one hand, physostigmine has been shown to improve performance during a visuospatial construction task (Muramoto *et al.* 1984). Yet in another study it also improved simple reaction time (Gustafson *et al.* 1987). The question of whether cholinesterase inhibition primarily affects memory or whether it affects other cognitive domains (particularly attention) will be further examined below.

Tacrine

The investigation of tetrahydroaminoacridine (tacrine or THA) has received widespread attention, not least because this compound is the only experimental cholinomimetic to receive Food and Drug Administration (FDA) approval for prescription use in the United States. Tacrine has a longer lasting action than physostigmine, although it may have additional modes of action in high doses. These include monoamine oxidase inhibition, interaction with muscarinic and nicotinic receptors, and potassium channel blockade (Eagger *et al.* 1991).

Interest in tacrine was precipitated by Summers *et al.* (1986), who reported a dramatic improvement in scores for the Names Learning Test (episodic memory and verbal associative learning) and the Orientation Test (orientation to time) in 14 AD patients taking this agent within a double-blind crossover trial. However, this study was criticized by the FDA for a variety of reasons. At the same time, several trials failed to detect an improvement in cognitive function following tacrine administration (Chatelier and Lacomblez 1990; Gauthier *et al.* 1990; Molloy *et al.* 1991), although methodological details of these trials have also been criticized (Levy 1994).

Two large double-blind studies subsequently reported improved cognitive function in response to tacrine, and the results of these trials were presented to the FDA as evidence for approval of a New Drug Application (NDA; see Whitehouse 1993). Unfortunately, one of these studies (Davis *et al.* 1992) did not provide detailed information on patterns of neuropsychological performance since the only cognitive outcome measure reported was the Alzheimer's Disease Assessment Scale (ADAS; Rosen *et al.* 1984). This represents global cognitive function by amalgamating subscores from different cognitive domains (spontaneous speech, naming, word list learning, word recognition, following commands, and visual construction).

More detailed neuropsychological information was provided by Sahakian *et al.* (1993) as part of the other study, first reported by Eagger *et al.* (1991). Tacrine had a modest but beneficial effect on choice reaction time (but not simple reaction time), and ability to follow a simple rule and to reverse that rule. On the other hand, tacrine had no significant effect on tests of visuospatial recognition, target searching, matching or construction, on tests of associative learning or verbal and non-verbal memory, and on WAIS-R Digit Span and Digit Symbol substitution. Sahakian *et al.* (1993) argued that tacrine improves attentional rather then mnemonic function in AD and that the cholinergic system is therefore involved in the control of attentional processes.

AD patients show a wide range of responses to tacrine. For example Eagger *et al.* (1991) reported that 44% of their tacrine patients were responders, that is to say they showed improvements of three or more MMSE points, 33% showed MMSE changes of 0–2 points, with MMSE scores declining in the remaining 23% patients. In an intriguing study, Alhainen and Riekkinen (1993) exposed 14 AD patients to a single dose of tacrine. These authors found that responders (as defined by Eagger *et al.* 1991) showed a more general improvement in cognitive function, including word list learning (Buschke Selective Reminding Test), vigilance (Continuous Performance Test), Trailmaking (errors for Part B), clock reading and clock setting. It should be noted, however, that the test–retest interval was only 120 minutes and that tacrine was administered by an open procedure. In spite of a comprehensive effort, there appears to be no way of identifying tacrine responders other than through response to tacrine itself.

Cholinergic agonists

Cholinergic agonists increase the effect of ACh itself, either directly or by sensitizing the receptor site. Nicotine is one such agent. Several studies have reported a reduction in nicotinic cholinergic receptors in AD (Perry *et al.* 1986, 1987). It is also clear from epidemiological studies that cigarette smoking has a protective effect against AD (Lee 1994). It is therefore of interest to examine the effects of nicotine administration on cognitive function in AD. Sahakian *et al.* (1989) demonstrated that subcutaneous injections of nicotine improved performance in attention and information processing (detection of particular digit sequences within a larger digit series), reaction time and tapping time, and critical flicker fusion (a measure of temporal resolution of the visual system and an indirect measure of cortical arousal). No effect of nicotine was found on short-term memory (WAIS-R Digit Span and a computerized version of the delayed response). These results were replicated by Jones *et al.* (1992). Both studies therefore provide further evidence that the cholinergic system is involved in attention and information processing. In this regard, we should note a positron emission tomography study by Nordberg *et al.* (1992), who found that tacrine increased the number of nicotinic cholinergic receptors in AD patients.

Other cholinergic agonists that have been investigated for use in AD include the muscarinic agent RS-86 (Spiegel *et al.* 1984), pilocarpine, arecoline, oxotremorine, and bethanecol. Unfortunately, none of these have been effective to date and some appear to be highly toxic.

Other pharmaceutical cholinergic strategies

Several other types of agent have been explored for improving cholinergic function in AD. One such class are the ACh release enhancers. Of particular interest is phosphatidylserine (BC-PS), a phospholipid which is thought to alter the lipid composition of neuronal membranes and which has been shown to increase ACh release from rat cortical slices (Pedata *et al.* 1989). This compound has been administered to individuals with age-associated memory impairment (Crook *et al.* 1991), where modest improvements in verbal memory (Wechsler Logical Memory, telephone numbers) and non-verbal memory (name–face acquisition, facial recognition, and object recall) were demonstrated in subjects with relatively poor cognitive performance at baseline. Placebo-controlled, double-blind studies with AD patients have been inconsistent however; Amaducci *et al.* (1988) demonstrated a treatment-related improvement in verbal category fluency and spatial memory (Corsi blocks), but Crook *et al.* (1992) found little or no effect of treatment on cognitive function.

There are other pharmaceutical agents thought to modulate ACh production that are currently being assessed in AD. These include beta carbolines, which influence GABA function, and odansetron, a 5-HT^3 inhibitor. Results of these trials are not available at the present time.

Transplantation of neural cholinergic tissue

Although cholinomimetic therapies have achieved some degree of success in AD, beneficial effects are invariably modest and transient. Cholinergic systems exist in regions of the brain that do not degenerate in AD, such as the brainstem, striatum, and thalamus. The presence of these systems prohibits the use of drug doses necessary to alter cholinergic function in the cortex or hippocampus for any length of time (Perry 1994). Furthermore, cholinomimetic agents interact with systemic cholinergic function to produce autonomic and glandular side effects. An important goal therefore is to develop compounds that target specific cholinergic receptors. So far, this has proved to be a formidable challenge (Whitehouse 1993).

A fundamental alternative is based on the possibility of transplanting embryonic basal forebrain cells into key degenerating areas in the AD brain. This approach would be analogous to the transplantation of dopamine-rich cells into the basal ganglia in Parkinson's disease, a strategy which is under intensive investigation (Lindvall 1991). It is now well documented that transplantation of fetal cholinergic cells can successfully reverse cognitive impairment induced by experimental surgery in animals (Sinden *et al.* 1992). The prospect of neural transplantation in AD has, however, evoked controversy among health-care professionals. Discussion of this is not within the remit of the present chapter, although it should be noted that intercranial procedures are unlikely to be feasible for any but a small number of AD patients (Levy 1994).

Nerve growth factor

One possible phenomenon mediating the action of neural grafts in animals is the stimulation of neurotropic factors. This raises the topic of nerve growth factor (NGF). The biology of NFG is complex and the reader is referred to Thoenen and Barde (1980) and Wilcock and Dawbarn (1994) for detailed reviews. Briefly, in the 1950s mouse sarcomas were found to secrete NFG. When these sarcomas were transplanted into chick embryos, they stimulated nerve fibre innovation. NFG was subsequently discovered to be released by the target tissues of sensory and sympathetic fibres, internalized by the relevant receptors, and transported back to the nucleus where it exerts a protective effect. When radiolabelled NFG was injected into the hippocampus or cortex, it labelled neurones in cholinergic projection groups of the septum, the diagonal band of Broca, and the nucleus basalis of Meynert (Seiler and Schwab 1984). Of particular interest therefore was the finding that administration of NFG to rat basal forebrain neurones results in increased cholinergic function (e.g. Honnegar and Lenoir 1982). Furthermore, administration of NFG via CSF has been shown partially to reverse atrophy of cholinergic neurones and spatial learning in ageing rats (Fischer *et al.* 1987) and primates (Tuszynski *et al.* 1990).

These lines of evidence suggest that the cholinergic deficit in AD might be associated with a reduction in NFG. So far, NFG levels appear to be similar in normal and AD brains (Wilcock and Dawbarn 1994), although the possibility remains that NFG is poorly transported within degenerating neurones in AD. An important question therefore is whether administration of NFG will improve cholinergic function in AD. There are two major difficulties surrounding the therapeutic use of this substance. First, NFG appears to increase amyloid precursor protein concentration in the brain (Mobley *et al.* 1988), raising the possibility that it might actually exacerbate abnormal amyloid deposition in AD. Second, NFG does not cross the blood–brain barrier. It must therefore be delivered directly to the cerebral ventricles, a procedure which is subject to similar medical and ethical difficulties as those surrounding neural transplantation. The technique is currently being explored in individual patients, although it is too early to comment on outcome at the present time.

NON-CHOLINERGIC TECHNIQUES

Attempts to manipulate functioning of the forebrain cholinergic projection system have formed the core biomedical strategy for therapeutic intervention in AD. It has been shown that certain cholinomimetic agents can retard the progression of cognitive impairment in this disease, although few would claim that these gains constitute a therapeutic breakthrough. One problem is that AD, like most neurodegenerative diseases, is a multi-system disorder. It is unlikely therefore that strategies aiming to replenish one transmitter or strategies that target a single brain system will be particularly effective. However, other neurochemical strategies are being explored. Some of these are summarized in Table 17.2 and are briefly reviewed in the final section.

Vascular agents

Vascular pathology is generally regarded as orthogonal to that of classical AD. Nevertheless, epidemiological research is beginning to blur the boundaries between AD and cognitive impairment associated with vascular pathology. It is therefore worth briefly noting that certain vasodilators have been administered as possible treatments for AD. These include the ergots co-dergocrine mesylate (Hydergine), which has little effect in AD and may even be harmful, and nicergoline, which has been shown to improve orientation (Battaglia *et al.* 1989). They also include calcium channel blocking agents, such as nimodipine. Other

TABLE 17.2 Non-cholinergic therapy in AD

Method	Action	Agents
Vasodilators	Increase cerebral blood perfusion	Hydergine Nicergoline Nimodipine Nicardipine
Neuropeptides	Act as neurotransmitters and modify the action of other neurotransmitters	Somatostatin ACTH Vasopressin
Opiate antagonism	Endogenous opiate system involved in learning and memory	Naloxone
Neurotropics	Stimulates nerve fibre innovation, modifies expression of neuroproteins	Nerve growth factor Oligonucleotides
Nootropics	Uncertain	Piracetam Oxiracetam

agents that can affect cerebral blood flow are certain antihypertensives and antithrombotics. An intriguing issue is the growing evidence that the use of non-steroidal anti-inflammatory drugs (for instance aspirin) may be protective in AD (Canadian Study of Health and Aging 1994).

Other non-cholinergic agents

Several alternative molecular strategies are being attempted in AD. Most are based on hypothesis-driven basic research, although some compounds appear to have beneficial effects on memory and vigilance in the absence of any clear explanatory model. Notable in this regard are the so-called neurotropics, such as piracetam and oxiracetam.

Studies have shown that neuropeptides, particularly somatostatin, adrenocorticotrophic hormone (ACTH), and vasopressin, are involved in learning and memory. In addition, some of these peptides appear to be reduced in AD (Whalley and Bailey 1994). These findings have led investigators to attempt experimental administration of neuropeptides in this disease. Results so far have been disappointing. A similar conclusion was reached regarding the use of opiate antagonists, in spite of an early demonstration by Reisberg *et al.* (1983*a*, *b*) that naloxone improves symptoms of AD.

A potentially exciting frontier in biomedical intervention concerns the possibility of direct manipulation of the genetic processes involved in the generation of AD neuropathology. For example oligonucleotides may be targeted to modify the biosynthetic pathway that generates amyloid precursor protein (Whalley and Bailey 1994). It is far too early, however, to comment on the use of these strategies within a clinical setting.

CONCLUSIONS

The past decade has witnessed an intensive effort to develop efficacious biomedical therapies for AD. This effort has largely been targeted at pharmacotherapy, although the possibility of transplanting acetylcholine-rich fetal tissue into the AD brain has been mooted. To date, the most intensive strategy has aimed to increase cholinergic function in AD, particularly by cholinesterase inhibition, although several other methods are under investigation. Cholinomimetic therapies have yielded modest improvements in verbal learning and memory. Studies have shown that these therapies can also improve psychomotor performance and attentional processes and there has been some debate as to whether these latter improvements constitute their primary cognitive effect. A series of 'next generation' cholinesterase inhibitors are currently under invesigation.

Several non-cholinergic agents are also being developed. Perhaps the most exciting of these are the neurotropics, such as oligonucleotides, which are intended to modify biosynthetic pathways involved in the generation of AD pathology. It is too early, however, to comment on the effects of these agents on cognitive function in AD.

ACKNOWLEDGEMENT

Financial support during the preparation of this chapter was provided by an Alzheimer's Disease Society Research Fellowship to the author.

REFERENCES

Alhainen, K. and Riekkinen, P. J. (1993). Discrimination of Alzheimer patients responding to cholinesterase inhibitor therapy. *Acta Neurologica Scandinavica*, **Suppl. 149**, 16–21.

Amaducci, L. (1988). Phosphatidylserine in the treatment of Alzheimer's disease: results of a multicenter study. *Psychopharmacology Bulletin*, **24**, 130–4.

Battaglia, A., Bruni, G., Ardia, A., and Sachetti, G. (1989). Nicergoline in mild to moderate dementia—a multi-centre double-blind placebo controlled study. *Journal of the American Geriatric Society*, **37**, 295–302.

Beller, S.A., Overall, J.E. and Swann, A.C. (1985). Efficacy of oral physostigmine in primary degenerative dementia. *Psychopharmacology*, **87**, 147–51.

Canadian Study of Health and Aging. (1994). The Canadian Study of Health and Aging: risk factors for Alzheimer's disease in Canada. *Neurology*, **44**, 2073–80.

Canal, N., Hachinski, V., McKhann, G., and Franceschi, M. (1993). *Guidelines for drug trials in memory disorders.* Raven Press, New York.

Chatelier, G. and Lacomblez, L. (1990). Tacrine (tetrahydroaminoacridine, THA) and lecithin in senile dementia of the Alzheimer type; a multicentre trial. Groupe Francaise d'Etude de la Tetrahydroamioacridine. *British Journal of Medicine*, **300**, 495–9.

Christie, J.E., Shering, A., Ferguson, J., and Glen, A.I.M. (1981). Physostigmine and arecholine: effects of intravenous infusions in Alzheimer's presenile dementia. *British Journal of Psychiatry*, **138**, 46–50.

Chui, H.C., Teng, E.L., Henderson, V.W., and Moy, A.C. (1985). Clinical subtypes of dementia of the Alzheimer type. *Neurology*, **35**, 1544–50.

Crook, T.H., Tinklenberg, J., Yesavage, J., Petrie, W., Nunzi, M.G., and Massari, D.C. (1991). Effects of phosphatidylserine in age-associated memory impairment. *Neurology*, **41**, 644–9.

Crook, T.H., Wells, P.W., and Massari, D.C. (1992). Effects of phosphatidylserine in Alzheimer's disease. *Psychopharmacology Bulletin*, **28**, 61–6.

Davis, K.L., Thal, L.J., Gamzu, E.R., Davis, C.S., Woolson, R.F., Gracon, S.I. *et al.* (1992). A double-blind, placebo-controlled multicenter study of tacrine for Alzheimer's disease. *New England Journal of Medicine*, **327**, 1253–9.

Eagger, S.A., Levy, R., and Sahakian, B.J. (1991). Tacrine in Alzheimer's disease. *Lancet*, **337**, 989–92.

Fischer, W., Wictorin, A., Bjorklund, A., Williams, L.R., Varon, S., and Gage, F.H. (1987). Amelioration of cholinergic neuronal atrophy and spatial memory impairment in aged rats by NFG. *Nature*, **329**, 65–7.

Folstein, M.F., Folstein, S.E., and McHugh, P.R. (1975). 'Mini-Mental State.' A practical method for grading the cognitive state of patients for the clinician. *Journal of Psychiatric Research*, **12**, 189–98.

Gauthier, S., Bouchard, R., Lamontagne, A., Bailey, P., Bergman, H., Ratner, J., *et al.* (1990). Tetrahydroaminoacridine– lecithin combination treatment in patients with intermediate stage Alzheimer's disease. Results of a Canadian double-blind, crossover, multicentre study. *New England Journal of Medicine*, **322**, 1272–6.

Gustafson, L., Edvinson, L., Dahlgren, N., Hagberg, B., Reisberg, B., Rosen, I., and Ferno, H. (1987). Intravenous physostigmine treatment of Alzheimer's disease evaluated by psychometric testing, regional blood flow (rCBF) measurement, and by EEG. *Psychopharmacology*, **93**, 31–5.

Heyman, A., Schmechel, D., Wilkinson, W., Rogers, H., Krishnam, R., Holloway, D. *et al.* (1987). Failure of long term high dose lecithin to retard progression of early-onset Alzheimer's disease. In *Alzheimer's disease: advances in basic research and therapies* (ed. R.J. Wurtman, S.H. Corkin, and J.H. Growdon), pp. 293–302. Centre for Brain Sciences and Metabolism Charitable Trust, Cambridge, MA.

Honnegar, P. and Lenoir, D. (1982). Nerve growth factor (NFG) stimulation of cholinergic telencephalic neurons in aggregating cell cultures. *Developmental Brain Research*, **3**, 229–38.

Imperato, A., Ramacci, M.T., and Angelucci, L. (1989). Acetyl-L-carnitine enhances acetylcholine release in the striatum and hippocampus of awake freely moving rats. *Neuroscience Letters*, **107**, 251–5.

Jones, G.M.M., Sahakian, B.J., Levy, R., Warburton, D.M., and Gray, J. (1992). Effects of acute subcutaneous nicotine on attention, information processing and short-term memory in Alzheimer's disease. *Psychopharmacology*, **108**, 485–94.

Lee, P.N. (1994). Smoking and Alzheimer's disease: a review of the epidemiological evidence. *Neuroepidemiology*, **13**, 131–44.

Levy, R. (1994). Cholinergic treatment of Alzheimer's disease. In *Dementia* (ed. A. Burns and R. Levy), pp. 511–18. Chapman and Hall Medical, London.

Lindvall, O. (1991). Prospects of transplantation in human neurodegenerative diseases. *Trends in Neurosciences*, **14**, 376–84.

Little, A., Levy, R., Chauqui-Kidd, P., and Hand, D. (1985). A double-blind, placebo controlled trial of high dose lecithin in Alzheimer's disease. *Journal of Neurology, Neurosurgery and Psychiatry*, **48**, 736–42.

Livingston, G.A., Sax, K.B., McClenahan, Z., Blumenthal, E., Foley, K., Willison, J., *et al.* (1991). Acetyl-l-carnitine in dementia. *International Journal of Geriatric Psychiatry*, **6**, 853–60.

McKhann, G., Drachman, D., Folstein, M., Katzman, R., Price, D., and Stadlan, E.M. (1984). Clinical diagnosis of Alzheimer's disease: Report of the NINCDS–ADRDA Work Group. *Neurology*, **34**, 939–44.

Marek, K.L., Bowen, D.M., Sims, N.R., and Davison, A.N. (1982). Stimulation of acetylcholine synthesis by blockade of pre-synaptic muscarinic inhibitory autoreceptors: observations in rat and human brain preparations and comparison with the effect of choline. *Life Sciences*, **30**, 1517–24.

Mayeux, R., Stern, Y., and Spanton, S. (1985). Heterogeneity in dementia of the Alzheimer type: evidence of subgroups. *Neurology*, **35**, 453–61.

Mobley, W.C., Neve, R.L., Pruisner, S.B., and McKinley, M.P. (1988). Nerve growth factor increases mRNA levels for the prion protein and the beta-amyloid protein precursor in the developing hamster brain. *Proceedings of the National Academy of Science, USA*, **85**, 9811–15.

Molloy, D.W., Guyatt, G.H., Wilson, D.B., Duke, R., Rees, L., and Singer, J. (1991). Effect of tetrahydroaminoacridine on cognition, function and behaviour in Alzheimer's disease. *Canadian Medical Association Journal*, **144**, 29–34.

Muramoto, O., Sugishita, M., and Ando, K. (1984). Cholinergic system and constructional praxis: a further study of physostigmine in Alzheimer's disease. *Journal of Neurology, Neurosurgery and Psychiatry*, **47**, 484–9.

Nordberg, A., Lilja, A., Lundqvist, H., Hartvig, P., Amberla, K., Viitanen, M., *et al.* (1992). Tacrine restores cholinergic nicotinic receptors and glucose metabolism in Alzheimer patients as visualised by positron emission tomography. *Neurobiology of Aging*, **13**, 747–58.

Pedata, F., Giovannelli, G., Spignoli, G., and Pepeu, G. (1985). Phosphatidylserine increases acetylcholine release from cortical slices in aged rats. *Neurobiology of Aging*, **6**, 337–9.

Perry, E.K. (1994). Cholinergic component of cognitive impairment in Alzheimer's disease. In *Dementia* (ed. A. Burns and R. Levy), pp. 143–58. Chapman and Hall Medical, London.

Perry, E.K., Perry, R.H., Smith, C.J., Purohit, J., Bonham, P., Dick, D., *et al.* (1986). Cholinergic receptors in cognitive disorders. *Canadian Journal of Neurological Science*, **13**, 521–7.

Perry, E.K., Perry, R.H., Smith, C.J., Dick, D., Candy, J., Edwardson, J.A., *et al.* (1987). Nicotine receptor abnormalities in Alzheimer's and Parkinson's diseases. *Journal of Neurology, Neurosurgery and Psychiatry*, **50**, 806–9.

Reisberg, B., Ferris, S.H., Anand, R., and de Leon, M.J. (1983*a*). Effects of naloxone in senile dementia: a double blind trial (letter). *New England Journal of Medicine*, **308**, 721–2.

Reisberg, B., London, E., Ferris, S.H., *et al.* (1983*b*). Novel pharmacologic approaches to the treatment of senile dementia of the Alzheimer's type (SDAT). *Psychopharmacology Bulletin*, **19**, 220–5.

Richards, M., Folstein, M., Albert, M., Miller, L., Bylsma, F., Lafleche, G. *et al.* (1993). Multicenter study of predictors of disease course in Alzheimer's disease (the 'Predictors Study'). II. Neurological, psychiatric, and demographic influences on baseline measures of disease severity. *Alzheimer Disease and Associated Disorders*, **7**, 22–32.

Rosen, W.G., Mohs, R.C., and Davis, K.L. (1984). A new rating scale for Alzheimer's disease. *American Journal of Psychiatry*, **141**, 1356–64.

Sahakian, B.J., Jones, G., Levy, R., Gray, J., and Warburton, D. (1989). The effects of nicotine on attention, information processing, and short-term memory in patients with dementia of the Alzheimer type. *British Journal of Psychiatry*, **154**, 797–800.

Sahakian, B.J., Owen, A.M., Morant, N.J., Eagger, S.A., Boddington, S., Crayton, L., *et al.* (1993). Further analysis of the cognitive effects of tetrahydroaminoacridine (THA) in Alzheimer's disease: assessment of attentional and mnemonic function using CANTAB. *Psychopharmacology*, **110**, 395–410.

Sano, M., Bell, K., Cote, L., Dooneief, G., Lawton, A., Legler, L., *et al.* (1992). Double-blind parallel design pilot study of acetyl levocarnitine in patients with Alzheimer's disease. *Archives of Neurology*, **49**, 1137–41.

Sano, M., Bell, K., Marder, K., Stricks, L., Stern, Y., and Mayeux, R. (1993). Safety and efficacy of oral physostigmine in the treatment of Alzheimer's disease. *Clinical Neuropharmacology*, **16**, 61–9.

Seiler, M. and Schwab, M.E. (1984). Specific retrograde transport of nerve growth factor (NFG) from neocortex to nucleus basalis in the rat. *Brain Research*, **300**, 33–9.

Siegfried, K.R. (1991). Some considerations on the methodology of clinical trials with anti-dementia compounds in patients with Alzheimer's disease. In *Dementia: molecules, methods and measures* (ed. I. Hindmarch, H. Hippius, and G.K. Wilcock), pp. 47–60. John Wiley and Sons, Chichester.

Sinden, J.D., Marsden, K.M., and Hodges, H. (1992). Neural transplantation and recovery of function: animal studies. In *Recovery from brain damage: reflections and directions* (ed. F.D. Rose and D.A. Johnson), pp. 35–65. Plenum, New York.

Spagnoli, A., Lucca, U., Menasce, G., Bandera, L., Gizza, G., Forloni, G. *et al.* (1991). Long-term acetyl-l-carnitine treatment in Alzheimer's disease. *Neurology*, **41**, 1726–32.

Spiegel, R., Azcona, A., and Wettstein, A. (1987). First results with RS86, an orally active muscarinic agonist in healthy subjects and in patients with dementia. In

Alzheimer's disease: advances in basic research and therapy (ed. R. Wurtman, S. Corkin, and J. Growdon), pp. 391–405. Center for Brain Sciences and Metabolism Charitable Trust, Cambridge, MA.

Stern, Y., Sano, M., and Mayeux, R. (1987). Effects of oral physostigmine in Alzheimer's disease. *Annals of Neurology*, **22**, 306–10.

Stern, Y., Sano, M., Mayeux, R. (1988). Long-term administration of oral physostigmine in Alzheimer's disease. *Neurology*, **38**, 1837–41.

Summers, W.K., Majovski, L.V., Marsh, G.M., Tachiki, K., and Kling, A. (1986). Oral tetrahydroaminoacridine in long-term treatment of senile dementia, Alzheimer type. *New England Journal of Medicine,* **315**, 1241–5.

Thal, L.J., Fuld, P.A., Masur, D.M., and Sharpless, N.S. (1983). Oral physostigmine and lecithin improve memory in Alzheimer's disease. *Annals of Neurology*, **13**, 491–6.

Thoenen, H. and Barde, Y. A. (1980). Physiology of nerve growth factor. *Physiology Reviews*, **60**, 1284–335.

Tuszynski, M.H., U, H. S., Amaral, D.G., and Gage, F.H. (1990). Nerve growth factor infusion in the primate brain reduces lesion-induced cholinergic neuronal degeneration. *Journal of Neuroscience,* **10**, 3604–14.

Whalley, L. and Bailey, S. (1994). Non-cholinergic therapies of dementia. In *Dementia* (ed. A. Burns and R. Levy), pp. 493–509. Chapman and Hall Medical, London.

Whitehouse, P.J. (1993). Cholinergic therapy in dementia. *Acta Neurologica Scandinavica,* **Suppl. 149**, 42–5.

Wilcock, G.K. (1993). End points, duration, and side effects. In *Aging,* Vol. 39: *Guidelines for drug trials in memory disorders* (ed. N. Canal, V.C. Hachinski, G. McKhann, and M. Francheschi), pp. 115–24. Raven Press, New York.

Wilcock, G.K. and Dawbarn, D. (1994). Nerve growth factor and other biological treatments: an overview. In *Dementia* (ed. A. Burns and R. Levy), pp. 477–91. Chapman and Hall Medical, London.

Index

Note: page numbers in *italics* refer to figures and tables.